POVERTY, U. S. A.

THE HISTORICAL RECORD

ADVISORY EDITOR: David J. Rothman

Professor of History, Columbia University

ON BEHALF
OF THE INSANE POOR

Selected Reports

DOROTHEA L. DIX

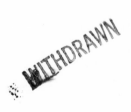

Arno Press & The New York Times
NEW YORK   1971

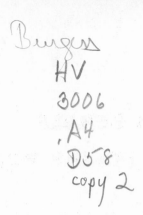
Reprint Edition 1971 by Arno Press Inc.

LC# 78—137163
ISBN 0—405—03101—7

POVERTY, U.S.A.: THE HISTORICAL RECORD
ISBN for complete set: 0-405-03090-8

Manufactured in the United States of America

CONTENTS

(in chronological order)

Memorial Soliciting Adequate Appropriations for the Construction of a State Hospital for the Insane in the State of Mississippi. February, 1850.

Memorial of Miss D. L. Dix, to the Honorable the General Assembly in behalf of the Insane of Maryland. February 25, 1852.

MEMORIAL

MASSACHUSETTS

1843

MEMORIAL

To the Legislature of Massachusetts.

GENTLEMEN,

I RESPECTFULLY ask to present this Memorial, believing that the *cause*, which actuates to and sanctions so unusual a movement, presents no equivocal claim to public consideration and sympathy. Surrendering to calm and deep convictions of duty my habitual views of what is womanly and becoming, I proceed briefly to explain what has conducted me before you unsolicited and unsustained, trusting, while I do so, that the memorialist will be speedily forgotten in the memorial.

About two years since leisure afforded opportunity, and duty prompted me to visit several prisons and alms-houses in the vicinity of this metropolis. I found, near Boston, in the Jails and Asylums for the poor, a numerous class brought into unsuitable connexion with criminals and the general mass of Paupers. I refer to Idiots and Insane persons, dwelling in circumstances not only adverse to their own physical and moral improvement, but productive of extreme disadvantages to all other persons brought into association with them. I applied myself diligently to trace the causes of these evils, and sought to supply remedies. As one obstacle was surmounted, fresh difficulties appeared. Every new investigation has given depth to the conviction that it is only by decided, prompt, and vigorous legislation the evils to which I refer, and which I shall proceed more fully to illustrate, can be remedied. I shall be obliged to speak with great plainness, and to reveal many things revolting to the taste, and from which my woman's nature shrinks with peculiar sensitiveness. But truth is the highest consideration. *I tell what I have seen*—painful and shocking as the details often are—that from them you may feel more deeply the imperative obligation which lies upon you to prevent the possibility of a repetition or continuance of such outrages upon humanity. If I inflict pain upon you, and move you to horror, it is to acquaint you with sufferings which you have the power to alleviate, and make you hasten to the relief of the victims of legalized barbarity.

I come to present the strong claims of suffering humanity. I come to place before the Legislature of Massachusetts the condition of the miserable, the desolate, the outcast. I come as the advocate of helpless, forgotten, insane and idiotic men and women ; of beings, sunk to a condition from which the most unconcerned would start with real horror ; of beings wretched in our Prisons, and more wretched in our Alms-Houses. And I cannot suppose it needful to employ earnest persuasion, or stubborn argument, in order to arrest and fix attention upon a subject, only the more strongly pressing in its claims, because it is revolting and disgusting in its details.

I must confine myself to few examples, but am ready to furnish other and more complete details, if required. If my pictures are displeasing, coarse, and severe, my subjects, it must be recollected, offer no tranquil, refined, or composing features. The condition of human beings, reduced to the extremest states of degradation and misery, cannot be exhibited in softened language, or adorn a polished page.

I proceed, Gentlemen, briefly to call your attention to the *present* state of Insane Persons confined within this Commonwealth, in *cages, closets, cellars, stalls, pens ! Chained, naked, beaten with rods,* and *lashed* into obedience !

As I state cold, severe *facts,* I feel obliged to refer to persons, and definitely to indicate localities. But it is upon my subject, not upon localities or individuals, I desire to fix attention ; and I would speak as kindly as possible of all Wardens, Keepers, and other responsible officers, believing that *most* of these have erred not through hardness of heart and wilful cruelty, so much as want of skill and knowledge, and want of consideration. Familiarity with suffering, it is said, blunts the sensibilities, and where neglect once finds a footing other injuries are multiplied. This is not all, for it may justly and strongly be added that, from the deficiency of adequate means to meet the wants of these cases, it has been an absolute impossibility to do justice in this matter. Prisons are not constructed in view of being converted into County Hospitals, and Alms-Houses are not founded as receptacles for the Insane. And yet, in the face of justice and common sense, Wardens are by law compelled to receive, and the Masters of Alms-Houses not to refuse, Insane and Idiotic subjects in all stages of mental disease and privation.

It is the Commonwealth, not its integral parts, that is accountable for most of the abuses which have lately, and do still exist. I repeat it, it is defective legislation which perpetuates and multiplies these abuses.

In illustration of my subject, I offer the following extracts from my Note-Book and Journal:—

Springfield. In the jail, one lunatic woman, furiously mad, a state pauper, improperly situated, both in regard to the prisoners, the keepers, and herself. It is a case of extreme self-forgetfulness and oblivion to all the decencies of life; to describe which, would be to repeat only the grossest scenes. She is much worse since leaving Worcester. In the almshouse of the same town is a woman apparently only needing judicious care, and some well-chosen employment, to make it unnecessary to confine her in solitude, in a dreary unfurnished room. Her appeals for employment and companionship are most touching, but the mistress replied, 'she had no time to attend to her.'

Northampton. In the jail, quite lately, was a young man violently mad, who had not, as I was informed at the prison, come under medical care, and not been returned from any hospital. In the almshouse, the cases of insanity are now unmarked by abuse, and afford evidence of judicious care by the keepers.

Williamsburg. The almshouse has several insane, not under suitable treatment. No apparent intentional abuse.

Rutland. Appearance and report of the insane in the almshouse not satisfactory.

Sterling. A terrible case; manageable in a hospital; at present as well controlled perhaps as circumstances in a case so extreme allow. An almshouse, but wholly wrong in relation to the poor crazy woman, to the paupers generally, and to her keepers.

Burlington. A woman, declared to be very insane; decent room and bed; but not allowed to rise oftener, the mistress said, 'than every other day : it is too much trouble.'

Concord. A woman from the hospital in a cage in the almshouse. In the jail several, decently cared for in general, but not properly placed in a prison. Violent, noisy, unmanageable most of the time.

Lincoln. A woman in a cage.

Medford. One idiotic subject chained, and one in a close stall for 17 years.

Pepperell. One often doubly chained, hand and foot; another violent; several peaceable now.

Brookfield. One man caged, comfortable.

Granville. One often closely confined; now losing the use of his limbs from want of exercise.

Charlemont. One man caged.

Savoy. One man caged.

Lenox. Two in the jail ; against whose unfit condition there, the jailor protests.

Dedham. The insane disadvantageously placed in the jail. In the almshouse, two females in stalls, situated in the main building ; lie in wooden bunks filled with straw ; always shut up. One of these subjects is supposed curable. The overseers of the poor have declined giving her a trial at the hospital, as I was informed, on account of expense.

Franklin. One man chained ; decent.

Taunton. One woman caged.

Plymouth. One man stall-caged, from Worcester hospital.

Scituate. One man and one woman stall-caged.

Bridgewater. Three idiots ; never removed from one room.

Barnstable. Four females in pens and stalls ; two chained certainly, I think all. Jail, one idiot.

Welfleet. Three insane ; one man and one woman chained, the latter in a bad condition.

Brewster. One woman violently mad, solitary : could not see her, the master and mistress being absent, and the paupers in charge having strict orders to admit no one.

Rochester. Seven insane ; at present none caged.

Milford. Two insane, not now caged.

Cohasset. One idiot, one insane ; most miserable condition.

Plympton. One insane, three idiots ; condition wretched.

Besides the above, I have seen many who, part of the year, are chained or caged. The use of cages all but universal ; hardly a town but can refer to some not distant period of using them : chains are less common : negligences frequent : wilful abuse less frequent than sufferings proceeding from ignorance, or want of consideration. I encountered during the last three months many poor creatures wandering reckless and unprotected through the country. Innumerable accounts have been sent me of persons who had roved away unwatched and unsearched after ; and I have heard that responsible persons, controlling the almshouses, have not thought themselves culpable in sending away from their shelter, to cast upon the chances of remote relief, insane men and women. These, left on the highways, unfriended and incompetent to control or direct their own movements, sometimes have found refuge in the hospital, and others have not been traced. But I cannot particularize ; in traversing the state I have found hundreds of insane persons in every variety of circumstance and condition ; many whose situation could not and need not be improved ; a less number, but that very large, whose lives are the saddest pictures of human suffering and degradation. I give a few illustrations; but description fades before reality.

Danvers. November; visited the almshouse; a large building, much out of repair; understand a new one is in contemplation. Here are rom fifty-six to sixty inmates; one idiotic; three insane; one of the latter in close confinement at all times.

Long before reaching the house, wild shouts, snatches of rude songs, imprecations, and obscene language, fell upon the ear, proceeding from the occupant of a low building, rather remote from the principal building to which my course was directed. Found the mistress, and was conducted to the place, which was called '*the home*' of the *forlorn* maniac, a young woman, exhibiting a condition of neglect and misery blotting out the faintest idea of comfort, and outraging every sentiment of decency. She had been, I learnt, " a respectable person; industrious and worthy; disappointments and trials shook her mind, and finally laid prostrate reason and self-control; she became a maniac for life! She had been at Worcester Hospital for a considerable time, and had been returned as incurable." The mistress told me she understood that, while there, she was " comfortable and decent." Alas! what a change was here exhibited! She had passed from one degree of violence and degradation to another, in swift progress; there she stood, clinging to, or beating upon, the bars of her caged apartment, the contracted size of which afforded space only for increasing accumulations of filth, a *foul* spectacle; there she stood with naked arms and dishevelled hair; the unwashed frame invested with fragments of unclean garments, the air so extremely offensive, though ventilation was afforded on all sides save one, that it was not possible to remain beyond a few moments without retreating for recovery to the outward air. Irritation of body, produced by utter filth and exposure, incited her to the horrid process of tearing off her skin by inches; her face, neck, and person, were thus disfigured to hideousness; she held up a fragment just rent off; to my exclamation of horror, the mistress replied, " oh, we can't help it; half the skin is off sometimes; we can do nothing with her; and it makes no difference what she eats, for she consumes her own filth as readily as the food which is brought her."

It is now January; a fortnight since, two visitors reported that most wretched outcast as " wallowing in dirty straw, in a place yet more dirty, and without clothing, without fire. Worse cared for than the brutes, and wholly lost to consciousness of decency!" Is the whole story told? What was seen, is; what is reported is not. These gross exposures are not for the pained sight of one alone; all, all, coarse, brutal men, wondering, neglected children, old and young, each and all, witness this lowest, foulest state of miserable humanity. And who protects her, that worse than Paria outcast, from other wrongs and blacker outrages? I do not *know* that such *have been.* I do know that they are to be dreaded, and that they are not guarded against.

Some may say these things cannot be remedied; these furious maniacs are not to be raised from these base conditions. I *know* they are; could give *many* examples; let *one* suffice. A young woman, a pauper, in a distant town, *Sandisfield,* was for years a raging maniac. A cage, chains, and *the whip,* were the agents for controlling her, united with harsh tones and profane language. Annually, with others (the town's poor) she was put up at auction, and bid off at the lowest price which was declared for her. One year, not long past, an old man came forward in the number of applicants for the poor wretch; he was taunted and ridiculed; "what would he and his old wife do with such a mere beast?" "My wife says yes," replied he, "and I shall take her." She was given to his charge; he conveyed her home; she was washed, neatly dressed, and placed in a decent bed-room, furnished for comfort and opening into the kitchen. How altered her condition! As yet *the chains* were not off. The first week she was somewhat restless, at times violent, but the quiet kind ways of the old people wrought a change; she received her food decently; forsook acts of violence, and no longer uttered blasphemous or indecent language; after a week, the chain was lengthened, and she was received as a companion into the kitchen. Soon she engaged in trivial employments. "After a fortnight," said the old man, "I knocked off the chains and made her a free woman." She is at times excited, but not violently; they are careful of her diet; they keep her very clean; she calls them "father" and "mother." Go there now and you will find her "clothed," and though not perfectly in her "right mind," so far restored as to be a safe and comfortable inmate.

Newburyport. Visited the almshouse in June last; eighty inmates; seven insane, one idiotic. Commodious and neat house; several of the partially insane apparently very comfortable; two very improperly situated, namely, an insane man, not considered incurable, in an out-building, whose room opened upon what was called 'the dead room,' affording in lieu of companionship with the living, a contemplation of corpses! The other subject was a woman in a *cellar.* I desired to see her; much reluctance was shown. I pressed the request; the Master of the House stated that she was *in the cellar;* that she was *dangerous to be approached;* that 'she had lately attacked his wife ;' and *was often naked*. I persisted ; 'if you will not go with me, give me the keys and I will go alone.' Thus importuned, the outer doors were opened. I descended the stairs from within ; a strange, unnatural noise seemed to proceed from beneath our feet ; at the moment I did not much regard it. My conductor proceeded to remove a padlock, while my eye explored the wide space in quest of the poor woman. All for a moment was still. But judge my horror and amazement, when a door to a closet *beneath* the *staircase* was opened, revealing in the imperfect light a female apparently wasted to a skeleton, partially wrapped in blankets, furnished for the narrow bed on which she was sitting ; her countenance furrowed, not by age, but suffering, was the image of distress ; in that contracted space, unlighted, unventilated, she poured forth the wailings of despair : mournfully she extended her arms and appealed to me, " why am I consigned to hell ? dark—dark—I used to pray, I used to read the Bible—I have done no crime in my heart ; I had friends, why have all forsaken me !—my God ! my God ! why hast *thou* forsaken me !" Those groans, those wailings come up daily, mingling, with how many others, a perpetual and sad memorial. When the good Lord shall require an account of our stewardship, what shall all and each answer !

Perhaps it will be inquired how long, how many days or hours was she imprisoned in these confined limits ? *For years !* In another part of the cellar were other small closets, only better, because higher through the entire length, into one of which she by turns was transferred, so as to afford opportunity for fresh whitewashing, &c.

Saugus. December 24 ; thermometer below zero ; drove to the poorhouse ; was conducted to the master's family-room by himself ; walls garnished with handcuffs and chains, not less than five pair of the former ; did not inquire how or on whom applied ; thirteen pauper inmates ; one insane man ; one woman insane ; one idiotic man ; asked to see them ; the two men were shortly led in ; appeared pretty decent and comfortable. Requested to see the other insane subject ; was denied decidedly ; urged the request, and finally secured a reluctant assent. Was led through an outer passage into a lower room, occupied by the paupers ; crowded ; not neat ; ascended a rather low flight of stairs upon an open entry, through the floor of which was introduced a stove pipe, carried along a *few feet*, about six inches above the floor, through which it was reconveyed below. From this entry opens a room of moderate size, having a sashed-window ; floor, I think, painted ; apartment ENTIRELY unfurnished ; no chair, table, nor bed ; neither, what is seldom missing, a bundle of straw or lock of hay ; cold, very cold ; the first movement of my conductor was to throw open a window, a measure imperatively necessary for those who entered. *On the floor* sat a woman, her limbs immovably contracted, so that the knees were brought upward to the chin ; the face was concealed ; the head rested on the folded arms ; for clothing she appeared to have been furnished with *fragments* of many discharged garments ; these were folded about her, yet they little benefitted her, if one might judge by the constant shuddering which almost convulsed her poor crippled frame. Woful was this scene ; language is feeble to record the misery she was suffering and had suffered ! In reply to my inquiry if she could not change her position, I was answered by the master in the negative, and told that the contraction of limbs was occasioned by " neglect and exposure in former years," but *since she had been crazy*, and before she fell under the charge, as I inferred, of her present *guardians*. Poor wretch ! she, like many others, was an example of what humanity becomes when the temple of reason falls in ruins, leaving the mortal part to injury and neglect, and showing how much can be endured of privation, exposure, and disease, without extinguishing the lamp of life.

Passing out, the man pointed to a something, revealed to more than one sense, which he called " her bed ; and we throw some blankets over her at night." Possibly this is done ; others, like myself, might be pardoned a doubt, if they could have seen all I saw, and heard abroad all I heard. The *bed*, so called, was about *three* feet long, and from a half to three-quarters of a yard wide ; of old ticking or tow cloth was the case ; the contents might have been a *full handful* of hay or straw. My attendant's exclamations on my leaving the house were emphatic, and can hardly be repeated.

The above case recalls another of equal neglect or abuse. Asking my way to the almshouse in Berkeley, which had been repeatedly spoken of as greatly neglected, I was answered as to the direction, and informed that there were " plenty of insane people and idiots there." " Well taken care of ? " " Oh, well enough for such sort of creatures ? " " Any violently insane ? " " Yes ; my sister's son is there, a real tiger. I kept him here at my house awhile, but it was too much trouble to go on ; so I carried him there." " Is he comfortably provided for ? " " Well enough." " Has he decent clothes ? " " Good enough ; wouldn't wear them if he had more." " Food ? " " Good enough ; good enough for him." " One more question, has he the comfort of a fire ? " " Fire ! fire, indeed ! what does a crazy man need of fire ? red-hot iron wants fire as much as he ! " And such are sincerely the ideas of not a few persons in regard to the actual wants of the insane. Less regarded than the lowest brutes! no wonder they sink even lower.

Ipswich. Have visited the prison three several times; visited the almshouse once. In the latter are several cases of insanity; three especially distressing, situated in a miserable out-building, detached from the family-house, and confined in stalls or pens; three individuals, one of which is apparently very insensible to the deplorable circumstances which surround him, and perhaps not likely to comprehend privations or benefits. Not so the person directly opposite to him, who looks up wildly, anxiously by turns, through those strong bars. Cheerless sight! strange companionship for the mind flitting and coming by turns to some perception of persons and things. He too is one of the returned incurables. His history is a sad one; I have not had all the particulars, but it shows distinctly, what the most prosperous and affluent may come to be. I understand his connexions are excellent and respectable; his natural abilities in youth were superior; he removed from Essex county to Albany, and was established there as the editor of a popular newspaper, in course of time he was chosen a senator for that section of the state, and of course was a Judge in the Court of Errors.

Vicissitudes followed, and insanity closed the scene. He was conveyed to Worcester; after a considerable period, either to give place to some new patient, or because the County objected to the continued expense, he being declared incurable, was removed to Salem jail; thence to Ipswich jail; associated with the prisoners there, partaking the same food, and clad in like apparel. After a time the town complained of the expense of keeping him in jail; it was cheaper in the almshouse; to the almshouse he was conveyed, and there perhaps must abide. How sad a fate! I found him in a quiet state; though at times was told that he is greatly excited; what wonder, with such a companion before him; such cruel scenes within! I perceived in him some little confusion as I paused before the stall, against the bars of which he was leaning; he was not so lost to propriety but that a little disorder of the bed-clothes, &c. embarrassed him. I passed on, but he asked, in a moment, earnestly, "Is the lady gone—gone quite away?" I returned; he gazed a moment without answering my inquiry if he wished to see me? "And have you too lost all your dear friends?" Perhaps my mourning apparel excited his inquiry. 'Not all.' "Have you any dear father and mother to love you?" and then he sighed and then laughed and traversed the limited stall. Immediately adjacent to this stall was one occupied by a *simple* girl, who was "put there to be out of harm's way." A cruel lot! for this privation of a sound mind. A madman on the one hand, not so much separated as to secure decency, another almost opposite, and no screen ! I do not know how it is argued, that mad persons and idiots may be dealt with as if no spark of recollection ever lights up the mind; the observation and experience of those, who have had charge of Hospitals, show opposite conclusions.

Violence and severity do but exasperate the Insane : the only availing influence is kindness and firmness. It is amazing what these will produce. How many examples might illustrate this position : I refer to one recently exhibited in Barre. The town Paupers are disposed of annually to some family who, for a stipulated sum agree to take charge of them. One of them, a young woman, was shown to me well clothed, neat, quiet, and employed at needle-work. Is it possible that this is the same being who, but last year, was a raving madwoman, exhibiting every degree of violence in action and speech ; a very tigress wrought to fury ; caged, chained, beaten, loaded with injuries, and exhibiting the passions which an iron rule might be expected to stimulate and sustain. It is the same person ; another family hold her in charge who better understand human nature and human influences ; she is no longer chained, caged, and beaten ; but if excited, a pair of mittens drawn over the hands secures from mischief. Where will she be next year, after the annual sale ?

It is not the insane subject alone who illustrates the power of the all prevailing law of kindness. A poor idiotic young man, a year or two since, used to follow me at times through the prison as I was distributing books and papers : at first he appeared totally stupid, but cheerful expressions, a smile, a trifling gift, seemed gradually to light up the void temple of the intellect, and by slow degrees some faint images of thought passed before the mental vision. He would ask for books, though he could not read. I indulged his fancy and he would appear to experience delight in examining them ; and kept them with a singular care. If I read the Bible, he was reverently, wonderingly attentive ; if I talked, he listened with a half-conscious aspect. One morning I passed more hurriedly than usual, and did not speak particularly to him. "Me, me, me a book." I returned ; " good morning, Jemmy ; so you will have a book today ? well, keep it carefully." Suddenly turning aside he took the bread brought for his breakfast, and passing it with a hurried earnestness through the bars of his iron door—" Here's bread, a'nt you hungry ? " Never may I forget the tone and grateful affectionate aspect of that poor idiot. How much might we do to bring back or restore the mind, if we but knew how to touch the instrument with a skilful hand !

My first visit to Ipswich prison was in March, 1842. The

day was cold and stormy. The Turnkey very obligingly conducted me through the various departments. Pausing before the iron door of a room in the jail, he said, "we have here a crazy man, whose case seems hard, for he has sense enough to know he is in a prison, and associated with prisoners. He was a physician in this county, and was educated at Cambridge, I believe; it was there, or at one of the New-England colleges. Should you like to see him?" I objected that it might be unwelcome to the sufferer; but urged, went in. The apartment was very much out of order, neglected, and unclean; there was no fire; it had been forgotten amidst the press of other duties. A man, a prisoner waiting trial, was sitting near a bed where the Insane man lay, rolled in dirty blankets. The Turnkey told him my name, and he broke forth into a most touching appeal, that I would procure his liberation by prompt application to the highest State authorities. I soon retired, but communicated his condition to an official person before leaving the town, in the hope he might be rendered more comfortable. Shortly I received from this Insane person, through my esteemed friend, Dr. Bell, several letters, from which I venture to make a few extracts. They are written from Ipswich where is the general County receptacle for insane persons. I may remark that he has at different times been under skilful treatment, both at Charlestown and Worcester; but being, long since, pronounced incurable, and his property being expended, he became chargeable to the town or county, and was removed, first to Salem jail, thence to that at Ipswich by the desire of the High Sheriff, who requested the Commissioners to remove him to Ipswich as a more retired spot, where he would be less likely to cause disturbance." In his paroxysms of violence, his shouts and turbulence disturb a whole neighborhood. These still occur. I give the extracts literally :—"Respected lady : since your heavenly visit my time has passed in perfect quietude, and for the last week I have been entirely alone; the room has been cleansed and whitewashed, and is now quite decent. I have read your books and papers with pleasure and profit, and retain them subject to your order. You say, in your note, others shall be sent if desired, and if any particular subject has interest it shall be procured. Your kindness is felt and highly appreciated," &c. In another letter he writes, " You express confidence that I have self-control, and self-respect. I have, and, were I free and in good circumstances, could command as much as any man." In a third he says, " Your kind note, with more books and papers was received on the 8th, and I immediately addressed to you a letter superscribed to Dr. Bell; but having discovered the letters on your seal, I suppose them the initials of your name, and now address you directly," &c. &c.

The original letters may be seen. I have produced these extracts, and stated facts of personal history, in order that a judgment may be formed from few of many examples, as to the justness of incarcerating lunatics in all and every stage of insanity, for an indefinite period, or for life, in dreary prisons, and in connection with every class of criminals who may be lodged successively under the same roof, and in the same apartments. I have shown, from two examples, to what condition men may be brought, not through crime, but misfortune, and that misfortune embracing the heaviest calamity to which human nature is exposed. In the touching language of scripture may these captives cry out—"Have pity upon me! have pity upon me! for the hand of the Lord hath smitten me." "My kinsfolk have failed, and my own familiar friend hath forgotten me."

The last visit to the Ipswich prison was the third week in December. Twenty-two Insane persons and Idiots: general condition gradually improved within the last year. All suffer for want of air and exercise. The Turnkey, while disposed to discharge kindly the duties of his office, is so crowded with business, as to be positively unable to give any but the most general attention to the Insane department. Some of the subjects are invariably confined in small dreary cells, insufficiently warmed and ventilated. Here one sees them traversing the narrow dens with ceaseless rapidity, or dashing from side to side like caged tigers, perfectly furious, through the invariable condition of unalleviated confinement. The case of one *simple* boy is peculiarly hard. December 6, 1841, he was committed to the house of correction, East Cambridge, from Charlestown, as an *Insane* or *Idiotic* boy. He was unoffending, and competent to perform a variety of light labors under direction, and was often allowed a good deal of freedom in the open air. September 6, 1842, he was directed to pull some weeds, (which indulgence his harmless disposition permitted) without the prison walls, merely, I believe, for the sake of giving him a little employment. He escaped, it was thought, rather through sudden waywardness than any distinct purpose. From that time nothing was heard of him till in the latter part of December, while at Ipswich, in the common room, occupied by a portion of the lunatics not furiously mad, I heard some one say, "I know her, I know her," and with a joyous laugh John hastened towards me. "I'm so glad to see you! so glad to see you! I can't stay here long; I want to go out," &c. It seems he had wandered to Salem, and was committed as an Insane or *Idiot* boy. I cannot but assert that most of the Idiotic subjects in the prisons in Massachusetts are unjustly committed, being wholly incapaple of doing harm, and none manifesting any disposition either to injure others or to exercise mischievous propensities. I ask an investigation into this subject for the sake of many whose association with prisoners and criminals, and also with persons in almost every stage of insanity, is as useless and unnecessary, as it is cruel and ill-judged. If it were proper, I might place in your hands a volume, rather than give a page, illustrating these premises.

Sudbury. First week in September last I directed my way to the poor-farm there. Approaching, as I supposed, that place, all uncertainty vanished, as to which, of several dwellings in view, the course should be directed. The terrible screams and imprecations, impure language and amazing blasphemies, of a maniac, now, as often heretofore, indicated the place sought after. I know not how to proceed! the English language affords no combinations fit for describing the condition of the happy wretch there confined. In a stall, built under a woodshed on the road, was a naked man, defiled with filth, furiously tossing through the bars and about the cage, portions of straw (the only furnishing of his prison) already trampled to chaff. The mass of filth within, diffused wide abroad the most noisome stench. I have never witnessed paroxysms of madness so appalling; it seemed as if the ancient doctrine of the possession of demons was here illustrated. I hastened to the house overwhelmed with horror. The mistress informed me that ten days since he had been brought from Worcester Hospital, where the town did not choose any longer to meet the expenses of maintaining him; that he had been "dreadful noisy and dangerous to go near," ever since; it was hard work to give him food at any rate, for what was not immediately dashed at those who carried it, was cast down upon the festering mass within. "He's a dreadful care; worse than all the people and work on the farm beside." Have you any other insane persons? "Yes; this man's sister has been crazy here for several years; she does nothing but take on about him; and may-be she'll grow as bad as he." I went into the adjoining room to see this unhappy creature; in a low chair, wearing an air of deepest despondence, sat a female no longer young; her hair fell uncombed upon her shoulders; her whole air revealed woe, unmitigated woe! She regarded me coldly and uneasily; I spoke a few words of sympathy and kindness; she fixed her gaze for a few moments steadily upon me, then grasping my hand, and bursting into a passionate flood of tears, repeatedly kissed it, exclaiming in a voice broken by sobs, "O, my poor brother, my poor brother; hark, hear him! hear him!" then relapsing into apathetic calmness, she neither spoke nor moved, but the tears again flowed fast, as I went away. I avoided passing the maniac's cage ; but there, with strange curiosity and eager exclamations, were gathered, at a safe distance, the children of the establishment, little boys and girls, receiving their early lessons in hardness of heart and vice ; but the demoralizing influences were not confined to children.

The same day revealed two scenes of extreme exposure and unjustifiable neglect, such as I could not have supposed the whole New-England States could furnish.

Wayland. Visited the almshouse. There, as in Sudbury, caged in a wood-shed, and also *fully exposed* upon the *public* road, was seen a man at that time less violent, but equally debased by exposure and irritation. He then wore a portion of clothing, though the mistress remarked that he was " more likely to be naked than not ;" and added that he was "less noisy than usual." I spoke to him, but received no answer ; a wild, strange gaze, and impatient movement of the hand, motioned us away ; he refused to speak, rejected food, and wrapped over his head a torn coverlet ; want of accommodations for the imperative calls of nature had converted the cage into a place of utter offence. "My husband cleans him out once a week or so ; but it's a hard matter to master him sometimes. He does better since the last time he was broken in." I learnt that the confinement and cold together, had so affected his limbs that he was often powerless to rise ; " you see him," said my conductress, " in his best state." *His best state !* what then was the *worst* ?

—— *Westford.* Not many miles distant from Wayland is a sad spectacle ; was told by the family who kept the poorhouse, that they had twenty-six paupers ; one idiot ; one simple ; and one insane, an incurable case from Worcester hospital. I requested to see her, but was answered that she " wasn't fit to be seen ; she was naked, and made so much trouble they did not know how to get along." I hesitated but a moment ; I must see her, I said. I cannot adopt descriptions of the condition of the insane secondarily ; what I assert for fact, I must see for myself. On this I was conducted above stairs into an apartment of decent size, pleasant aspect from abroad, and tolerably comfortable in its general appearance ; but the inmates !—grant I may never look upon another such scene ! A young woman, whose person was partially covered with portions of a blanket, sat upon the floor ; her hair dishevelled ; her naked arms crossed languidly over the breast ; a distracted, unsteady eye, and low, murmuring voice, betraying both mental and physical disquiet. *About the waist was a chain*, the extremity of which was fastened into the wall of the house. As I entered she raised her eyes, blushed, moved uneasily, endeavoring at the same time to draw about her the insufficient fragments of the blanket. I knelt beside her and asked if she did not wish to be dressed? "Yes; I want some clothes." "But you'll tear 'em all up, you know you will," interposed her attendant. "No, I won't, I won't tear them off;" and she tried to rise, but the waist-encircling chain threw her back, and she did not renew the effort, but bursting into a wild shrill laugh, pointed to it, exclaiming, "see there, see there, nice clothes!" Hot tears might not dissolve that iron bondage, imposed, to all appearance, most needlessly. As I left the room the poor creature said, "I want my gown!" The response from the attendant might have roused to indignation one not dispossesed of reason, and owning self-control.

Groton. A few rods removed from the poorhouse is a wooden building upon the road-side, constructed of heavy board and plank; it contains one room, unfurnished, except so far as a bundle of straw constitutes furnishing. There is no window, save an opening half the size of a sash, and closed by a board shutter; in one corner is some brick-work surrounding an iron stove, which in cold weather serves for warming the room. The occupant of this dreary abode is a young man, who has been declared incurably insane. He can move a measured distance in his prison; that is, so far as a strong, heavy chain, depending from an *iron collar which invests his neck*, permits. In fine weather, and it was pleasant when I was there in June last, the door is thrown open, at once giving admission to light and air, and affording some little variety to the solitary in watching the passers-by. But that portion of the year which allows of open doors is not the chiefest part; and it may be conceived, without drafting much on the imagination, what is the condition of one who, for days, and weeks, and months, sits in darkness and alone, without employment, without object. It may be supposed that paroxysms of frenzy are often exhibited, and that the tranquil state is rare in comparison with that which incites to violence. This I was told is the fact.

I may here remark that severe measures, in enforcing rule, have in many places been openly revealed. I have not seen chastisement administered by stripes, and in but few instances have I seen the *rods* and *whips*, but I have seen blows inflicted, both passionately and repeatedly.

I have been asked if I have investigated the causes of insanity? I have not; but I have been told that this most calamitous overthrow of reason, often is the result of a life of sin; it is sometimes, but rarely, added, they must take the consequences; they deserve no better care! Shall man be more just than God ; he who causes his sun, and refreshing rains, and life-giving influence, to fall alike on the good and the evil ? Is not the total wreck of reason, a state of distraction, and the loss of all that makes life cherished a retribution, sufficiently heavy, without adding to consequences so appalling, every indignity that can bring still lower the wretched sufferer ? Have pity upon those who, while they were supposed to lie hid in secret sins, "have been scattered under *a dark veil of forgetfulness ;* over whom is spread a heavy night, and who unto themselves are more grievous than the darkness."

Fitchburg. In November visited the almshouse : inquired the number of insane ? was answered, several ; but two in close confinement ; one idiotic subject. Saw an insane woman in a dreary neglected apartment, unemployed and alone. Idleness and solitude weaken, it is said, the sane mind, much more must it hasten the downfall of that which is already trembling at the foundations. From this apartment I was conducted to an out-building, a portion of which was inclosed, so as to unite shelter, confinement, and solitude. The first space was a sort of entry, in which was a window ; beyond, a close partition with doors indicated where was the insane man I had wished to see. He had been returned from the hospital as incurable ; I asked if he was violent or dangerous ? 'No.' Is he clothed ? 'Yes.' Why keep him shut in this close confinement ? 'O my husband is afraid he'll run away, then the overseers won't like it ; he'll get to Worcester, and then the town will have money to pay." He must come out, I wish to see him. The opened door disclosed a squalid place, dark, and *furnished* with straw. The crazy man raised himself slowly from the floor upon which he was couched, and with unsteady steps came towards me. His look was feeble and sad, but calm and gentle.

"Give me those books, oh give me those books !" and with trembling eagerness he reached for some books I had carried in my hand : "do give them to me, I want them," said he with kindling earnestness. You could not use them, friend ; you cannot see there ; "O give them to me, do ;" and he raised his hand and bent a little forward, lowering his voice ; "*I'll pick a little hole in the plank and let in some of God's light.*"

The master came round. "Why cannot you take this man abroad to work on the farm, he is harmless ; air and exercise will help to recover him." The answer was in substance the same as that first given ; but he added, "I've been talking with our overseers, and I've proposed getting from the blacksmith an iron collar and chain, then I can have him out by the house." An iron collar and chain ! "Yes, I had a cousin up in Vermont, crazy as a wild-cat, and I got a collar made for him, *and he liked it.*" Liked it! how did he manifest his pleasure? "Why he left off trying to run away. I kept the alms-house at Groton : there was a man there from the Hospital : I built an out-house for him, and the blacksmith made him an iron collar and chain, so we had him fast, and the overseers approved it, and—" I here interrupted him. I have seen that poor creature at Groton in his doubly iron bondage, and you must allow me to say that as I understand you remain but one year in the same place, and you may find insane subjects in all, I am confident, if overseers permit such a multiplication of collars and chains, the public will not long sanction such barbarities; but if you had at Groton any argument for this measure in the violent state of the unfortunate subject, how can you justify such treatment of a person quiet and not dangerous as is this poor man ? I beg you to forbear the chains, and treat him as you yourself would like to be treated in like fallen circumstances.

Bolton. Late in December, 1842; thermometer 4° above zero; visited the almshouse; neat and comfortable establishment; two insane women, one in the house associated with the family, the other "*out of doors.*" The day following was expected a young man from Worcester Hospital, incurably insane; fears were expressed of finding him "dreadful hard to manage." I asked to see the subject who was "out of doors ; " and following the mistress of the house through the deep snow, shuddering and benumbed by the piercing cold, several hundred yards, we came in rear of the barn to a small building, which might have afforded a degree of comfortable shelter, but it did not. About two thirds of the interior was filled with wood and peat; the other third was divided into two parts, one about six feet square contained a cylinder stove, in which was no fire, the rusty pipe seeming to threaten, in its decay, either suffocation by smoke, which by and by we nearly realized, or conflagration of the building, together with destruction of its poor crazy inmate. My companion uttered an exclamation at finding no fire, and busied herself to light one, while I explored, as the deficient light permitted, the cage which occupied the undescribed portion of the building. "Oh, I'm so cold, so cold," was uttered in plaintive tones by a woman within the cage; "oh, so cold, so cold ! " And well might she be cold; the stout, hardy, driver of the sleigh had declared 'twas too hard for a man to stand the wind and snow that day, yet here was a woman caged and imprisoned without fire or clothes, not naked indeed, for one thin cotton garment partly covered her, and part of a blanket was gathered about the shoulders; there she stood, shivering in that dreary place, the grey locks falling in disorder about the face gave a wild expression to the pallid features; untended and comfortless, she might call aloud, none could hear; she might die, and there be none to close the eye. But death would have been a blessing here. "Well, you shall have a fire, Axey; I've been so busy getting ready for the funeral!" One of the paupers lay dead. "Oh, I want some clothes," rejoined the lunatic; "I'm so cold." "Well, Axey, you shall have some as soon as the children come from school; I've had so much to do." "I want to go out, do let me out!" "Yes, as soon as I get time," answered the respondent. "Why do you keep her here?" I asked, "she appears harmless and quiet." "Well, I mean to take her up to the house pretty soon; the people that used to have care here, kept her shut up all the year; but it *is* cold here, and we take her to the house in hard weather; the only danger is her running away; I've been meaning to, this good while." The poor creature listened eagerly, "oh, I won't run away, do take me out!" "Well, I will in a few days." Now the smoke from the kindling fire became so dense that a new anxiety struck the captive; "oh, I shall smother, I'm afraid; don't fill that up, I'm afraid." Pretty soon I moved to go away; "stop, did you walk?" "No." "Did you ride?" "Yes." "Do take me with you, do, I'm so cold. Do you know my sisters? they live in this town; I want to see them so much; do let me go!" and shivering with eagerness to get out, as with the biting cold, she rapidly tried the bars of the cage.

The mistress seemed a kind person; her tones and manner to the lunatic were kind; but how difficult to unite all the cares of her household, and neglect none! Here was not wilful abuse, but great, very great, suffering through undesigned negligence. We need an Asylum for this class, the incurable, where conflicting duties shall not admit of such examples of privations and misery.

One is continually amazed at the tenacity of life in these persons. In conditions that wring the heart to behold, it is hard to comprehend that days rather than years should not conclude the measure of their griefs and miseries. Picture her condition! place yourselves in that dreary cage, remote from the inhabited dwelling, alone by day and by night, without fire, without clothes, *except when remembered;* without object or employment; weeks and months passing on in drear succession, not a blank, but with keen life to suffering; with kindred, but deserted by them; and you shall not lose the memory of that time when they loved you, and you in turn loved them, but now no act or voice of kindness makes sunshine in the heart. Has fancy realized this to you? It *may* be the state of some of those you cherish! Who shall be sure his own hearth-stone shall not be desolate? nay, who shall say his own mountain stands strong, his lamp of reason shall not go out in darkness! To how many has this become a heart-rending reality! If for selfish ends only, should not effectual Legislation here interpose?

Shelburne. November last; I found no poorhouse, and but few paupers; these were distributed in private families. I had heard, before visiting this place, of the bad condition of a lunatic pauper. The case seemed to be pretty well known throughout the county. Receiving a direction by which I might find him, I reached a house of most respectable appearance; every thing without and within indicating abundance and prosperity. Concluding I must have mistaken my way, I prudently inquired where the insane person might be found? was readily answered, "here." I desired to see him; and after some difficulties raised and set aside, I was conducted into the yard, where was a small building of rough boards imperfectly joined; through these crevices was admitted what portion of heaven's light and air was allowed by man to his fellow-man. This shanty or shell, inclosing a cage, might have been eight or ten feet square, I think it did not exceed; a narrow passage within allowed to pass in front of the cage. It was very cold; the air within was burthened with the most noisome vapors, and Desolation with Misery seemed here to have settled their abode. All was still, save now and then a low groan. The person who conducted me tried, with a stick, to rouse the inmate; I intreated her to desist; the twilight of the place making it difficult to discern any thing within the cage; there at last I saw a human being, partially extended, cast upon his back amidst a mass of filth, the sole furnishing, whether for comfort or necessity which the place afforded; there he lay, ghastly, with upturned, glazed eyes, and fixed gaze, heavy breathings, interrupted only by faint groans, which seemed symptomatic of an approaching termination of his sufferings. Not so, thought the mistress; "he has all sorts of ways; he'll soon rouse up and be noisy enough; he'll scream and beat about the place like any wild beast, half the time." "And cannot you make him more comfortable? can he not have some clean, dry place, and a fire?" "As for clean, it will do no good; he's cleaned out now and then; but what's the use for such a creature? his own brother tried him once, but got sick enough of the bargain." "But a fire, there is space even here, for a small box stove?" "If he had a fire he'd only pull off his clothes, so it's no use." "But you say your husband takes care of him, and he is shut in here in almost total darkness, so that seems a less evil than that he should lie there to perish in that horrible condition." I made no impression; it was plain that to keep him securely confined from escape was the chief object. "How do you give him his food? I see no means for introducing any thing here?" "O," pointing to the floor, "one of the bars is cut shorter there, we push it through there." "There? impossible! you cannot do that; you would not treat your lowest dumb animals with that disregard *to decency!*" "As for what he eats, or where he eats, it makes no difference to him, he'd as soon swallow one thing as another."

Newton. It was a cold morning in October last, that I visited the almshouse. The building itself is ill adapted for the purposes to which it is appropriated; the town, I understand have in consideration a more advantageous location, and propose to erect more commodious dwellings. The mistress of the house informed me that they had several insane inmates, some of them very bad. In reply to my request to see them, she objected "that they were not fit—that they were not cleaned—that they were very crazy," &c. Urging my request more decidedly, she said they should be got ready, if I would wait. Still no order was given which would hasten my object. I renewed the subject, when, with manifest unwillingness, she called to a colored man, a cripple, who with several others of the poor were employed in the yard, to go and get a woman up—naming her. I waited some time at the kitchen door to see what all this was to produce. The man slowly proceeded to the remote part of the wood-shed where, part being divided from the open space, were two small rooms, in the outer of which he slept and lived, as I understood; there was his furniture; and there his charge! Opening into this room only, was the second, which was occupied by a woman not old, and furiously mad: it contained a wooden bunk filled with filthy straw, the room itself a counterpart to the lodging place; inexpressibly disgusting and loathsome was all: but the inmate herself was even more horribly repelling; she rushed out, as far as the chains would allow, almost in a state of nudity, exposed to a dozen persons, and vociferating at the top of her voice; pouring forth such a flood of indecent language as might corrupt even Newgate. I entreated the man, who still was there, to go out and close the door. He refused; that was *his place!* Sick, horror-struck, and almost incapable of retreating, I gained the outward air, and hastened to see the other subject, to remove from a scene so outraging all decency and humanity. In the apartment over that last described was a crazy man, I was told. I ascended the stairs in the wood-shed, and passing through a small room stood at the entrance of the one occupied; occupied with what? The furniture was a wooden box or bunk containing straw, and

something I was told was a man, I could not tell, as likely it
might have been a wild animal, half buried in the offensive
mass that made his bed; his countenance concealed by long
tangled hair and unshorn beard. He lay sleeping. Filth,
neglect and misery reigned there. I begged he might not be
roused. If sleep could visit a wretch so forlorn, how merciless to break the slumber! Protruding from the foot of
the box was——, nay, it could not be the feet ; yet from
these stumps, these maimed members were swinging chains,
fastened to the side of the building. I descended; the master
of the house briefly stated the history of these two victims of
wretchedness. The old man had been crazy above twenty
years. As, till within a late period, the town had owned no
farm for the poor, this man with others had been annually put
up at auction. I hope there is nothing offensive in the idea of
these *annual sales* of old men and women, the sick, the
infirm, and the helpless, the middle-aged and children ; why
should we not *sell* people as well as otherwise blot out human
rights, it is only being *consistent*, surely not worse than chain-
ing and caging naked Lunatics upon public roads, or burying
them in closets and cellars ? But,as I was saying, the crazy man
was annually sold to some new master, and a few winters since,
being kept in an out-house, the people within being warmed
and clothed, 'did not reckon how cold it was,' and so his feet froze.
Were chains now the more necessary ? he cannot run. But he
might *crawl* forth, and in his transports of frenzy "do some
damage."

That young woman ; her lot is most appalling! who shall
dare describe it! who shall have courage or hardness to write
her history ? That young woman was the child of respectable,
hard-working parents. The girl became insane ; the father, a
farmer with small means, from a narrow income had placed her
at the State Hospital. There, said my informer, she remained
as long as he could by any means pay her expenses. Then,
then only, he resigned her to the care of the town, to those who
are, in the eye of the law, the guardians of the poor and
needy ; she was placed with the other town-paupers, and given
in charge to a man. I assert boldly, as truly, that I have given
but a *faint representation* of what she was, and what was her
condition as I saw her last autumn. Written language is weak
to declare it.

Could we in fancy place ourselves in the situation of some of
these poor wretches, bereft of reason, deserted of friends, hopeless ; troubles without, and more dreary troubles within, overwhelming the wreck of the mind as ' a wide breaking in of the
waters,'—how should we, as the terrible illusion was cast off,

not only offer the thank-offering of prayer, that so mighty a destruction had not overwhelmed our mental nature, but as an offering more acceptable devote ourselves to alleviate that state from which we are so mercifully spared.

It may not appear much more credible than the fact above stated, that a few months since, a young woman in a state of complete insanity, was confined entirely naked in a pen or stall in a barn ; there, unfurnished with clothes, without bed, and without fire, she was left—but not alone ; profligate men and idle boys had access to the den, whenever curiosity or vulgarity prompted. She is now removed into the house with other paupers ; and for this humanizing benefit she was indebted to the remonstrances, in the first instance, *of an insane man !*

Another town now owns a poorhouse, which I visited, and am glad to testify to the present comfortable state of the inmates ; but there the only provision the house affords for an insane person, should one, as is not improbable, be conveyed there, is a closet in the cellar, formed by the arch upon which the chimney rests ; this has a close door, not only securing the prisoner, but excluding what of light and pure air might else find admission.

Abuses assuredly cannot always or altogether be guarded against ; but if in the civil and social relations all shall have "done what they could," no ampler justification will be demanded at the Great Tribunal.

Of the dangers and mischiefs sometimes following the location of insane persons in our almhouses, I will record but one more example. In Worcester, has for several years resided a young woman, a lunatic pauper of decent life and respectable family. I have seen her as she usually appeared, listless and silent, almost or quite sunk into a state of dementia, sitting one amidst the family, 'but not of them.' A few weeks since, revisiting that almshouse, judge my horror and amazement to see her negligently bearing in her arms a young infant, of which I was told she was the unconscious parent ! Who was the father, none could or would declare. Disqualified for the performance of maternal cares and duties, regarding the helpless little creature with a perplexed, or indifferent gaze, she sat a silent, but O how eloquent, a pleader for the protection of others of her neglected and outraged sex ! Details of that black story would not strengthen the cause ; needs it a weightier plea, than the sight of that forlorn creature and her wailing infant ? Poor little child, more than orphan from birth, in this unfriendly world ! a demented Mother—a Father, on whom the sun might blush or refuse to shine !

Men of Massachusetts, I beg, I implore, I demand, pity

and protection, for these of my suffering, outraged sex !—
Fathers, Husbands, Brothers, I would supplicate you for this
boon — but what do I say? I dishonor you, divest you at
once of christianity and humanity—does this appeal imply
distrust.   If it comes burthened with a doubt of your righteousness in this Legislation, then blot it out; while I declare
confidence in your honor, not less than your humanity.   Here
you will put away the cold, calculating spirit of selfishness and
self-seeking ; lay off the armor of local strife and political opposition ; here and now, for once, forgetful of the earthly and
perishable, come up to these halls and consecrate them with one
heart and one mind to works of righteousness and just judgment.   Become the benefactors of your race, the just guardians
of the solemn rights you hold in trust.   Raise up the fallen ;
succor the desolate ; restore the outcast ; defend the helpless ;
and for your eternal and great reward, receive the benediction....
" Well done, good and faithful servants, become rulers over
many things ! "
But, gentlemen, I do not come to quicken your sensibilities
into short-lived action, to pour forth passionate exclamation, nor
yet to move your indignation against those, whose misfortune,
not fault, it surely is to hold in charge these poor demented
creatures, and whose whole of domestic economy, or prison
discipline, is absolutely overthrown by such proximity of conflicting circumstances, and opposite conditions of mind and
character.   Allow me to illustrate this position by a few examples ; it were easy to produce hundreds.
The master of one of the best regulated almshouses, viz.
that of Plymouth, where every arrangement shows that the
comfort of the sick, the aged, and the infirm, is suitably cared
for, and the amendment of the unworthy is studied and advanced, said, as we stood opposite a latticed stall, where was
confined a madman, that the hours of the day were few, when
the whole household was not distracted from employment by
screams, and turbulent stampings, and every form of violence,
which the voice or muscular force could produce.   This unfortunate being was one of the " returned incurables," since whose
last admission to the almshouse, they were no longer secure of
peace for the aged, or decency for the young ; it was morally
impossible to do justice to the sane and insane in such improper
vicinity to each other.   The conviction is continually deepened
that Hospitals are the only places where insane persons can be
at once humanely and properly controlled.   Poorhouses, converted into madhouses, cease to effect the purposes for which
they were established, and instead of being asylums for the
aged, the homeless, and the friendless, and places of refuge for

orphaned or neglected childhood, are transformed into perpetual bedlams.

This crying evil and abuse of institutions, is not confined to our almshouses. The warden of a populous prison near this metropolis, populous, not with criminals only, but with the insane in almost every stage of insanity, and the idiotic in descending states from silly and simple, to helpless and speechless, has declared that, since their admission under the Rev. Stat. of 1835, page 382, "the prison has often more resembled the infernal regions than any place on earth!" and, what with the excitement inevitably produced by the crowded state of the prisons, and multiplying causes, not subject to much modification, there has been neither peace nor order one hour of the twenty-four; if ten were quiet, the residue were probably raving. Almost without interval might, and *must*, these be heard, blaspheming and furious, and to the last degree impure and indecent; uttering language, from which the base and the profligate have turned shuddering aside, and the abandoned have shrunk abashed. I myself, with many beside, can bear sad witness to these things.

Such cases of transcendent madness have not been few in this prison. Admission for a portion of them, not already having been discharged as incurable from the State Hospital, has been sought with importunity, and pressed with obstinate perseverance, often without success or advantage; and it has not been, till application has followed application, and petition succeeded petition, that the Judge of Probate, absolutely wearied by the 'continual coming,' has sometimes granted warrants for removal. It cannot be overlooked that in this delay or refusal was more of just deliberation than hardness, for it is well known that, in the present crowded state of the Hospital, every new patient displaces one who has for a longer or shorter time received the benefit of that noble institution.

A few months since, through exceeding effort, an inmate of this prison, whose contaminating influence for two years had been the dread and curse of all persons who came within her sphere, whether incidentally, or compelled by imprisonment, or by daily duty, was removed to Worcester. She had set at defiance all efforts for controlling the contaminating violence of her excited passions; every variety of blasphemous expression; every form of polluting phraseology, was poured forth in torrents, sweeping away every decent thought, and giving reality to that blackness of darkness, which it is said might convert a heaven into a hell; there, day after day, month after month, were the warden and his own immediate household; the subordinate officials, and casual visitors; young women detained as

witnesses ; men, women, and children, waiting trial or under
sentence ; debtors and criminals ; the neighborhood, and almost the whole town ; subjected to this monstrous offence—*and
no help !* the *law* permitted her there, and there she remained
till July last, when, after an application to the Judge, so determined, that all refusal was refused, a warrant was granted
for her transfer to the State Hospital. I saw her there two
weeks since ; what a change ! decent, orderly, neatly dressed ;
capable of light employment ; partaking with others her daily
meals. Decorously, and without any manifestation of passion,
moving about, not a rational woman by any means, but no
longer a nuisance, rending off her garments and tainting the
moral atmosphere with every pollution ; she exhibited how
much could be done for the most unsettled and apparently the
most hopeless cases, by being placed in a situation adapted to
the wants and necessities of her condition. Transformed from
a very Tisiphone, she is now a controllable woman. But this
most wonderful change may not be lasting ; she is liable to
be returned to the prison, as have been others, and then, no
question, but in a short time like scenes will distract and torment
all in a vicinity so much to be dreaded.

Already has been transferred from Worcester to Concord a
furious man, last July conveyed to the Hospital from Cambridge, whose violence is second only to that of the subject
above described. While our *Revised Statutes* permit the incarceration of madmen and madwomen, epilectics and idiots in
prisons, all responsible officers should, in ordinary justice, be ex-
onerated from obligation to maintain prison discipline. And
the fact is conclusive, if the injustice to prison officers is great,
it is equally great towards prisoners ; an additional penalty to
a legal sentence pronounced in a Court of Justice, which might,
we should think, in all the prisons we have visited, serve as a
sound plea for false imprisonment. If reform is intended to be
united with punishment, there never was a greater absurdity
than to look for moral restoration under such circumstances ;
and if that is left out of view, we know no rendering of the law
which sanctions such a cruel and oppressive aggravation of the
circumstances of imprisonment, as to expose these prisoners day
and night to the indescribable horrors of such association.

The greatest evils, in regard to the insane and idiots in the
prisons of this Commonwealth, are found at Ipswich and Cambridge, and distinguish these places only, as I believe, because
the numbers are larger, being more than twenty in each. Ipswich has the advantage over Cambridge in having fewer furious
subjects, and in the construction of the buildings, though these
are so bad as to have afforded cause for presentment by the

Grand Jury some time since. It is said that the new County House,in progress of building,will meet the exigencies of the case. If it is meant that the wing in the new prison, to be appropriated to the insane, will provide accommodation for all the insane and idiotic paupers in the county, 1 can only say that it could receive no more than can be gathered in the three towns of Salem, Newburyport, and Ipswich, supposing these are to be removed ; there being in Ipswich twenty-two in the prison, and eight in the almshouse ; in Salem almshouse, seventeen uniformly crazy, and two part of the time deranged ; and in that of Newburyport eleven, including idiots.   Here at once are sixty.   The returns of 1842 exhibit an aggregate of one hundred thirty-five.   Provision is made in the new prison for fifty-seven of this class, leaving seventy-eight unprovided for, except in the almshouses.   From such a fate, so far as Danvers, Saugus, East Bradford, and some other towns in the county, reveal conditions of insane subjects, we pray they may be exempt.

1 have the verbal and written testimony of many officers of this Commonwealth, who are respectable alike for their integrity and the fidelity with which they discharge their official duties, and whose opinions, based on experience, are entitled to consideration, that the occupation of prisons for the detention of lunatics and of idiots is, under all circumstances, an evil, subversive alike of good order, strict discipline, and good morals.   I transcribe a few passages which will place this mischief in its true light.   The Sheriff of Plymouth county writes as follows :—"I am decidedly of the opinion that the county jail is a very improper place for lunatics and idiots.   The last summer its bad effects were fully realized here, not only by the prisoners in jail, but the disturbance extended to the inhabitants dwelling in the neighborhood.   A foreigner was sentenced by a Justice of the Peace, to thirty days' confinement in the house of correction.   He was to all appearance a lunatic, or madman. He destroyed every article in his room, even to his wearing apparel, his noise and disturbance was incessant for hours, day and night.   I consider prisons places for the safe keeping of prisoners, and all these are equally entitled to humane treatment from their keepers, without regard to the cause of commitment.   We have in jails no conveniences to make the situation of lunatics and idiots much more decent than would be necessary for the brute creation, and impossible to prevent the disturbance of the inmates under the same roof."

In relation to the confinement of the insane in prisons the Sheriff of Hampshire county writes as follows :—

" I concur fully in the sentiments entertained by you in relation to this unwise,not to say inhuman, provision of our law (see

Rev. Stat. 382) authorizing the commitment of lunatics to our Jails and Houses of Correction. Our Jails preclude occupation, and our Houses of Correction cannot admit of that variety of pursuit, and its requisite supervision, so indispensable to these unfortunates.

"Indeed this feature of our law seems to me a relic of that ancient barbarism which regarded misfortune as a crime, and those bereft of reason as also bereft of all sensibility ; as having forfeited not only all title to compassion but to *humanity*, and consigned them without a tear of sympathy, or twinge of remorse, or even a suspicion of injustice to the companionship of the vicious, the custody of the coarse and ignorant, and the horrors of the hopelsss dungeon. I cannot persuade myself that any thing more than a motion by any member of our Legislature is necessary to effect an immediate repeal of this odious provision."

The Sheriff of Berkshire says, conclusively, that "Jails and Houses of Correction *cannot* be so managed as to render them suitable places of confinement for that unfortunate class of persons, who are the subjects of your inquiries, and who, never having violated the law, should not be ranked with felons, or confined within the same walls with them. Jailors and Overseers of Houses of Correction, whenever well qualified for the management of criminals, do not usually possess those peculiar qualifications required in those to whom should be entrusted the care of lunatics."

A letter from the surgeon and physician of the Prison Hospital at Cambridge, whose observation and experience has laid the foundation of his opinions, and hence has a title to speak with authority, affords the following views. "On this subject it seems to me, there can be but one opinion. No one can be more impressed than I am with the great injustice done to the insane by confining them in Jails and Houses of Correction. It must be revolting to the better feelings of every one to see the innocent and unfortunate insane occupying apartments with, or consigned to those occupied by the criminal. Some of the insane are conscious of the circumstances in which they are placed, and feel the degradation. They exclaim sometimes in their ravings, and sometimes in their lucid intervals, "What have *I* done that I must be shut up in Jail ?" and "why do you not let me out ?" This state of things unquestionably retards the recovery of the few who do recover their reason under such circumstances, and may render those permanently insane, who, under other circumstances might have been restored to their right mind. There is also in our Jails very little opportunity for the classification of the insane. The quiet and orderly must in many cases occupy the same rooms with the restless and noisy, another great hindrance to recovery.

"*Injustice* is also done to the *convicts ;* it is certainly very wrong that they should be doomed day after day, and night after night, to listen to the ravings of madmen and madwomen. This is a kind of punishment, that is not recognised by our statutes ; and is what the criminal ought not to be called upon to undergo. The confinement of the criminal and of the insane in the same building is subversive of that good order and discipline which should be observed in every well-regulated prison. I do most sincerely hope that more permanent provision will be made for the Pauper Insane by the State, either to restore Worcester Insane Asylum to what it was originally designed to be, or else make some just appropriation for the benefit of this very unfortunate class of our 'fellow beings'."

From the efficient Sheriff of Middlesex county, I have a letter upon this subject, from which I make such extracts as my limits permit :—"I do not consider it right, just, or humane, to hold for safe keeping, in the county jails and houses of correction, persons classing as lunatics or idiots. Our prisons are not constructed with a view to the proper accommodation of this class of persons ; their interior arrangements are such as to render it very difficult, if not impossible, to extend to such persons that care and constant oversight which their peculiarly unfortunate condition absolutely demands ; and besides, the occupation of prisons for lunatics is unquestionably subversive of discipline, comfort, and good order. Prisoners are thereby subjected to unjust aggravation of necessary confinement, by being exposed to an almost constant disquiet from the restless or raving lunatic. You inquire whether "it may not justly be said, that the qualifications for wardenship, or for the offices of overseer, do not usually embrace qualifications for the management of lunatics, whether regarded as curable or incurably lost to reason ?" and also, whether "the government of jails and houses of correction for the detention or punishment of offenders and criminals, can suitably be united with the government and discipline fitted for the most unfortunate and friendless of the human race, viz : pauper lunatics and idiots, a class not condemned by the laws, and I must add not mercifully protected by them ?" The first of the preceding questions I answer in the *affirmative ;* the last *negatively*."

A communication from the warden of the Cambridge prison affords the following opinions, results of his experience :—"As to the expediency or propriety of holding for safe keeping, in the jails or houses of correction, insane persons or idiots, I must say that I consider it both inexpedient and decidedly wrong that the insane, or idiots, or any other persons, should be confined in prisons, except those who have been convicted for crimes, or who are so strongly suspected that it is necessary they should be holden for safe keeping until they can be tried for the offences for which they stand charged. Any person having the least experience in prison-keeping, must, I think, be fully sensible of the demoralizing and pernicious influences insane persons must have on the order and discipline of a prison, nor can it be doubted that the punishment of all sane persons is very much enhanced and aggravated by their exposure to the ravings of the insane. Neither can the keepers or other officers of prisons be selected with a view to their fitness to take care of the insane, consequently they are in want of those qualifications which make them suitable for the management of such persons, be they curable or incurable."

From the Sheriff of Dukes county I have testimony, corresponding to that elsewhere received, and from which I am obliged to make extracts, when the entire letters would be valuable:—" I beg leave to say that I am decidedly of opinion that such confinement, even if it were in some cases " expedient," is not in accordance with the principles of sound enlightened philanthropy. Humanity shudders at the thought that those whom God in his providence has bereft of the light of reason, should be confined within the narrow bounds of a prison, deprived of the enjoyment of the pure air of heaven ; of necessary exercise ; of the comforts to which they have been used, comforts which their peculiar circumstances render so necessary ; and made companions of felons, and the worthless outcasts of society.

" With proper care and attention, lunatics may not only be made comfortable, but in many instances restored again to society with sound minds. But this care and attention cannot be expected from those who have charge of prisons, worthy men though many of them be ; it requires a union of qualifications rarely found in one individual, to manage successfully those from whom, that which chiefly distinguishes man from the brute creation, is taken away.

" I conclude with expressing the hope that the wisdom of our Legislature may devise a remedy for the evils now attending the unfortunate pauper lunatic and idiot."

The warden of one of the best conducted prisons in this or any other country, I refer to that at South Boston, writes:—" I affirm, most decisively, that jails and houses of correction are not fit places for the safe keeping of lunatics and idiots, and, as far as my experience goes, the officers are not qualified to take charge of lunatics."

The master of the Plymouth almshouse writes, in a letter containing many clear views,—" I hope to hear people are awake on this subject, and trust they will not rest till they have compelled the public to provide suitable places for that unfortunate class of demented persons. They should never be received in almshouses."

It is not few but many, it is not a part but the whole, who bear unqualified testimony to this evil. A voice strong and deep comes up from every almshouse and prison in Massachusetts where the insane are or have been, protesting against such evils as have been illustrated in the preceding pages.

Gentlemen, I commit to you this sacred cause. Your action upon this subject will affect the present and future condition of hundreds and of thousands.

In this legislation, as in all things, may you exercise that " wisdom which is the breath of the power of God."

Respectfully submitted,

D. L. DIX.

85 MT. VERNON ST. BOSTON.
January, 1843.

BOSTON : PRINTED BY MUNROE & FRANCIS.

MEMORIAL

NEW YORK

1844

MEMORIAL.

—

TO THE HONORABLE THE LEGISLATURE OF THE STATE OF NEW-YORK.

Gentlemen—

Your attention is solicited to the condition of many indigent and pauper insane persons in the county-houses of this State elsewhere. Your petitioner asks to present their wants and their claims, regarding this unfortunate class, not as being properly the charge of those towns and counties where their lot may have fallen, but as Wards of the State, made so by the most terrible calamity that can assail human nature—a shattered intellect, a total incapacity for self-care and self-government.

Notwithstanding the liberal appropriations for the relief of this class by the establishment of the State curative asylum at Utica, large numbers are yet unprovided for. Many whose cases offer every hope of recovery, if brought under remedial treatment, are sinking in the prime of life into irrecoverable insanity; others, whose condition exhibits nothing to encourage hope of benefit from being placed in a curative asylum, are permitted to fall into states of the most shocking and brutalizing degradation—pitiable objects, at once sources of greatest discomfort to all brought within their vicinity, and exposed to exciting irritation from the reckless sports of the idle and vicious. But this is not the darkest view of their condition; these most unfriended and wretched beings are often subject to more horrible circumstances. Fidelity to my cause compels me, however revolting the topic, to speak more explicitly. I state, therefore, that both idiots and insane women are exposed to the basest vice, and become mothers without consciousness of maternity, and without capacity in any way to provide for their offspring, or to exercise those cares which are instinctive with the lowest brute animals. Is this a condition of things to be tolerated in a christian land, in the very heart of a community claiming to take rank for elevation of moral principles and high-minded justice ? I am persuaded it is unnecessary to dwell upon this subject ; it must be enough that these evils are known to exist, for legislation to guard against their continuance. It may be well to say that the broadest evidence, sustained by appalling facts, can be adduced, substantiating these monstrous offences. Special details here would be out of place ; suffice it, that an investigating committee, though governed by no nice sensibilities, would shrink before half their task should be accomplished.

I will not consume time by narrating individual histories, which, however they might rouse your indignation, or awaken your sensibilities, will, I believe, not be needed to strengthen a cause so evidently claiming your very serious consideration and efficient action. I shall, as briefly as possible, refer to those institutions in the State, where are found both sufficient and defective provision for all classes of the insane, that from such statements you may determine what additional establishments are required.

The Asylums at Utica and at Bloomingdale afford insufficient accommodations for the reception of even the curable insane ; large numbers of both classes are accumulated in the county alms-houses, and in private dwellings. Of the condition, generally, of such as are retained by their own families, I am unprepared to speak ; were it proper to visit these as a stranger, time would not have afforded opportunity. Ten weeks of uninterrupted travelling has barely sufficed to ascertain the general condition of those in county-houses ; but inquiry in towns through which I have passed, has been met by information of one or several cases in each neighborhood ; sometimes these have been represented as hopelessly insane, returned from hospitals ; but oftener such as have received no skilful care or remedial medical treatment; and in not few instances subject to the application of a severe discipline, almost too terrible to be described. The cases are not many where this has appeared to be the result of wilful brutality, so much as a consequent of ignorance and great perplexity under unaccustomed trials. Few persons, however well-disposed and patient of trouble, have tact and discretion in managing a raving madman, or a perverse maniac.

I am spared the pain of describing the jails of New-York as containing, like those of Massachusetts, receptacles for the insane, or dungeons occupied not by criminals, but by those whom misfortune, not
guilt, has brought low. Against that monstrous abuse, your just laws
have effectually guarded ; nearly every county-house however, has its
" crazy-house," its " crazy-cells," or its " crazy-dungeons " and " crazy-cellar," as that of Albany, for example.

The county and city of New-York have made liberal and ample provision for their pauper lunatics, in establishing upon Blackwell's island
a hospital capable of receiving four hundred patients. This is considered a branch of the Alms-house establishment, which is in the city. At
the time of my visit, this hospital contained about three hundred patients, curable and incurable. This institution, so honorable to the city,
went into operation in 1839, and received from the alms-house all such
as were considered fit subjects for removal. About twenty-five, princi-
pally idiots in the lowest state of imbecility, remain at Bellevue.
The prominent defect of the asylum at Blackwell's island, seemed to
me the want of a sufficient number of competent attendants, and sufficient employment, and out-door exercise for the patients. I was told, in
answer to a remark on the advantages of household labor for a portion
of those heretofore accustomed to active life, that " under present arrangements this was impossible, as women of the vilest class from the
prison were employed to perform most of the work of the establishment, and it would not answer to expose the patients to their debasing
conduct, and profane language " ! This plan of accomplishing the domestic labor of the hospital is so very objectionable, that it cannot, it is
believed, be long suffered. New institutions often have great difficulties to overcome in course of being carried into operation ; it is not to
be supposed that the responsible officers of the New-York Asylum, will
be satisfied that it should hold a secondary rank in its internal or more
general form of administration.

The alms-house at Bellevue is placed on a much better system of
moral discipline than formerly. The house of refuge for juvenile offenders appeared to be conducted in the most unexceptionable manner.
The farm schools on Long island, belonging to the city, and connected
with the alms-house, are models of order and good government, and illustrate the solid advantages of separating the juvenile from the adult
poor. Connected with these extensive establishments and the alms-
house in the city, is a hospital on Blackwell's island for the children

and infants, who are sick and feeble. The plan of these judicious and humane establishments, can only be appreciated by those who have compared the results they afford, with those which flow from the more prevailing and most pernicious system of indiscriminate alms-house association of the old with the young. A partial division is ineffectual to prevent evil; to be productive of substantial good, it must be complete—then will alms-houses cease to be primary schools for jails and State prisons.

ALBANY COUNTY ALMS-HOUSE, at *Albany*, as I saw it in November, 1842, presented scenes of horrible neglect and misery, which even now I shudder to recall, and I rejoice, that a late visit in December, 1843, afforded evidence of many favorable changes, especially in the "dungeons" so called, and the "crazy cellar;" yet there even now, one finds many friendless creatures whose condition urges a sufficient and early provision, by the State, for their relief.

It was on the afternoon of a severely cold day in November of 1842, that I visited the alms-house at Albany. Inquiring of the master who held charge of the establishment, the number of the insane then in close confinement, I was answered, " There are plenty of them ; somewhere about twenty." " Will you let me see them ? " " No, you can't, they're naked, in the crazy cellar." " Are all in the same apartment then ? " " No, not all, but you can't see them." " Excuse me, but I must see the women's apartment. It is to learn the condition of the insane here, that I have come." At length a direction was given, and I was conducted by the mistress of the house into a court-yard, and the person holding charge over the insane women was summoned to attend me. Ascending a flight of stairs, conducting from without, to the second story of a large building, I entered an apartment not clean, not ventilated, and over-heated : here were several females chiefly in a state of dementia ; they were decently dressed, but otherwise exhibited personal neglect ; the beds were sufficiently comfortable ; the hot air, foul with noisome vapors, produced a sense of suffocation and sickness impossible to be long endured by one unaccustomed to such an atmosphere. I delayed here but few moments, and asked to be conducted to the dungeons : " dungeons," repeated the attendant, eyeing me closely. " Yes, the dungeons, I have heard there are dungeons here ; I am in haste, oblige me by losing no time." She still hesitated, when speaking more decidedly I said, " I must go, friend, and that immediately :" whereupon she led the way over the outer staircase, across the common court-yard, and descending into a spacious cellar kitchen, crowded by a most disorderly and profane set of men, women, and children, emerged on the opposite side upon a yard enclosed by a high board fence, and opening on the left upon still another enclosed space, surrounding a wooden building. We here encountered the man who kept the keys of this place, and who appeared to have charge of the building. I do not hesitate to say that he was unfit for the office. I was told both these persons were " paupers from Canada," and their phraseology did not contradict the information. A noisy altercation ensued, made up of coarse oaths and expletives, unmatched except in Newgate or on Blackwell's island. I again interposed, and at length induced the *turnkey* to produce his keys. Detaining my first companion, I followed through the opened doors, and ascending a flight of steps found myself in a passage not very narrow, on each side of which were " the dungeons " or cells. These were totally dark and unventilated, and there was *then* no provision for drying or warming them. To describe the scenes which were revealed as these loathsome dens were successively thrown open is impossible. Those who have read the reports of the Hospital Commissioners to the British Parliament, exposing the condition of the wretched inmates of the private mad-houses in England, may conceive an idea of what existed in the alms-house at Albany a year since. The keeper unlocking the first door on the left, vociferated to the poor wretch there confined, to " come out to the light and be seen." The horrible stench emitted from this dreadful place compelled me repeatedly to retreat to the outer air to recover from overpowering sickness. When I could so far command myself as to observe this dungeon and its occupant, God forgive me (if it was sinful,) the vehement indignation that rose towards the inhabitants of a city and county, who could suffer such abominations as these to exist ;—towards all official persons holding direct or indirect responsibility, who could permit these brutalizing conditions of the most helpless of human beings, and towards a country ever vain-glorious of its liberty, and of its civil, social, and religious institutions. I affirm that the dungeons of Spielberg and of Chillon, and the prisons of the Court of the Inquisition before their destruction, afforded no more heart-rending spectacles than the dungeons (not subterranean) of the Albany alms-house, at the time referred to. Language is feeble to represent them, and the mind shudders with disgust and horror in the act of recalling the state of the unfortunate insane there incarcerated.

In the cell first opened was a madman ; the fierce command of his keeper brought him to the door—a hideous object ; matted locks, unshorn-beard, a wild wan countenance, yet more disfigured by vilest uncleanness, in a state of entire nudity, save the irritating incrustations derived from that dungeon reeking with loathsome filth : here, without light, without pure air, without warmth, without cleansing, without *anything* to secure decency or comfort, here was a human being, forlorn, abject, and disgusting it is true, but not the less a human being—nay more, an immortal being, though now the mind had fallen in ruins, and the soul was clothed in darkness. And who was he — this neglected, brutalized wretch — a burglar, a murderer, a miscreant, who, for base foul crimes had been condemned by the justice of outraged laws, and the righteous indignation of his fellow-men to expiate offences, by exclusion from his race, by privations and sufferings, extreme, yet not exceeding in measure the enormities of his misdeeds ? No, this was no criminal outcast, who was here festering in filth, wearing out the warp of life in dreariest solitude and darkness— no, this was no criminal, but "*only a crazy man !*" Of him in the touching language of Scripture could it be said : " My brethren are far from me, and mine acquaintance are verily estranged from me ; my kinsfolk have failed, and my familiar friends have forgotten me : my bone cleaveth unto my skin and my flesh. Have pity upon me—have pity upon me, for the hand of God hath touched me ! "

I turned from this miserable scene only to witness another, yet more pitiable. A woman, of what age one could not conjecture, so disfigured was she by neglect and suffering, occupied a dungeon on the right. The keeper harshly summoned her " to come out," but she only moved feebly amidst the filthy straw which was the only furnishing of the place ; her moans and low cries indicated both mental anguish and physical pain. In vain they tried to force her forward—she seemed powerless to raise herself upright ; she, too, was unclothed ; and here alone in sickness and want, with no pure air, no pleasant warmth, no light, (those unmeasured gifts of God, alike shared by "the good and the evil, the just and the unjust,") no friendly hand to chafe the aching limbs, no kind voice to raise and cheer—there she lay on that loathsome plank, miserable beyond words to represent. I know nothing of her history, whether forsaken by able kindred, or reluctantly given over to the *public charity* by indigent parents, or taken in, a wandering, demented creature ; I only know that I found and left her reduced to a condition upon which not one who reads this page, could look but with unmitigated horror ! Do you turn with inexpressible disgust from these details ? It is worse to witness the reality. Is your refinement shocked by such statements ? There is but one remedy—prevent the possibility of such monstrous abuses by providing hospitals and asylums where vigilant inspection, and faithful care, shall protect and minister to those who, in losing reason, can no longer protect themselves ; who, as young, feeble infants, are helpless and unconscious ; who, through the calamity of insanity, become in the most peculiar manner the charge of those whose " light has not gone out."

Turning from the dungeons, the keeper said, " come to the crazy-cellar, you'll get noise enough there." I objected, that the master of the house had said, they were in no condition to be visited. "Oh, come, he knows nothing about them. The woman there told him, three weeks ago, that the dungeons were too cold for those people you saw, but he's forgot all about them—he's something else to think of—come, this is the way." I hesitated, but the idea that possibly I might learn facts which should lead to a change for the sufferers, led me on ; reaching the cellar—within which, just then, all was quiet—the keeper entered, and "for the sake of exercise," began by knocking one down, and so went on to rouse the whole company ; there were twelve or four-teen men here, sufficiently clothed for decency—some extended on the floor, others *chained to their beds*—all exhibiting a disgusting and miserable appearance : in an adjoining apartment were others in like circumstances. In March last, some gentlemen visited this same cellar, and returned expressing horror, that " such things could be tolerated, or that they ever could have existed in any civilized country."

I revisited this county house a few weeks since ; there had been a change of masters. The present overseer evidently has qualifications which enable him to secure a very improved order of things throughout the establishment; he has to contend against the great defects of the present system, and prominent evils must of course exist. Five hundred paupers of every age and various conditions, (a large proportion of these able-bodied foreigners, who here are idle for want of work, which the county does not provide, as well as idle in many cases from choice,) compose this family or rather community. Considering the very crowded state of the house, and all the difficulties to be encountered, a surprising degree of order and cleanliness are *now* secured. But inevitably this is a soil where the vices will take

root and flourish. I visited "the dungeons," and found but two females
in confinement there ; by comparison only could they be called comfortable. A stove is now placed in the passage, I cannot say it seemed to afford any great advantage to the insane in the cells ; in these
apartments were bunks, beds and bed-clothing. The apparel was
slight and required attention ; but the fact is, the inmates ought
to be transferred to a hospital where they can receive appropriate care. In the crowded "crazy cellar" I found improved accommodations, better beds, &c. One man " poor George," had just deceased, and his coffin was borne past as I stood at the entrance of
this dreary place ; surely the angel of death here performed a most
blessed ministration. Several men were chained to the beds or the
floor ; a general quiet prevailed. I noticed that the master " our boss"
was welcomed as a friend, and no doubt, so far as he had the power,
the condition of these friendless insane was made comfortable. The
time has past, however, for society to sanction such provision for this
class of the poor.

RENSSELAER COUNTY HOUSE, in *Troy*, about two miles from the
city, is composed of extensive buildings, constructed on a much more
judicious plan than most houses of this class. I understand that at no
distant time, here, as in many other places, very gross abuses have
existed, but at present the establishment appears in excellent condition. It is said that the insane have suffered both personal injuries
and neglect. I saw none in the cells. One young woman was confined in a comfortable apartment, but in a state of furious madness.
The room was evidently not left without care. A young man not long
insane, appeared a subject for a curative institution ; but the mother
was poor, and some objections I was told had been made by the county
officers to incurring the expense. The house throughout exhibited a remarkable attention to neatness ; it was not the neatness and order consequent on a weekly arrangement, but the result of daily and constant
care. The cells for " the crazy inmates" are said to be in very bad
condition ; I did not see them. The county are liberal in providing
supplies of clothing and furniture for the various departments, and except for the insane, it is one of the most complete establishments in
the State ; it has the faults common to all these institutions, arising
from a defective system.

SCHENECTADY COUNTY HOUSE, at *Schenectady*, is at the *present*
time in excellent condition, having advantage of one of those efficient,

active housekeepers, whose ready capabilities put things, and keep them, in right order. By kindness, encouragement, and decision, the comfort of the house is admirably maintained ; ample supplies of good beds and bed-clothing ; clean and well arranged rooms ; carefully mended apparel, and cut with due regard to convenience and economy when new ; food not only supplied in sufficient quantity, but wholesome and properly cooked, all these characterize the Schenectady alms house ; nothing is wasted, and nothing needed which is not supplied ; but here classification of the adults is less complete than at Troy, from deficiency of room. All the children for the same reason, are associated with the adults. But one insane person was found in close confinement ; not neglected ; her history would be out of place here, but will no doubt be made public.

SARATOGA COUNTY HOUSE, near *Ballston*, presented neat and comfortably arranged apartments ; the poor were neatly clothed, and the children taught by a " hired teacher." The house has a larger number of occupants in the winter than can be well provided with lodging-rooms. It was expected that when the State Lunatic Asylum was opened, all the insane would be sent from this place to Utica ; but so soon as the terms of admission were made known, and it was found that they could not be received " without cost to the county," the plan was abandoned, and consequently here are many, both men and women, in various stages of insanity, some curable probably, others affording no favorable symptoms, and all very improperly situated. The upper apartments occupied by these persons, are not so well arranged and attended as they might be, even under all the disadvantages inevitable upon being connected with an alms-house. They are said to be less objectionable than before the present master was appointed. The cells in the " cellar basement" " by the wash room," are neither ventilated nor do they admit light uniformly ; here I found two females in the worst possible condition personally. I cannot say that any who were appointed to take charge of them, wilfully neglected or abused them. I can but speak of the circumstances in which I found them ; and leave it for others to determine where blame should primarily be attached. Each cell contained a little straw ; it was said that one patient was so furious that she destroyed every thing upon which she could place her hands ; and I had ample evidence of her destructive propensities during the short time I was there. In answer to some remark implying great disapprobation of the cells as places of confinement for these maniacs, I was answered that it was strange I "should find fault, for the mother of one of the insane women came to see her sometimes, and she did'nt complain; and the doctor, when he came, did'nt complain; and why should a stranger care any thing about it? She was no better than a brute beast, and the place was good enough for such an ugly creature." I quote literally, from the person having daily care of these poor maniacs.

The family who have charge of the house at large, have effected, I was told, very important reforms from the earlier condition of the alms-house.

The county jail at Ballston was in very excellent order, highly credit-able to the warden and his family.

I heard in this county of the extreme wretchedness of several insane persons in private families, but did not visit them.

WASHINGTON COUNTY HOUSE, at *Argyle*, is well built, in good repair, and *at the present time* well conducted. The school is taught by a hired instructress, and the children looked after, at all times, with a care very unusual in alms-houses.

The family were respectably clothed, the apartments suitably furnished, the food of excellent quality, and prepared in a wholesome manner. The great want of free ventilation in the lodging rooms was manifest upon the countenances of many; one evidence was afforded, by the remark that the "children were so pale and feeble when they got up in the morning that they seemed about to faint, and that they had to be nursed up in the spring with *bitters* and strengthening things, to keep them along at all." The mistress added, "that she sometimes thought they would all be sick, sleeping so many in one room." I hinted that a supply of pure air would probably be the most effectual tonic.

In this establishment I found above twenty insane men and women, besides several "simple, silly, and idiotic." The men were in most cases confined by *fetters, with chains and balls*, to prevent their escape from the premises, and were thus allowed to leave their cells or little apartments in an outbuilding. "By adopting this plan," said the master, "I am able to give them air and exercise, otherwise I should have to keep them constantly shut up." Several females, who were in a very

tranquil state, were in the main building, in all respects neat and comfortable ; and of this I am quite confident, that however revolting were
some methods of restraint, they were adopted because at the time, they
were supposed to be the only modes of controlling the violent, or detaining the vagrant. A considerable number of women, most of them
apparently classing as incurables, were " behind the pickets," in an
outbuilding ; here was a passage of sufficient width for exercise, both
lighted and warmed ; upon this the cells opened, these with two exceptions, were comfortable, in good repair, white-washed, and furnished with good beds and well supplied with bed-clothing. The noisy
here of course, disturbed the quiet; the restless excited the more tranquil, and annoyed the feeble. One woman who had a propensity for
rending her clothes, and destroying any thing she could seize, was held
in restraint by a very singular apparatus ; I should not commend its
use to others. This consisted of an iron collar investing the throat,
through which, at the place where it was united in front, passed a
small iron bolt or bar, from this depended an iron triangle, the sides of
which might measure about sixteen or eighteen inches ; iron wristlets
were attached to the corners, and so the hands held in confinement,
and as far apart as the length of the base of the triangle. If the hands
and arms were suddenly elevated, pressure upon the apex of the triangle at the point of connection at the throat, produced a sense of suffocation, and why not complete strangulation, it was not easy to see.
I suggested a muff and belt for the hands and waist, as securing the
necessary restraint in a less objectionable form, but they had none and
had never seen any. I must repeat it as my full belief, that, however
unsuitable the condition of the insane at this alms-house, I cannot
think any blame should attach to the master of the establishment. It
was evidently his desire to do what was right, so far as he knew how,
in the management of those committed to his care. I saw in Argyle,
an insane and most wretched being, in a state of great excitement, and in very painful circumstances ; difficult to manage, and
seldom in a tranquil state : addicted to the most offensive language and
habits, she had exhausted the patience of the former keepers at the
alms-house, and abuse, violent measures, and neglect followed. Her
sisters, too poor to support her unassisted, laboring for daily bread
with the needle, begged to take her to their own home, and solicited
aid from the county. I found them humbly and earnestly toiling to
fulfil their duties, patiently performing the most difficult and revolting
offices, and trying to meet expenses which their situation rendered

both uncertain and painful. I carefully inquired into the facts of the case, and learned that the county officers had said " it would cost less to keep her at the poor-house, and they had no right to expend the public money by such appropriation."

I trust the appeal made in hope of changing their views was not unavailing, and that the devoted sisters receive at least *fifty cents* per week regularly paid, for their hard work of duty.

The jail at Sandy-Hill, is in a poor condition, and little used. That at Salem is better built and kept in order.

WARREN COUNTY-HOUSE, at *Warrensburgh*, is well situated, but the buildings are not constructed for convenient classification. Some repairs were in progress. Greater care was called for in several departments. The insane, when requiring to be kept in close confinement, occupied cages, or spaces divided from the common room of the poor, by perpendicular wooden bars ; the objections to such arrangements are too obvious for comment. At the time of my visit there were none in a very excited state. The family having charge of the poor were well spoken of in the vicinity ; they certainly are not accountable for all the deficiencies in the establishment.

The county jail at Caldwell was inconvenient and not suitable for comfort or the secure detention of the prisoners. It has recently been destroyed by fire.

ESSEX COUNTY POOR-HOUSE, near *Essex* and *Westport*. That portion of the dwelling occupied by the family having charge of the establishment, neat to exactness, and comfortable without deficiency. The apartments of the poor, ill-arranged, ill-furnished, ill-kept, (except two,) and very inconvenient. No hospital apartments ; no suitable provision for the children, though when sent to school, a teacher was hired to instruct them ; no proper classification of the inmates on the lower floor. The neglect manifested here did not produce much suffering I imagine, but it did not show that regard to decency and propriety which would be creditable to a county-house,—or is deemed fit in any family. The floors, wood-work, walls, and beds were *greatly* neglected. Some apology was offered for the " confusion of the rooms," on account of some repairs in progress ; carpenter's work however, is clean work, and this was not the occasion of the various defects observable. I learnt in different parts of the county, that dissatisfaction existed in regard to the deficient furnishing of the house, and perhaps by this time the superintendent may have supplied some pressing wants. I am sure the people of Essex county are not parsimonious where suffering is to be relieved, or the care of the poor and infirm is to be considered. Perhaps if less sums were charged for the removal of the poor from their respective towns, there would be less objection to making appropriations for additional conveniences, putting up additional buildings, and furnishing them for more decent and respectable accommodation. There were here no proper apartments for the insane, and at the time of my visit, there were none of this class confined " in the cells." These I did not go "below" to see. They were described as "very cold, damp, and dreary, and not fit for a dog to house in." It did not seem necessary to add any testimony of mine to verify such a description; since with but little variation the same account was derived from a variety of sources, and confirmed on the premises. I believe that the master and mistress of the house are humane people, and would desire to treat kindly any person laboring under this calamitous visitation who should be sent to their care. I am aware that some remarks respecting this and other like establishments may seem to contradict each other; but as in private families may be often seen attention to some things, and remarkable negligencies in other departments, it is not singular that these should be noticed in yet broader contrast in a county poor-house.

CLINTON COUNTY HOUSE at Plattsburgh, is not a good building, and much out of repair; it is not large enough for the numbers thronging to it in the winter. It is distinguished by a remarkable neatness throughout. I visited this place on a stormy day, at an unexpected and unseasonable hour; it was doubly gratifying to notice a place of so much comfort and quiet, made so by the uncommon care and capability of the master and mistress of the house. Here the sick were in well arranged apartments, and well attended; the household suitably and neatly clothed; garments well made, and in *good repair*; clean beds, bedsteads, and bed-clothing; clean tables, chairs and floors; clean walls and clean windows, showing that neither the application of white-wash, or water and the scrubbing brush were spared. The kitchen in good order.

There were here at the time of my visit in October, no insane in close confinement. I saw in the house, seated quietly by the fire, an insane man, who formerly, before the present master of the house was appointed, was kept chained to a post in the barn, in a state of complete nudity, " receiving" said my informant, " no other care than to have his food tossed to him like a dog—and not always cooked." The poor wretch had been released for a considerable period ; was washed, dressed, and taken into the house, where he partook of his meals with others of the family. He occasionally rendered some little assistance in bringing wood and water. Great care was requisite in managing him : he was subject to outbreaks of violence, and really was an unsafe inmate ; a proper subject for hospital treatment, or for an asylum adapted for such cases. This crazy man bore marks of former " lashes of the cow-skin, applied to drive the —l out of him," as was significantly said.

An insane female was assisting about some household work, and though often much excited was still kept pretty tranquil a large part of the time, by patient care. In most families I have found such cases subject to close confinement.

Compassion was deeply moved at seeing a little girl, about nine or ten years of age, who suffered the fourfold calamity of being blind, deaf, dumb, and insane. I can conceive no condition so pitiable as that of this unfortunate little creature, the chief movements of whose broken mind, were exhibited in restlessness, and violent efforts to escape, and unnatural screams of terror. No gentleness or kindness seemed to sooth her, or to inspire confidence. Various methods had been tried to promote her comfort, but with little success. She would rend her garments and bed clothing to pieces, and seemed most content when she could bury herself in a heap of straw ; when food was presented, she swallowed it with avidity, and seemed indifferent to its kind or quality. It was necessary to watch her with great care. To promote her comfort at one time, she was removed from the cells and placed with other persons in a large room, fastened by a small chain to the floor, to prevent her from falling upon the heated stove. She resists control, and perpetually struggles to escape. If left at large in mild weather, for a few minutes, she gropes her way, or rather rushes off avoiding by some invisible instinct violent falls, and conceals herself beneath a bush or fence : when brought back she resists violently, and utters the most vehement outcries. I took her hand gently, but she fell into the wildest paroxysm, which passed by, only when she had concealed herself in the straw in her cell. The utmost care was taken to keep her clean, and to do all for her comfort that her unhappy condition permitted.

There is at this house no provision for the insane who are at any time too violent to be permitted at large, except low, dismal cells, fit for no use, and which should never be employed for any persons of this class. The true remedy will be found in State asylums, on a cheap, but comfortable plan for the incurables.

FRANKLIN COUNTY-HOUSE, at *Malone*, fifty miles from Plattsburgh, is at present under so good administration, that it is to be hoped a change of its present master will be avoided, for years to come. The defects of the present system are, however, apparent here quite as much as elsewhere. The house is crowded with inmates beyond its capacity for either health or convenient accommodation. There is no proper provision for the insane, who need separation, by occasion of their violence, from the other members of the household. There can be no really suitable arrangements planned for them in county houses.

There are few insane in the alms-house at Malone. These are kept pretty comfortably ; yet I say this by comparison with many found in worse conditions. I heard in this section of the country of many recent cases of insanity ; several of much suffering. It was not seldom replied, when I questioned why these, and also others in remote counties, were not sent to the hospital at Utica, that they could send but one or two from any county ; and assurance has repeatedly been given that some of these would have been sent, if it had not been officially declared that only a specified number would be received from each county. In many instances, no doubt, this was a true reason ; in others it was made an excuse for not incurring the expense necessary for removal, and board at the Asylum. It is frequent to hear of whippings and other severe measures ; and many have yet to learn that the all-prevailing law of kindness, has a truer influence than brute force or vehement language. Of one truth may all be sure ; if, for a time, the former appear ineffective, the latter not only never accomplishes the end aimed at, but aggravates the malady while it enhances the sufferings of the unfortunate maniac.

ST. LAWRENCE COUNTY-HOUSE, at *Canton*, consists of several excellently constructed buildings, in many respects adapted for convenience and classification. The apartments were well arranged, decently ordered, and comfortably furnished. There was a general attention to

neatness throughout all these, and also more than usual attention to
furnishing those able to work, with employment. The children's school
was taught by a young woman hired for the purpose. There is here, as
at nearly every alms-house in the country, great neglect of the moral
and religious instruction of the poor. I will not decide where this fault
rests; it is not with the master and mistress of these houses, whose
whole time is necessarily engrossed with other important cares. It may
be hoped that both the county-house schools, and the inmates generally,
will receive inspection and instruction at suitable times, and no longer
be regarded as excepted from the consideration of communities in the
vicinity, because " it is the poor-house establishment." To the poor
was the gospel preached in the days of the Saviour, and we have no reason to believe that these cease to need the benign influences of christianity. The excuses often offered for these neglects are unworthy and
trivial. The insane poor at Canton occupy chiefly a building constructed for their use; it may be well warmed and completely ventilated, but it exhibited defects which would make those interested in
this subject solicitous for other provision for all this class.

JEFFERSON COUNTY-HOUSE, at *Watertown*, is remarkably well built,
and judiciously situated in a pleasant and healthful section of the county. It is constructed on a more commodious plan than many, though
often too much crowded in the winter. No sufficient plan for employing the inmates, who are able for work, has been devised. The children
require much more care than they can easily receive ; here, as in other
places, often acquiring and confirming indolent habits. The time
which is given to school instruction is less here, throughout the year,
than is usual in alms-houses. The house is generally neatly kept, and
a complete change was going on throughout the establishment, prepa-
ratory for winter arrangements. The building appropriated to the
insane, was clean, well lighted, well warmed, and sufficiently ventilated. Here are to be found demented persons of both sexes ; some
traversing the long passage in front of the " cells or dungeons," some
seated, others standing. Again others in close confinement in the cells,
the doors of which were composed of wooden bars, affording a distinct
view within. Part of the inmates were quiet, others raving ; part
clothed ; part in a state of nudity ; all exposed to any who chose to
observe them, whether men or women. So far as general daily care
was regarded, none seemed to suffer neglect, but I have no confidence
that this may not occur. A man and woman, themselves paupers, took

charge of all the cells, and really appeared heartily interested for the unfortunate creatures so dependant on their continued good offices ; yet were these subject, by many contingencies, to serious evils and sufferings.

LEWIS COUNTY-HOUSE, at *Lowville*, is small, ill built, and in no way suited for the use to which it is appropriated. It is uncommonly deficient in ventilation, and in being purified by frequent applications of lime-wash, and scrubbing. The inmates appeared to be abundantly supplied with food ; and to have suitable apparel, if it had only had the advantage of more frequent washings. The overheated and crowded rooms gave the idea of great discomfort, though no discontent was manifest on the part of the occupants ; and it is quite likely they would not feel under obligation to any who should insist on a more suitable conduct of their domestic affairs. There are no tolerable apartments for the insane ; and at the time I was there, none were in close confinement. In fact, for such as these, there is no provision at all. Several crazy persons were associated with the family at large. I understand that the farm and the dairy are well conducted. Justice to the master and mistress of such an establishment seems to require new and wholly different buildings. Certainly under the present circumstances they are very unjustly burthened with responsibilities, without fit means for securing good conduct or moral discipline. I have understood that this subject is likely to receive attention.

HAMILTON COUNTY is but partially settled, and till lately has been an almost unbroken extent of wilderness. It covers an area of one thousand and sixty-four square miles, has but seven small settlements, and but about two thousand inhabitants. I was able to learn nothing of the poor and insane. It is safe to infer that they are very few ; and I may add that the former certainly would not be likely to fall into a condition of much suffering.

OSWEGO COUNTY-HOUSE at *Mexico*, is a decent building, with the usual defects as an alms-house. A part appeared well arranged : lodging-rooms not in the order which should distinguish them from the superior care they should be supposed to receive. General aspect of the inmates negligent, and implying want of sufficient employment for those able to work. I impute no intentional neglect to the overseer of this house, and I ought not to omit the fact that several imbecile persons seemed to receive uncommon care in being kept comfortably clean.

There could not be said to be any provision for the insane here, separate from others of the family.   At the time of my visit in November, there were *none* of this class in close confinement.

I heard in this county of many cases of insanity in private families, requiring skilful care and remedial treatment ; and at Pulaski was made fully acquainted with the touching and melancholy history of an insane female now in the Oneida county-house at Rome ; the facts have reached me from various authorized sources, and are too horrible to record.   I have but too much evidence that here is not a solitary example of brutal outrage and protracted misery.   So far as the cause of humanity might be served by a disclosure of facts, it may become obligatory to produce evidence that such abominations exist.   I do confess, with the author of the Inferno that—

> " So by my *subject, is my power surpassed,*
> *Whate'er I say compared with truth seems weak !* "

WAYNE COUNTY-HOUSE at *Lyons,* is at the present time under excellent administration, good discipline, kind care, and neatness being secured to a considerable degree.   The master of this establishment was a sensible well-informed man, having a clear comprehension of his duties, and understanding in the discharge of them.   So complex are the arrangements in alms-houses which are made to serve so many purposes opposite in object and result, that one must be rather singularly endowed to meet every emergency.   The children here appeared under a supervision careful beyond what is usual.   The cells for the insane were to some extent rendered comfortable—that is to say—though not by any means fit for crazy men and women, which is part the fault of the county, they were taken care of daily, and by inference I should suppose at no time neglected, which may be ascribed to the fidelity of the master.   One circumstance especially pained me ; it was the situation of an insane girl, who though placed in a comfortable apartment and decently dressed, was attended by a woman whose ill-temper was apologized for from the fact of her probably having been disturbed through the night by the restlessness and cries of the young woman.   She was represented as being a good nurse, and no doubt had some excellent qualifications, but she was not a good nurse for a creature like this poor girl, placed so much in her power.   " This is no house for such rich folks as her's to send their children to ; it is for the poor, and they may take care of her for themselves."   " She is more ugly than crazy, and knows well enough what she is about."

I pointed to a large bruise on the temple of the weeping girl; the nurse did not deny that she had inflicted a blow, but persisted that the girl was "ugly and would'nt be still ! "

MONROE COUNTY-HOUSE, at *Rochester*, is large and in general well and neatly arranged. There is still need of much more careful classification. The expenditures in this county are enormous for the support of the poor, who chiefly are foreigners, and who crowd in, as winter advances, from all quarters ; and not only are the expenses great, but most liberally met. The quantity of fuel, provision and clothing distributed alone in the city of Rochester at public cost, and through private charities, must appear quite incredible to those not familiar with the facts. One is made to feel the great importance of framing effectual plans for diminishing pauperism, rather than by supplying present urgent wants, increase dependence, and diminish the self-reliance and self-respect which is felt by those in humble circumstances, who endeavor, by care and economy, to provide, at least in part, for themselves. In Rochester, Buffalo, Utica and Albany, (which I particularly designate as being constantly crowded with foreign paupers able to work, but saying they cannot procure it,) work-houses are loudly called for. These might be so conducted as not to injure the more industrious and capable members of the community, and yet ensure employment without other compensation than the whole support of the families throwing themselves thus on the public charge ; let them know certainly, that if they do not support themselves abroad, they will, by law, be required to do so in a work-house, and I think pauperism, in a few years, would dwindle down to cases of the aged, the infirm, and to children without parental guardians. At Rochester, the master was making arrangements for providing separate apartments for the children, so as to cut off, in part at least, communication with the adults : the plan here is less perfect than that at Buffalo, but must have substantial advantages. Here is a school taught by a young woman hired for the purpose.

The insane who were in close confinement, were in decent cells of pretty good size, furnished with a bed ; the ravings of the violent disturbed the sick, and maintained discomfort throughout "their quarter." Several insane men, according to very common usage, were dragging about *a chain and heavy iron ball* attached, these were united to the *fetters*, and used for such as not being shut up, were liable to escape. Of one it was said that " the exercise of dragging his ball and chain, had much improved his health ! "

No neglects were apparent in the Rochester county house at large ; and I am told it receives much attention from the authorized inspectors from the city. This is right ! It should not be supposed that a master is deficient in fidelity, because his establishment is often inspected. Too much vigilance cannot be exercised, especially in reference to those made wholly dependent on the care of others through sickness or insanity. Persons have no right to *assume* the fact of a good administration of these affairs ; the evidence should consist in frequent visitations and the closest observation. All responsible persons should be able to say, " I do not *believe* only, I *know* that all is right."

The jail at Rochester, cannot be commended for good conduct or efficient management in its internal arrangments or daily care. I did not see the warden of the prison, but I should not consider the subordinates fit persons for the trust they hold, except their duties are confined literally to the " turning of the keys." Older and more responsible persons would be likely to exert a more wholesome influence in the *upper*, as well as the *lower* department.

ORLEANS COUNTY HOUSE, at *Albion,* has many great defects. I do not know but the farm is well conducted, and the inmates well supplied with food. In winter they have over-heated apartments ; for such indeed are found almost universally, *except for the insane* ; but essential improvements might be made in the domestic arrangements. I saw here but one insane person, a woman, in close confinement, and in a wretched condition, yet by comparison better than many beside, in having wider space, light and air. She was in an apartment divided into two parts by wooden bars, and within a similar enclosure was a large iron stove ; the *fire had been forgotten* however, on that day ; the weather was cold and rough, the crazy woman was employed in pulling the straw from one side of the room where she made her bed, and pushing through the bars towards the cold stove, one straw after another to "make a fire and keep the cold away." The aspect of this poor crazy girl, covered with a single garment, and crouched on the floor, offered little to inspire interest, except that she was a suffering human creature, therefore needed sympathy ; she was unfriended, and therefore needed just and watchful guardians. I do not know that the omission of the fire was habitual, but the neglect should never occur ; one was kindled before I came away. It had been the custom to keep the " crazy people," below stairs in the cells or dungeons, which were dark and with little air ; but " they were so raving there, that they had concluded to build, in the kitchen occupied by the paupers, a cage, composed of upright bars of wood," this I saw nearly completed, and to this the girl above, on the first floor, was in a few days to be removed! so insane as to require a degree of retirement and shelter. One would believe that the family, if not the county officers, would have discovered the impropriety of such an arrangement. Here, constantly exposed to exciting noise and merriments, and often to the teazing tricks of the many occupants of the room, she would have no quiet, if indeed she allowed it to others. This was a case of hopeless insanity; and this, combined with gross exposures, in all probability, will be a life-long condition.

NIAGARA COUNTY-HOUSE, at Lockport, is well built, but till recently is not spoken of as being of good repute. The most obvious defect, was overheated rooms, thronged with idle men and women. One insane man from this house, who is at present in the Asylum at Utica, *bears upon his ancles the scars of fetters and chains, and on his feet evidence of exposure to frost and cold.* He evinces much emotion when reference is made to these facts, and not long since, when I saw him, wept like a child, as he told of his sufferings there. It is quite common for patients at the hospital, who have been exposed to injury and abuse, to chains and fetters, to " blows" and " floggings," to exhibit great excitement, if reference is made to their former condition.

ERIE COUNTY-HOUSE, at *Buffalo*, situated a short distance from the city, consists of a large and not well constructed building, where are the adult poor; this affords insufficient accomodation for the large numbers gathering here in the winter months. The house, at the time of my visit, required extensive repairs; but so far as care on the part of the master and mistress was considered, the domestic arrangements were highly creditable. I remarked the humane consideration shown to the aged, who were at their morning meal, apart from the other inmates, and received the special care due to advanced age and infirmity.

A substantial and convenient building on the premises is exclusively devoted to the children, who are superintended by an excellent matron, and have a good school taught by a hired teacher. The counties of New-York and Erie, at present, have the only completely distinct establishments for poor children that are to be found in the State.

The insane occupy a pretty comfortable, but very small building in rear of that appropriated to the other poor. I saw nothing, at the time I was there, to indicate that these insane were not receiving sufficient general care from their attendants; but still I must renew and repeat protestations against *all county* receptacles for the insane, and *all private* institutions for this class throughout the country : they *may possibly* be exempt from abuse and neglect, but are not likely to be, and if not very exceptionable one year, the county receptacles may, by change of officers, become so the following season. Persons fully acquainted with these subjects, and medical men having experience, offer enough substantial reasons why such should never, at this advanced day, find favor or toleration. I am told that, at a recent meeting of the supervisors and superintendents of Erie county, these gentlemen voted that the series of cells at the county alms-house, should be called the *County Hospital for the Insane !* It will require a great many votes to convert that little building, with its few cell-rooms, into a hospital, or even an asylum. This may remain a petty receptacle for some five or six incurables, but it never can be a curative establishment. At present this county-house has the advantage of a sensible and benevolent physician, who, while he perceives the essential disadvantages of the place, has earnestly addressed himself to diminish the evils resulting from so defective a system, and I perceive has, in a recent number of the Medical Journal, offered some pertinent remarks on the bad custom of converting alms-houses into houses of correction ; thus bringing into contact, the basest class—the most guilty members of society—with those whose chiefest misfortune is infirmity, or poverty, or friendlessness.

Chautauque County-House, near *Mayville*, is well situated, and apparently, at the present time, under good direction : the general aspect of the household indicated care for their comfort and regular discipline. The apartments were too much crowded, and there was an unusual number of idiotic, imbecile and deformed persons. There was a school for children, and a variety of work was furnished to some who were able to be employed. Provision for the insane much the same as in a majority of these houses. The cells in part divided by solid partitions, and in part by perpendicular wooden bars, were wretched in the extreme. Bare of furniture and receiving insufficent light and ventilation, they exhibited little beside misery and suffering.

I passed into two which were occupied. In one were two very crazy females. The eldest fancied herself a queen, and greatly resented the familiar manners of her companion, advancing energetically from words to blows, she inflicted bruises and wounds without mercy ; in fact, she proceeded to biting ; and when I proposed that they should be wholly separated, was answered, " we would be glad to do it, but have no more room." In the adjoining cell, which might be eight or ten feet square, was no furniture of any description. Upon the floor, covered with one slight garment, sat in a contracted posture, a miserable looking woman, perhaps forty years of age. The cell was dismal and offensive. The only companionship of this unfortunate person was that of the other insane and idiotic women, who were in a room upon which this one looked by means of the bars between which the light and air were admitted. One could discern in this solitary female nothing indicating that she had ever been other than the debased creature she now appeared. Yet it was told me by those who had known her in her conscious, bright years, that she had been one of " the best wives, housekeepers, and landladies in all the county ;" that she had been "a good neighbor, a good member of society, a good christian ; but that trouble and hard work had broken down her strength and destroyed her mind ;" and here I found her deserted of every friend, desolate of every consolation, possessed of no comforts. And so to abandon one who, while she had ability, was faithful in all the social and domestic relations—so to forsake her, was not regarded as an offence against humanity or religious obligation. She was crazy ; who could be expected to do any thing for her ? She must go to the poor house, there she must be kept alive and tended ; and there she is now, a living monument of the injustice of society and the neglect of kindred !

CATTARAUGUS COUNTY-HOUSE, at *Machias*, was in a good condition apparently, so far as the master was responsible. It is ill constructed for an alms-house. The insane were in wretched cells, and in a miserable condition in a small building on the premises, called the " block house." Several seemed to require immediate hospital treatment ; all needed a very different situation, and a degree of personal care and attention wholly incompatible with the other duties devolving on the master of the house. I do not propose to consume time by entering on numerous details of individual histories, however appealing these would be to your sympathy. The present actual condition appears to me sufficiently wretched to move you to action in their behalf, unaccompanied by the heart-touching narratives of real life, revealing deep sorrows and harsh abuses.

ALLEGANY COUNTY-HOUSE, at *Angelica*, is well situated, and in some respects offered a better appearance within than report accorded, except the condition of the insane, who were most miserably provided for in cells, and in a comfortless room in an out-building, significantly called "the crazy house." This was neither sufficiently cleaned, warmed, nor ventilated. The most furious were in small cells, others in an apartment upon which these opened, and to which they were exposed. One of the men was greatly excited, and in the cell adjoining, an aged woman was imploring to be let out to warm herself, and "because they torment me so through the bars; there's no rest, no rest here; oh the noise; I can't have this noise;" she exclaimed in troubled accents, "oh let me out just for a little while." The misery of this place is not describable; perhaps those who had charge to the utmost of their knowledge, with means furnished, did the best they were able. I am slow to form harsh judgments, and ought to add that it was here, too, that an insane man whose touching history was given by some benevolent persons who had interposed in his behalf, to rescue him from the violent personal abuse and injustice of a *brother;* it was at this same place that he was kindly treated and carefully nursed during a dangerous and painful illness, occasioned by a serious wound; and at length recovering, was received by those who were strangers to him, but christians, through the exercise of a most blessed charity.

STEUBEN COUNTY-HOUSE, at *Bath*, has not a good reputation through the neighboring counties. At the season of my visit, the superintendents and supervisors were there, in session. The house was certainly in that kind of good order which could not be the result of a special care at one season. It was said that a spirit of kindness was wanting towards the inmates. The out-buildings which were appropriated to the insane, were not in good condition, and here, especially in the case of two crazy men, I noticed great neglect. I confess I was not inspired with confidence in their general humane treatment; in fact, these should not have been in a county house, but no other asylum as yet is provided in the State for the neglected incurables.

CHEMUNG COUNTY-HOUSE, on *Newtown creek*, ten miles from Elmira, is a poorly constructed wooden building, but well managed on the part of its present overseer. The inmates generally appeared well clothed and comfortable. I found two insane men in an out-building, which in all respects was more convenient and better furnished, than any appropriated to this class of poor in the southern counties of the State. Both cells were warmed by means of a stove in the outer apartment, warmth, air, and light passing through the bars in front.

TIOGA COUNTY-HOUSE, a little north from *Owego*, is built of stone, it is too small, and constructed with little regard to convenience or classification. I found here two insane women in out-buildings, one in a small cell, in a most wretched state, and perfectly furious; her language and conduct made it utterly unfit that she should be in the immediate vicinity of others, yet, here children and all the family were alike exposed to the most demoralizing influences. I do not know that it could be expected of the master of the establishment to make other provision for her; and considering her extreme violence, persons unaccustomed to the charge of the insane would find it a very difficult task to promote her comfort, or secure her in a proper manner. I understand that many inhabitants of this county desire to abandon the alms-house system, and return to the old custom of "bidding off the poor annually to the lowest purchaser." Perhaps some changes at the county-house might restore it to more general favor.

BROOME COUNTY-HOUSE, at *Binghamton*, is out of repair, and greatly deficient in neatness and comfort in every respect. The walls required white-wash, the apartments generally, complete cleansing; the food was sufficient in quantity and quality, but very badly cooked; there was need of a strong, active, working-woman, entirely devoted to that part of the establishment occupied by the poor, in fact two would find ample employment. Here were found a very unusual number of infirm, aged, and imbecile poor; indeed the inmates all were of the class properly subjects of an alms-house charity. There were here no insane persons in close confinement; several idiots occupied together a portion of one building; *one gibbering, senseless creature, was the mother of a young infant.*

CORTLAND COUNTY-HOUSE, at *Cortland*, was in excellent order, clean and comfortable beds and bed-clothing, clean walls, clean floors, and clean furniture, and the whole remarkably well arranged, especially considering that the house was not built for the uses to which it is appropriated. The children here looked well, they were in school, and taught by one of the inmates, a plan not well conceived as it seems to me ; in the present case perhaps it was less objectionable than in some places, but where the numbers to be taught are sufficient, there should be a competent hired teacher. The cells in which were such of the insane as could not be trusted at large were clean, and in not *severe weather perhaps* sufficiently warmed by the stove-pipe conveyed along the passage, in front of these compartments. This establishment affords insufficient employment for the *able-bodied men* who resort here in the winter months.

TOMPKINS COUNTY-HOUSE, near *Ithaca*, was visited very hastily in November last. It is a large wooden building, of which I saw but part; yet so far as this might represent the condition of the whole, it was very respectable. It was clean, well aired and warmed, and wore an aspect of general good order. One insane person only was in close confinement ; this was a woman within a cage, built in a comfortable apartment on the second floor : this was thoroughly clean, well warmed and convenient. The poor creature was decently dressed, but very greatly excited, noisy and violent. A fit subject for an asylum. I did not learn her history.

This was the aspect of the Tompkins County House this autumn ; perhaps it was, so far as the sane poor were concerned, equally creditable last April, but I cannot feel justified to pass by a case which I *know* to be exact. In the spring of last year, 1843, an insane man was removed from this almshouse, *who had been chained for three years, and shockingly neglected*, and this so as to produce consequences almost too offensive to be spoken of; but if public institutions are not guarded from such shameful abuses, I do not know why they should not be fully exposed ; what people are not careful to prevent, they must not be too delicate to hear declared. In addition to *every personal neglect*, this poor man was so infected with *insects over the whole person,* that those who received him were compelled to burn every article of clothing he wore from the almshouse and furnish new. When opportunity afforded the means of cleanliness after this, he was found to be remarkably neat.

YATES COUNTY-HOUSE, in *Jerusalem*, near Penn-Yan, is partly built of stone. It is a very neat, well ordered establishment. I particularly noticed the excellent care bestowed upon the children ; these I found neat and clean, in a well-ordered school, taught by a hired instructress. There were several insane persons, but all at large with the family, though one was much excited—a subject for some suitable asylum.

ONTARIO COUNTY-HOUSE, *Canandaigua.* This is an extensive establishment, and I am told very expensive to the county ; it ought to present a better aspect. " The people, it is said, have certainly plenty to eat, are warm enough, and have clothes enough." All this is undeniably true ; but they are disorderly, dirty, and negligent of all the appliances for keeping clean and well ordered apartments. There was a want of method, of discipline, and of good regulations, apparent over all the house. The insane were in a portion of the establishment chiefly apart from the rest. Their cells and apartments might pass through some wholesome changes. I had no direct evidence that the patients suffered serious neglect or abuse. Light, air and warmth were admitted, and they were furnished with beds : but still I cannot think, that should the citizens of Canandaigua, or of the county at large, visit this establishment, they would approve its condition. I am told the farm is well conducted.

LIVINGSTON COUNTY-HOUSE, at *Geneseo,* bears a good reputation in adjacent counties, which is confirmed by its neatly ordered apartments, its good discipline, in short, the whole air and aspect of the place within doors. It is not constructed on a good plan, but these deficiencies are in part compensated by the good judgment and discretion of the master and mistress of the house. No insane confined here in cells.

WYOMING COUNTY as yet, has no county-house, but one is in progress of being built, to be opened, as I understand, next year. At present, the poor are boarded in a farmer's family in *Orangeville.* A case of the greatest neglect of an insane man came to my knowledge, I could not secure time to see him, but several of his former friends and neighbors described his condition as one of much suffering through want of common daily care. I could not learn that he had ever been in any hospital. He had once filled a respectable place in society ; became impoverished, and insane: for a considerable time was taken to the house of one of his brothers ; finally, the other refusing to share the expense and trouble, and the family becoming weary of the case, he was cast on the public charity. " By neglect, his limbs are so contracted, that he neither can stand or walk ;" " he lies upon a miserable pallet in a most miserable condition," crippled, untended, uncared for. May those who have cast him off, never know the biting sorrow of abandonment and unfriended helplessness.

GENESEE COUNTY-HOUSE, at *Bethany*, is a well built commodious house, and a model of neatness and exact order throughout. The children were well directed, clean, and not neglected in discipline. A visiter for an hour, would almost here forget the defects of the general system, so excellent are the domestic arrangements. No insane here in close confinement. No provision for insane persons.

SENECA COUNTY-HOUSE, at *Fayette*, an ill constructed wooden building; for the sick, affording no convenient hospital room, and no sufficient lodging rooms during the winter months for the numerous family. Cells for the violently insane are in the basement; several crazy women were in apartments on the second floor, and not neglected; rooms less correctly neat than might be desired. All insane persons, in county-houses are subject to vexatious and disturbing acts from many, who either share their apartments, or who meet them during the day. This is a universal source of disquiet, and cannot be controlled by the overseers of the house—at least only imperfectly. The master of the house at Fayette, a sensible, practical man, seemed fully aware of the disadvantages under which he was acting. There was no school for the children; they were at one time sent to the district school in the immediate vicinity, but parents objected to having their children associate " with the children of the paupers," and these were sent home. The county provided no teacher, and the house afforded no person supposed competent to teach. The children took their education therefore into their own hands, and were acquiring a sort of knowledge which years of careful instruction will fail to eradicate.

In the basement I saw a man who for ten years had been chained in a cage: here, untended in any decent manner, without clothes, beating to chaff the straw which was supplied for bed and covering—-raving often day and night, disturbing the slumbers of all the family, and uttering the most horrible imprecations, he was at once a torment to himself, and a source of indescribable disturbance to all beside. One day shortly after the present master took him in charge, word was hastily brought that John had broken his fetters and chain, had broken open his cage, and was then in the outer room below. The master hurried down filled with apprehension; he found the madman in the greatest delight at gaining his freedom; he danced, and sung, and declared that he had done with chains and would no longer live in his cage. When attempts were made to remove him, his entreaties were so earnest and promises so eloquent that he prevailed on the kind-hearted overseer, and had permission "if he would do no mischief, and not attempt to hurt any body," to stay out, an order being at the same time given for him to be washed, shaved, and dressed.   Nothing could exceed John's transports.   The owner was necessarily absent from home through the day ; returning, John was the first to meet and salute him with the news that he had kept his promise and " no harm had come."   Several cases of this sort have come to my knowledge.   It cannot be regarded as safe to have these very excitable persons at large and unattended, and there certainly is great cruelty in keeping them chained and shut up like wild beasts.   For these things there is but one effectual remedy.

CAYUGA COUNTY-HOUSE, near *Auburn*, has not long since undergone a complete change in its domestic administration ; from being a most discreditable establishment, it has become subject to order, wholesome discipline, and careful supervision.   Mixed classes make it difficult to secure comfort to the more respectable of the inmates ; and double the labor of household care.   The provision for the insane though better than in many counties ; is not suitable ; it is but lately that the most extreme neglect of this class existed here ; but I remarked that cleanliness was now exacted of those who were appointed to take charge of the rooms.   This county has been very liberal in sending the insane poor to the Asylum at Utica.   The farm is said to be in excellent order and in good cultivation.

ONONDAGA COUNTY-HOUSE is at *Syracuse.*   I regret to refer to this establishment, since I cannot describe it advantageously in any respect. It compares very ill with most county-houses in general appearance, and arrangement.   All the apartments needed complete cleansing by white-washing, scrubbing, and the renewing of much of the bed clothing.   The aspect of the whole place was that of discomfort ; the sick needed more efficient care ; the aged and blind more attention ; the children some person to have them in sole charge ; and the insane needed every thing.   I found the women in cells in wretched conditions. I will not attempt to enter upon the description of them ; it was such as should never be suffered under any circumstances, and such as no apology can excuse.   *Possibly* at the time of my visit, there was a more than usual omission of care through the house.   I ought to say that the " hired girl" was absent, and the mistress had for several days been indisposed.   But when there are not persons enough to accomplish work properly, the deficiency should be supplied ; it is no excuse that the helpless and dependent be left to suffer through want of care, because there are not enough in the house to perform necessary labor.

I have been informed that the farm is well conducted : also that it is in contemplation to build a more suitable house in a more convenient situation. This is greatly needed. I am very slow to censure those who have personal charge of county-houses ; they have great difficulties to meet, complex duties to perform, and it must, to those who exercise fidelity, be at all times a very laborious charge both abroad and within doors. There will be less need of apology for defects when suitable houses are constructed, and a wholesome system adopted. The county-house of Onondaga ranks very low in other counties ; but I incline to think its moral condition greatly better than in former years ; for many deficiencies the superintendents are responsible rather than their overseer.

MADISON COUNTY-HOUSE, at *Eaton* is well built and well situated ; it has a good farm advantageously managed. The internal arrangements are not good ; the apartments are not well divided, nor well kept. The apparel of all the inmates was in remarkably good order ; a part of the lodging rooms were suitably furnished. A very excellent new building has lately been constructed of stone, which is designed as a hospital for the sick ; this is a department rarely found in county-houses, and always needed. There was wanting in this house a more careful discipline, order, method ; especially was there needed an overseer of the children, who should require cleanness, orderly habits, and maintain discipline at table and elsewhere. The mistress of the house has a most laborious life, and evidently too much care, with too little assistance.

Those of the insane kept constantly confined, are in cells, in the basement. Mercifully there were but three of these poor creatures. They *" are taken out once a week to be cleaned," " and to have fresh straw put into the cells !"* These are raving lunatics : others, not violent above stairs, were mingling with the family, some of them assisting in household labor.;

ONEIDA COUNTY-HOUSE, at *Rome*, is now, perhaps, in a better condition than at any former period since its establishment, but it is so very defective, that if I describe it as it really is, it will scarce be credited that a whole community so respectable as the citizens of Oneida county, and annually making such liberal appropriations for the suppor of the poor, should permit the existence of an institution bearing so vile repute as this. From Clinton county to Chautauque, from Columbia to Niagara, are proclaimed the late and long-passed immoralities of Oneida county-house. I feel confident I have heard hundreds refer to this subject, and never one voice in favor. It is said, that for a year or more, greater care has been exerted to maintain in some sort moral discipline, but the construction of the buildings does not permit classification to much extent. The rooms were out of repair, but several were kept neat. Most of these greatly needed the application of whitewash, and a new supply of beds, bedsteads, and bed clothing. Wearing apparel was more decent. The master desired the complete separation of the children from the adults, but had not the means to effect so wholesome an arrangement. The *present* master of the house and his wife, evidently desire to perform their duty towards the inmates.

Those of the insane who need close confinement, are in miserable narrow cells, which open upon a small yard. Here I found one man and two women, the latter neglected, and all very improperly placed. I left them in the yard. The history of these unfortunate females is shocking to relate. No more than brief allusion can be made to it. *They have here become mothers !* They, like others here, have formerly been exposed to the lowest vices. These shameless immoralities, these monstrous neglects are suffered. One would deem it time for State legislation to interpose, when county administration is so torpid, and county superintendents so culpably indifferent and inefficient. Oneida, Herkimer, Greene, and Orange county-houses, and ten or twelve beside, have reputations to earn, which till gained, leave their names only *synonyms* for foul crime and base licentiousness. To the guardianship of the State I commend with earnest importunity, the idiotic and insane who, in the overthrow of reason, are no longer accountable beings. Here are about twenty insane. The master of the house has made repeated application for changes in the buildings.

HERKIMER COUNTY-HOUSE is very badly situated, immediately adjacent to a tavern, and on the bank of the canal, near *German-Flats.* It is a miserable building, with about an acre of land attached. I am informed that it is proposed to purchase a farm in a more suitable place, and to erect suitable buildings. The present establishment is in very ill repute, and one of the most disorderly in the State. It was very much neglected, and most of the apartments out of order in all respects when

I saw them. The cells for the insane were most wretched. The exposures of the idiotic I need not name. The results the same as at Rome. A teacher was hired at the expense of the county for the children's school. All these were in a most neglected state personally. Several were suffering from opthalmia. I was not at the house during school hours, and do not know but they were well taught.

FULTON COUNTY has at present no alms-house. I have understood that the poor are boarded in farmer's families. I have received but little definite information.

MONTGOMERY COUNTY-HOUSE, at *Fonda,* near the Erie canal, is not well situated. It is a respectable building, in very neat order, and well arranged for the comfort of the inmates. *It is lately* that this house has come into more correct moral discipline. It is too much crowded in winter, as are most such houses. The insane require hospital treatment, or the shelter of an asylum.

SCHOHARIE COUNTY-HOUSE, at *Middleburgh,* can be described only by negatives, save that quite recently there has been appointed a competent master and mistress, to whom no fault is to be attributed for the indescribably bad state of the entire establishment. It is deficient in every thing necessary to secure comfort, decency, or order. Discipline is entirely out of the question ; it might properly be referred to the Grand Jury, who certainly would present it as a nuisance. No insane shut up.

OTSEGO COUNTY-HOUSE, at *Cooperstown,* has been, and is now, I am told, an expensive establishment. If it was subject to closer moral discipline, it would be a satisfaction to believe the money was applied to good or to a better purpose. Apparel, furniture, and beds were liberally furnished ; also, provisions and fuel. The lodging rooms often contain from fifty to sixty occupants, " so crowded as completely to cover the floors." The insane were in various parts of the buildings, and in *open pens* on the premises. I was assured there were none in the *dark* cells at the time I was there. One crazy woman, whose history I forbear, was *soon to be a mother.* She was with some others in a decent apartment. In a range of *pens,* beyond the court yard, were some crazy men and women. These *pens,* the first I have seen for *human* creatures, were built of rough boards, so high as to prevent escape, and with this exception, were on the plan of pig-pens, such as are commonly seen upon the premises of a farm house. The retreats at the rear, pent-houses perhaps they are called, or kennels, were stuffed with straw. I was not there at feeding hours! This county, I ought to add, has been very liberal in placing a portion of the insane poor in the asylum at Utica.

DELAWARE COUNTY-HOUSE, at *Delhi,* is an excellently managed place, where the sick, the aged, and the infirm *now* find a respectable and comfortable retreat: persons able to perform labor are not considered subjects for this alms-house. The mistress zealously superintends the domestic concerns, cuts, makes and mends the wearing apparel, assisted by persons under her direction; maintains a clean house throughout; above, below, and around, the "daily care" is manifest. This really was a *home* for the homeless and feeble. Here was an aspect of comfort, of content; of discipline without severity, and industry without excessive labor. Here the insane, as might be inferred, were kindly and carefully tended: yet, with all the care, which was not to be doubted, and kindness, which was evident, in the intercourse between them and "the boss," "our good boss," with all this to reconcile me, I still assert that county poor houses are not and cannot be fit places for the insane. Several here were chained by the ancle to the floor, that they need not be injured, or do mischief at the fire, and that they need not be shut up in cells and dungeons, or that they need not escape from the house and be exposed to perish in the cold and snow, at this inclement season. Here there could be no persons exclusively devoted to taking charge over them; and without this special care, and a building adapted to their peculiar condition, they either *must be chained,* or must be shut into cells or cages. And who is confident they will there always have a humane master, or if humane, that he will have the tact to manage them without harshness, and protect them from injury and outrage. It is not that one person, or two, or three, by unusual negligence has been permitted exposure to wrong; *it is the many, the very many* of these most dependent beings exposed to horrible and monstrous abuses of power, and neglect of responsibility, which impels me, in the most earnest manner, to urge ample provision for insane persons of both sexes; provision by the State, in safe asylums and hospitals closely inspected.

SULLIVAN COUNTY-HOUSE, at *Monticello,* was hastily visited, yet not so hastily as to prevent observation of a thorough neatness, a comfortable arrangement for the inmates; for example, lodging rooms not over crowded, furnished with comfortable beds and bed-clothing, convenient furniture, white-washed walls, well scrubbed floors, neat ap parel : the sick not forgotten, and the insane as well taken care of *as the provision made for them by the county* permitted. Some were able to be in the family-rooms, others were not at large, one woman was in a decent room in an out-building *chained*, but dressed, warmed and, I believe, otherwise well cared for. An insane man was performing some work in the yard. These required asylum care and protection ; indeed it would be greatly best for all.

ULSTER COUNTY-HOUSE, at *New-Paltz*, or county houses, for there are five occupied as dwellings, and parted by considerable distances ; beside these are various out-buildings, for the shops, children's school room, and usual barns and out-houses of a large farming establishment. Generally these were in excellent order, well arranged, and comfortable ; uncommonly neat, and well ventilated. The wearing apparel was respectable, and the poor were orderly and decent in their general demeanor. Children well attended to. Food good in quality, ample in quantity, and well prepared. I found an insane woman *chained* to the floor in a good apartment : those acquainted with the case, believed she might be restored under proper medical treatment. Beside this female, were other insane and idiotic persons in different parts of the establishment. I should have excepted one building from the list of those in proper order—this was at the most remote part of the grounds appropriated to the buildings, and was occupied by persons in various conditions of idiocy, imbecility and insanity ; very great neglect was visible here, which was more remarked, perhaps, from being in so broad contrast from the first visited divisions. The buildings are all of wood, and subject to serious objections in regard to domestic arrangements, especially during the winter season.

GREENE COUNTY-HOUSE, at *Cairo*, is well built, but not large enough for the occupants, nor as commodiously constructed as need requires. This establishment, lately one of the very worst in the State in regard to morals, is now under charge of a master and mistress, whose energetic supervision has effected so great and beneficial changes, that I feel much regret to offer any comments reflecting on their method of conducting its internal affairs. Many of the apartments are well arranged ; an attempt has been made to render a few of the sick comfortable, by apppropriating a room for their sole use. Portions of the house were clean, and part of the furniture for the lodging rooms in fit condition ; more liberal applications of lime-wash, and thorough cleaning of floors and tables was needed in most parts. The day room for the men was excessively crowded, over heated, not ventilated, and at present used also as a lodging room; every thing here was in very bad condition; one young man very feeble, suffering from a severe wound, needed every thing that could promote ease and recovery, and yet had nothing which his condition demanded; an insane man, *chained* in the same room was as improperly situated, and not clean.

An attempt had been made to classify part of the inmates, but want of room made this impossible to the extent required in a place where were congregated so large a proportion of vicious and insubordinate people. It is quite time that the authorized officers of the alms-house at Cairo, should make appropriations for furnishing in a more decent manner some of the lodging rooms; also a portion of the inmates with new apparel, which they should be required to keep in some sort clean; and a new building should be appropriated wholly to the children. These appeared to receive much judicious care, but all this is insufficient, while they have daily before them evil influences and corrupting example. Those of the insane who were confined in a miserable out-building, are in most wretched conditions; I do not mean abused by those who have direct charge of them; I have no reason to think this is the case *now*, but the place is not fit for a kennel for dogs, much less for the dwelling of infirm and imbecile men and women, and raving maniacs. Indignation, disgust and compassion, mingled, while examining this wretched place. One conclusion is certain, the county might furnish means for separating the insane men and women effectually and entirely; it is true, they do not occupy one cell or room wholly in common, because the furious are locked into cells, but these are exposed, and I may be spared, I trust, the necessity of specifying all the horrors and disgusting consequences of their being congregrated as I found them. This receptacle is a disgrace, alike to the alms-house, to the county, and to the State. The master of the house might effect some trival changes for the better; the county might have had a decent set of apartments constructed, and more properly conducted; but the State ought not to trust the insane to the evils and miseries almost inevitable upon county, or private superintendence and provision.

I saw much at the county-house at Cairo to commend, and was the more disposed to appreciate this, from knowing how debased was its state before the change above alluded to; but I saw also, much that shocked and pained me, and much that I trust has by this time in part at least, found remedy.

COLUMBIA COUNTY-HOUSE, at *Ghent,* is a populous, well kept establishment; somewhat crowded, but many disadvantages are avoided by judicious arrangements. Very liberal provision is here made for the poor, but, as elsewhere, a work-house department is loudly called for. The sick and aged here receive much attention; children are not neglected, either in school or out, and are as much as possible kept apart from the family at large. It must not be supposed that all even of substantial evils, are here overcome. Quite another alms-house system must be adopted in order to extinguish these. I am glad to say that, while the citizens of Columbia county desire economy in the conduct of the county poor-house, it is not any part of their plan to reduce expenses to the lowest possible rate. It seems to me little creditable to the officers of any such establishment to be able to say their poor are supported at the cost of only *three cents and three-fourths* of a cent per diem, as one reports; or at *thirty cents* per week as another records. We are not surprized, when such results of financial management are exhibited, to find the insane "cast out." But these are *exceptions* to the much mcre general rule of liberal expenditure. The prominent defects of county-houses in the State of New-York do not result from parsimonious restrictions and stinted appropriations.

The insane at Ghent occupy a department connected with the main building but partially. This was in respectable order, decently clean and furnished. A yard enclosed for exercise, in good weather, was appropriated to such of the inmates as were able to leave their rooms, or whom it was safe to trust. The wearing apparel and bed-clothing were sufficient. Besides these cases, I saw several insane men and women in the main building, who were so easily controlled that it was thought safe to associate them with the family at large. I saw nothing at this house, with all its advantages over some others, to dispose me to regard this as a desirable place for any of this class.

DUTCHESS COUNTY-HOUSE, at *Poughkeepsie,* is a model of neatness, order, and good discipline. The household arrangements are excellent; the kitchens and cellars complete in every part. I have seen nothing in the State so good as these. In some respects the county-house near Whiteplains, in Westchester, has the advantage. The buildings there are all of stone, and safer from the danger of conflagration; also they are better situated in regard to immediate vicinity to a large town. This must, at Poughkeepsie, be considered as undesirable at least, if it be not productive of serious annoyances.

Every apartment in the alms-house at Poughkeepsie was unexceptionally clean, well furnished, and neatly arranged. Great credit is due to those who have the immediate charge of this house, for so thorough supervision, and energetic administration of its affairs. Such of the insane as· were highly excited were in clean, decent rooms. Their well kept lodging rooms, opening upon one larger, where they could have more space, when tranquil enough to be let out. The women were in another part of the house, quite apart at all times from this division.

The state of this establishment has not always been so good as now ; but in the improvements annually made, it is gratifying to discover the increasing vigilance exercised to secure respectably conducted institutions ; and efforts to have them answer the important ends to society, which they ought always to propose.

The jail at Poughkeepsie was as remarkably well kept and neat as the alms-house.

WESTCHESTER COUNTY-HOUSE, near *Whiteplains*, consists of buildings solidly and handsomely constructed of stone, and adapted to receive more than two hundred persons. The interior plan of the buildings, though good, cannot be regarded as a model. Those at Flatbush, Kings county, are on a better plan, but not free from defects. " Seven hundred and seventy-five paupers," according to the last report, " have been relieved the past year in and out of the house." " Many of the inmates, able to work, have been employed on the farm, and in constructing two hundred and twenty rods of heavy substantial wall ; ditching, capping and filling up two hundred rods of deep ditch. All the necessary work of the house has been done by the inmates : as shoemaking, clothing, bedding, pails, brooms, without extra expense." The house is well furnished, and provided with all needed accommodations. The expenses last year were seven thousand four hundred dollars, besides nearly three thousand paid for out-residents.

The school for the children is taught by one of the paupers, and it is said to be faithfully conducted ; if so, I can see no good reason why the teacher should not be paid for this service by the county, over and above his clothes and board. I could form no opinion of the moral influences exerted here.

The department for the lunatics contains thirty inmates, and deserves something better than the name of receptacle. Neither pains nor expense have been spared here in providing for the comfort, order, and security of the inmates. In neatness throughout every part, I know nothing in the State which I can bring into comparison, except the Asylums at Utica and Bloomingdale. An air of cheerfulness even, pervades some of the rooms ; so white, so clean, so supplied with comfortable beds, and the inmates so cleanly dressed, so clean in their persons. If any thing could ever reconcile me to subordinate institutions, this certainly would do so ; but nothing can, I know too much of liabilites and realities. A physician attends once or twice a week, and I cannot suppose neglects this part of the alms-house establishment, yet I think he would be ready to allow that a hospital wholly devoted to curative treatment, would be the fitter place for such as are not incurable ; and that in all cases, *practised* and *paid attendants* are to be preferred before those considered as paupers. I know that sometimes one may secure the services of such as are of good characters and dispositions in a poor-house, who are able of body to perform the various labor requisite ; but if competent, for all this they are " worthy of their hire," and should be withdrawn from the class of those called dependants on public charity. It did not appear to me accordant with the best modes of managing excitable patients, to order their diet upon the plan here adopted, though this I am bound to suppose has not been done entirely without consideration. Several of the patients, in both male and female departments, would have been better and happier for more employment, though at times they are supplied with something answering this end, I think.

A pleasant temperature is maintained in all the apartments by means of hot air conveyed round the sides of the rooms through iron pipes ; ventilation is not overlooked. There is an abundant use of pure water. The aspect of the attendants was prepossessing. In fine, this asylum, constructed at great expense, and *now* conducted with care, does honor to the humanity and liberal-mindedness of the citizens of Westchester. They cannot guard it too vigilantly, or hold over it a watch too scrutinizingly investigating. It is hoped due caution will be exercised in dividing curable patients from those whose malady is confirmed ; and it is hoped too, while this just accord of much that is excellent is rendered to this institution, that other counties will not adopt the plan, unless the State fails to supply what humanity claims, and justice exacts.

RICHMOND COUNTY-HOUSE, near *Fort-Richmond*, on Staten island, affords a comfortable retreat for the aged, the infirm, and the sick. All the rooms exhibited decent and kindly care, and attention to order and general discipline. The buildings are not particularly good, but neither are they so defective as to fail in securing many important objects. This was like the county-house at Delhi, most strictly an alms-house; a place where the poor, who are disabled, the sick, aged, and infirm, and unprotected children find refuge: and not so much the resort of able-bodied, able-to-work people as are most "poor-houses." No insane confined here.

SUFFOLK COUNTY, *Long island,* has no county-house. A various provision is here made for the poor. In some towns they are "bid off" annually, on the old system, in others "boarded out," in one, or in several families. And again, in other towns they are to be found in "poor-houses," usually having a farm attached. At Coram in Brookhaven, Suffolk county, is a very respectable establishment for the poor; whose general appearance exhibited care and good attendance. There were here several insane persons, but not generally requiring close confinement; these were clean and well clothed.

Not distant many miles from Riverhead, is a "poor's farm," where general wants are well supplied. I was not able to reach this place, but seven or eight individuals described it from personal knowledge, and frequent visits. The house is small, and admits of no classification, and but little division; some additions seemed very much required. Here is a young man regarded as incurably insane; he was at a hospital for a considerable time, till his case being thought hopeless, he was brought here by the overseers of the poor. He is kept in a small building, consisting of a single apartment put up expressly for him in the yard, "because he is dangerous to be at large, and his screams disturb the people in the house;" here his shouts and violent proxysms do not so rack the sick and the aged; and here like a caged tiger he is kept successive months and years. "He has no fire; has never had here;" "he can keep warm enough in winter by beating about his cell." I suggested that there must be periods of quietness and inaction, and at such times, at least, there was danger of his suffering severely in cold weather. They answered there was no room for a stove, and if one should be put there he would burn up the building. I then proposed that if the room was too small to admit a safe division for a stove, a new one should be built, and that it was cruel in the extreme to leave him thus. I only elicited the reply that "he was warm enough."

At Smithtown are a few paupers chargeable to the county; these are "boarded out." There is here also a farm and dwelling owned by the town, where those having "their residence" in that town, are provided for. The number of the poor thus supported here is small.

In the town of Huntingdon is a small farm appropriated to the town's poor. The dwelling is small, inconvenient, and out of repair; it is a most discreditable and wretched establishment, but I should add that there is now reason to expect a speedy and complete reform; and in place of neglect, confusion, utter discomfort, and wretched apartments, most wretchedly furnished, where vice consorts with misery, and indolence with incapacity, we may hope for a new order of things. The children here most moved my compassion—little neglected creatures, wholly unattended to, by the confession of the mistress herself, and though having food and some clothing, otherwise were veriest outcasts from care and kindness. The incompetence of the mistress of the house for the duties assumed, was apparent every where in every thing. I know this is strong language, but it is borne out by facts, and the overseers of the town of Huntingdon very well know there are objections to present arrangements, which I do not feel called upon to state here explicitly. No insane persons are in this poor-house; a saving mercy for which I am devoutly thankful.

QUEEN'S COUNTY also has no general county-house; though there is an establishment at South-Hempstead, where the county poor are provided for, also one where are the town's poor. I found it quite impossible, through limited time, to visit every town in this county or in Suffolk. Much money is expended in both, for the relief of the poor, but after all with very unsatisfactory results.

I find it a most unwelcome duty to speak of establishments discreditable to the towns and counties from which their support is derived. I well know from personal conversations, that many of the respectable citizens of South-Hempstead greatly disapprove the manner in which their town poor, as well as the county poor, are supported and managed. I have reason to believe also, that the county superintendents are very much dissatisfied with the present arrangements for the poor in the county at large. Many of the evils and abuses now existing, I have strong hope will, before another year, have found remedy.

The *town poor* of South Hempstead, of whom there were but
fifteen, at the time of my visit in December, were " sold," " bid off,"
" or let," to a resident in the town, the landlord of a miserable tavern.
This man was addicted to intemperance, and found favor with the
paupers by small allowances of rum, with additions of snuff and tobacco. I went to his house and asked to see the family making at the
same time the usual inquiries. He replied surlily, that they lived at
some distance from his own house, that he had not much to do with
them, that his wife knew about them all. He professed not to know
either their numbers, age or condition. The wife came, but her information was equally insufficient, and I directed to be taken to the
house where the poor lived ; which was distant about one-eighth of a
mile from the tavern. This was a small building of one story, in a
state of wretched dilapidation. The fifteen inmates of various ages, of
both sexes, and various colors, presented a spectacle of squalid neglect, and one might say of poverty also : dirty in person and apparel,
in rooms equally exceptionable ; the little provision for lodging, was of
the worst description. One miserable creature, whether colored or
white, crazy or idiotic, I could not clearly make out, was rolled in
some ragged, dirty blankets in a bunk in a horrible state of neglect.
An aged black woman whose limbs were enveloped in a quantity
of rags, to serve the place both of shoes and stockings, was feebly
trying to quiet the cries of a young child. The only sufficient supplies
about the place for the wants of life were food and air, and even here,
there was of the last too much, pouring in through the holes, and broken
windows, and floors. Confusion, disorder, and wretched life characterized the place. I was told that the mistress came down almost
every day to see them, but her visits were followed it seemed by no
very wholesome household arrangements. The history of the town's
poor of South-Hempstead, for years past has been worse rather than
better than it is at the present time. *One dollar* per week is paid for
each of the poor ; provisions in this quarter are cheap, and rents moderate. In Westchester county-house, the cost of each person to the
county is *fifty cents two mills and four-tenths a mill* per week ;
what a contrast of condition !

The county poor were some miles distant from the place last described, and distant also from all taverns. The appropriations for the support of this class was liberal; indeed the inhabitants of Long island
pay their taxes for the poor ungrudgingly, and in these relations are not

governed by a parsimonious spirit. Money enough is expended; the misfortune is, it is not well applied.

The house last referred to was not adapted for either convenient or comfortable arrangements. The inmates were negligently appareled, and not clean, nor were the lodging rooms properly furnished with decent beds and bed clothing. I was told that I had visited it at an unfortunate time. Perhaps so, but I fancy all times would have been equally so in my judgment of the place. Accidental disarrangement may always be perceived; habitual neglects mark themselves. The children were untidy and unwashed; the adults, with one exception, the same. The only insane person I saw, was a young woman of good aspect, neat, and actively employed; I suspect the most efficient member of the household. To those who have seen no well conducted establishments for the poor, this might have appeared less disadvantageously; but I could not consider it other than *greatly discreditable* to those who contribute to its support, and promoting at best but a negative good.

The towns of North-Hempstead and Oyster bay, having received a bequest of ten thousand dollars unitedly, for the support of their poor, purchased a farm in a section of the latter township, and have built an alms-house. This, amongst other reasons, is assigned as the cause of not building a county poor-house. From personal observation and inquiries, in Queens and Suffolk counties, I am not inclined to the opinion advanced by many, that the poor in small towns, are severally as well provided for as they would be in county houses. Each *plan* offers advantages and objections, but in neither is the obligation *to do this well*, set aside.

Kings County-House, at *Flatbush*, takes rank with the very best establishments of this sort in the State, in being the most complete in every department, and excellently conducted. The buildings are so extensive as to afford means for classification in an uncommon degree, and so also, for securing good order and discipline. The respective houses were thoroughly neat, apartments clean to exactness, commodiously arranged, well warmed, and supplied with pure air. The children were neatly dressed, and uncommonly well attended. Food as is usual, not only liberal in allowance, but also, what is not as common, wholesome in quality, and well cooked, and finally, served with neatness and in order. The hospital department for the sick and feeble, was in excellent condition; every thing was comfortable, nothing seemed omitted that comfort required, nor neglected that duty enforced.

The asylum or hospital for the insane, stood apart. It was well ordered for a county receptacle, but altogether inferior to that in Westchester. With all its arrangements for keeping the insane of both sexes, and with all the care of the attendants as I saw them at their stations, I did not feel that this department, by any means, met the wants of the class it was designed to benefit. I saw not the smallest evidence of abuse or neglect; on the contrary, kindness and attention, so far as wants were comprehended; but much must be wanting here, which a well governed institution, wholly devoted to the insane, would secure. I was told that the county officers proposed to build a larger establishment, finding their numbers exceeding their present accommodations. Here were twenty-five in confinement, early in December, and another to be brought that same day. One had deceased the day before.

ROCKLAND COUNTY-HOUSE, near *Clarkstown*, is in some respects decent and neat; not completely or thoroughly so, especially the outbuildings occupied by some sick, infirm, insane, and feeble persons, and children; this greatly needed an entire reform in cleansing, furnishing, and in the personal care of the occupants. A little sick child was very improperly situated, and though it may sound severe, I should say neglected; the person having charge of it, a feeble infirm woman, having hardly capacity to reach the cradle; I think indeed she was called crazy. The main building was clean and well ordered. I found through this, and the adjoining counties, that this alms-house was not thought to afford the needed comforts, such an asylum is supposed to furnish: of this, I could form but a qualified opinion. The master and mistress were persons of respectable appearance; I incline to believe they purpose what one said of them, " to do about right;" I should perhaps add, so far as their knowledge leads them.

ORANGE COUNTY-HOUSE, at *Goshen*, is a large and expensive estabblishment; till quite lately, it has ranked very low in respect to morals, so much so, that great dissatisfaction has been created in several towns, with the plan of an alms-house common to all the poor of the county; and though greater care and close supervision are now exerted, the prejudice is not effaced. Though capacious, the house is crowded; many of the lodging rooms are well arranged, and an attempt at classification has placed things on a better foundation than before the present master took charge ; here, as at Cairo, there was so much for the present newly appointed master to do, so great abuses to reform, so many rules to enforce, that to those who have been laboring for this, the place appears to much greater advantage than to one who sees it for the first time, and compares it with institutions better established, and longer subject to judicious government. There is want at this season, of sufficient employment for those who gather from various quarters in the cold months. A hospital for the sick is also needed ; and one, by the energetic exertions of the master, has been partly built of stone the present year, free of county cost. The county officers have declined making any appropriations for this object. The school is said to be well taught; it costs the county nothing, besides the board and clothes of one of its paupers. The rooms occupied by the colored people were comfortable, though like all in the main building, too full of occupants. And now I come to the departments for the insane ; one severally for the men, and one for the women. Difficulties surround me ; if I attempt to describe these, few will find it easy to receive the statement as a fair relation of facts ; those who perhaps mean to do, not wrong, for and by these most afflicted beings, will feel injured, and I surely am convinced, that any language I employ, will fail to reach and expose all the evils of their lot. I would that I had skill to place before the Honorable Legislature of New-York, with distinctness, and in all its REALITY, one such receptacle for madmen and madwomen as I see repeated in many places ; my cause would be gained. The persuasion of the actual, would have wrought what its faint description is feeble to effect.

The insane women who are too violent to be at large, in the county house at Goshen, are in dreary, narrow cells, opening upon a yet more dreary apartment, of which they at all times have a view from between the perpendicular bars of the cell-doors, utter filth and wretchedness found place here. Personally neglected, indescribably so, their mad ravings resounded through the building—now imprecations, now wild cries rent the air. I approached a cell, and spoke soothingly to the poor maniac; suddenly she ceased, then whispered low, "speak, oh speak again ;" and drawing about her unclothed person a blanket, she grew still, and moaned no more ; but as I was turning away, she gently murmured, " stay, stay." Out from her cell she could look, but it was to see a gibbering idiot, or a cowering imbecile, or perhaps a murmuring half demented creature, wandering languidly about the room. In an adjoining cell was another female, not noisy, but loathsomely disgusting in a neglected person, and equally neglected cell. This *may* not have been a uniform state of debasement; I have no reason, however, to believe it otherwise. The irresponsible attendant, chosen from the poor who are regarded as incompetent to take care of themselves, as is shown by their presence in an alms-house, had no special interest in these unfortunates, no moving stimulant to urge her to a faithful care of these so peculiarly dependent beings. Neither the master or mistress of the house would intentionally sanction neglect; yet they at this time have failed to secure in any sufficient degree the daily attendance, and daily watchful, kindly care these helpless creatures so imperatively need. The place appropriated to the insane men, squalid and disgusting, generally and particularly, had yet one redeeming view : it was apart from that occupied by the women. A foreigner as dirty and offensive as those over whom he held charge, was the only attendant I saw here. Chains secured some, feebleness detained others, and imbecility controlled the residue.

It is impossible to enter upon individual histories here, and I think that the plain facts, stating recent outward conditions, are sufficient to show that society at large is unfaithful to its moral and social obligations. Neglects and injuries are not confined to county-houses. I know of insane sons permanently shut up by fathers, without fire, without light, without aim or object to revive, to cheer, or to heal the wounded mind. I know of sisters and daughters subject to abusive language, to close confinement, and to " floggings with the horse-whip." I know of parents in their old age, sunk into imbecility, basely abused, and left to suffer ; and I know of many *cast out from dwellings,* to wander forth, and live or die, as the elements, less merciless than man, permit. Many are these histories ; dark, but true, and difficult to credit, which reach me in many parts—nay, almost every part of the country. They are not peculiar to New-York, nor to any section of these United States which I have traversed ; but it is not the affecting histories, or moving passages in the lives of the insane, upon which I fix my own thought, or to which I desire to draw the attention of the public. These are common to humanity, are the providential dispensations which all at one time or another in part share. It is upon the real outward state of those who are suffering from a malady, truly appalling in its consequences, that I wish to concentrate your thoughts ;

it is to the grave consideration, whether these wrongs are to be redressed, these abuses guarded against, these mischiefs arrested, that I would
draw you.   Tearful sensibility is short-lived, and its shallow fountains
are soon dried away ; deliberate conviction and judgment are permanent, and conduct to effective acts and to solid advantages.

Permit me, briefly, to refer to the prominent defects of the present
county-house system throughout the State.

These institutions are *compound* and *complex* in their plans and objects.   They are at one and the same time, *alms-houses*, or retreats
for the aged, the invalid, and helpless poor: *houses of correction* for
the vicious and abandoned ; *asylums for orphaned and neglected children ; receptacles for the insane and imbecile ;* extensive *farming*, and
more limited *manufacturing establishments.*   Beside, in addition to
being *mixed establishments*, they are not, one in ten or twenty counties, built in reference to these various objects.   They are not planned
to secure division and classification of the inmates.   They afford insufficient accommodations, both in " the day rooms," and in the lodging
apartments ; not being constructed with a view to securing convenient
arrangement or sound health.   They are almost universally deficient
in hospitals, or rooms especially appropriated to the sick, and to invalids.   They do not guard against the indiscriminate association of the
children with the adult poor.   The education of these children, with
rare exceptions, is conducted on a very defective plan.   The alms-
house schools, so far as I have learnt from frequent inquiries, are not
inspected by official persons, who visit and examine the other schools
of the county.   The moral and religious instruction of the poor at
large, in these institutions is either attended to at remote and uncertain
intervals, or entirely neglected.   The scriptural text, that to " the poor
the gospel is preached," that " good news of glad tidings," appears to
have failed in its application to alms-houses.   " We cannot afford it,"
says one ; " our subscriptions and donations are even now burthensome
in the support of foreign missions, to Asia and the South Sea islands."
" We have not time," say others, " we have in our town been wholly
engaged, for the last six months, by a revival."   " Why do you not
visit those degraded beings at your alms-house, and try to reclaim them
to goodness and virtue ?"   " Oh, I have no time for such things.   I am
an active member and secretary of the Moral Reform Society."   " How
can you refrain from interposing in behalf of those poor fettered maniacs, wearing out a terrible life in chains, shut out from the light of

the beautiful sky, and pining in friendless neglect ?"   " I assure you I have quite as much as I can do to work for the Anti-Slavery Fair.   I detest all abuses and oppressions, and have devoted myself to the cause of emancipation in the slave-holding States."   "And I," said another, " must lecture on freedom, and justice, and human rights.   We at the north must be zealous to rouse the citizens of the southern States from their apathy to the claims of suffering humanity."   These, and such like answers, to often renewed questionings, are given continually ; and to me they are evidence of our proneness to overlook the discharge of duties " nigh at hand ;" and to forget that " the good example " is better than the " reiterated precept."   Here *at home,* for a long time, have we ample fields of labor : to teach the gospel of the blessed Jesus by *word* and *life ;* to enlighten ignorance ; to stay the tide of vicious pauperism ; to succor the friendless, support the feeble ; to visit the afflicted ; to raise the depressed ; to lessen human suffering, and elevate human aims ; to redress wrongs ; rectify abuses ; unloose the chains of the maniac and bring release to those who pine in dark cells and dreary dungeons : having plucked the beam from our own eye, we can with a less pharisaical spirit, direct our efforts to clearing the mental vision of neighbor.

I have referred to some of the most obvious defects of county-houses. Considering the compound objects of these, it is surprising that so much good is found in them.   It is to be remembered that knowledge is the growth of a tedious experience.   The evils to which I have alluded, are felt and acknowledged by all those brought into direct acquaintance with the subject.   Greatly too much is required, both of the masters and mistresses of county-houses. Few men and women possess such varied and rare gifts as are called into exercise, in conducting these institutions.

The master must be, at one and the same time, an able practical *farmer ;* the *warden* of a *prison ;* the vigilant *superintendent* of a *community,* rather than of a family, composed of persons of different tempers, habits, and all ages.   He must *direct a school ; conduct* a various *manufacturing establishment ;* be the responsible *superintendent* of a *lunatic receptacle ;* a good *accountant ;* ready at *bargaining* with *trades-people,* and *acute* in *selling* to advantage surplus produce, and a *vigilant overseer* and *watchman.*   The mistress is expected to be an excellent *house-keeper ;* good *cook ;* quick *seamstress ;* skilled in *tailoring, mantuamaking ;* repairing garments ; competent in making up beds, bed clothing, and household linen. She must be vigilant in every department : in the laundry ; in the dairy ; in the sewing rooms ; in the kitchen. She must hold watch and ward, at all times, over a refractory and ill-assorted household. All these duties, and many beside, devolve on the master and mistress of a county-house. And I am constantly assured that, of all these, perplexing as are many of them, the care of the insane is the most difficult, and attended with fewest satisfactory results.

I respectfully suggest the adoption of an *improved system* for county alms-houses. I know that this subject is encompassed with difficulties, and that it is much easier to indicate mistakes, and to detect errors, than to rectify misjudgments or retrieve faults. To maintain public charities, so that there shall be no premium on pauperism, and so that vice shall be kept at bay, is still a problem in civilized society : we can only say that if all evils cannot be excluded, many may be abated ; if pauperism cannot be extinguished, the muddy fountains which generate it may be reduced.

The annual disbursements from the county treasuries in the State of New-York, for the support of the poor, is enormous ; some plan for diminishing these without trenching upon the just claims of those dependent, seems worthy of consideration. It is difficult to legislate upon this subject, so that all, in every section of this " Empire State," shall be equally benefitted, and none suffer disadvantages. Laws wholesome in their application at the north, might work contrary results at the south ; plans suited to the wants of the east, would be mischievous carried into effect at the west ; what might promote good on Long island, would perhaps show different results on the shores of Lake Erie. This State, as yet infant in age, though of gigantic growth, exhibits social phases accordant with its paradoxical combinations of immaturity and precocity. " Rest content," said to me not long since, one of your distinguished statesmen, "rest content, if these desired reforms are not all speedily wrought ; all will follow in time : the life of a State, is not as the life of a man ; with the *first*, thirty years is but a pulsation, with the *last*, it is the half almost of a whole life." The greatest good cannot I know, be suddenly accomplished, but is it not true wisdom by present energetic measures, to guard against growing evils : is it not better to eradicate the masterroot, and not rest satisfied with having merely pruned the fibrous offsets. The present plan of supporting the poor, was a great advance from that barbarous usage sb long prevailing this whole country, of "bidding them off," "letting them out," &c. The really necessary expenses of the poor, are, it appears to me, with very rare exceptions, cheerfully met throughout the State; but still it is felt that the taxes for these objects rise to the verge of excess. It might be well to examine impartially, the modes of expending these moneys. Possibly they would be reduced in many ways, *without touching* the *direct special* appropriations at county-houses. The charges of transporting the poor from place to place, for example, are very large, and this is made the ground of one argument with many towns, for not sending their poor to the county houses, or sending them reluctantly.

In Berlin, and other parts of Prussia, very little is expended in the *management of their poor system;* here in this country might be another saving; without trenching on the claims of poverty. But there is another and broader ground for consideration. Of those now annually supported in the State of New-York, in the county poor-houses, much the largest portion are foreigners; most of these are able-bodied men and women, with entire families, competent to perform labor, and many of these are not cast transiently upon the public charity, but hundreds of them resort annually as the cold season advances, to the county-poor houses. Here they remain till spring opens, from four to six months, and departing are seen again only as autumn approaches winter, when the fields have all been tilled and the harvest gathered. This especially is the case in the larger cities and towns of populous counties. In November of 1842, I was informed at the alms-house in Albany, that *four-fifths* of the inmates were foreigners, most of whom were able to perform full day-labor. In December 1843, the master told me the whole number of inmates was *five hundred,* a large proportion of whom are in health and competent to labor, " but for these," he added, " I have but little or no employment." These facts, with many which might be adduced, go to show the expediency of establishing work-houses in many counties, if not in every one of them. By the adoption of such establishments, under good regulations uniting kindness and necessary discipline, all, whether Americans or foreigners, might when able to work, be transferred from the alms-houses, to the houses of employment, and the former be reserved for the aged and infirm, for feeble persons, and young children. Well conducted alms-houses will be oftener found, when less crowded with able-bodied paupers, and when they cease to contain receptacles for the insane.

There is but one testimony throughout the land, from county officers respecting the unfitness of county alms-houses for the insane ; these results of a various, and not new experience, appear entitled to consideration.

Among the prominent objections to retaining insane patients in almshouses are these : burthened by crowding household cares, and with various objects connected with these institutions, the masters and mistress of them, have no time to bestow upon these very dependent beings ; had they time, they seldom have had opportunity of acquiring a knowledge of the proper modes of governing them ; or, if possessing tact for these duties, they are liable to removal themselves from their places at any renewed vibration of the pendulum of political parties.

The insane require a daily care, wholly different from that requisite for any other persons ; this only can be commanded in institutions founded expressly for their reception.

In alms-houses, if violent, their outcries and noise disturb the slumbers of the household, and continually disquiet the sick and infirm.

If blasphemous and indecent, their presence is mischievous and demoralizing.

They are themselves exposed to the teazing tricks and injurious treatment of many whose chief pleasure consists in exciting and irritating them.

They are liable to great neglects, and to the most terrible outrages.

The most shocking abuses may exist towards them, without the power on their part, of claiming or finding redress. It is well known, that *recovery is very rare in alms-houses, where confinement in cells, and rigorous methods of government, are enforced:* it is also well known that a large majority of the insane in this State, and in the United States generally, are either in narrow circumstances, or wholly dependent on public charity ; it is not wise therefore, to provide curative institutions, where those who give hope of recovery may be brought under skilful treatment ; and asylums, where those in whom the malady has become settled, may find kindness and protection. The expense of institutions *appropriate* for the *cure* and the *care* of *the insane,* may be sustained by the State at less cost, than any creditable hospitals can be by the counties severally.

Of lunatics and idiots I have seen in the county-houses of the State of New-York about *fifteen hundred ;* of the same classes in private families, I know comparatively but little, and can produce no statistics ; but I believe we may fairly estimate all of these classes in the State as numbering about three thousand. A part of these, both the idiots and the insane, would in no sort be benefitted by change of place—but a great number are suffering more terribly than language can describe, for want of appropriate care, and accommodations adapted to their peculiar necessities, and their entire dependence on others for all that can ameliorate the miseries of their earthly life.

I find in the very able report of the Trustees of the New-York State Lunatic Asylum, for 1841, the following important remark, sound in its text, and demanding serious consideration. " *The incurables should not be received or retained, to the exclusion of the curables ;* and of *the latter class, recent cases should always be accommodated rather than old ones :*" and in a subjoined note is added, " *too much importance cannot be attached to this distinction ;* ample confirmation of this view of the subject, is quoted at length in the appendix.

Dr. Bell, the justly distinguished and honored superintendent of the M'Lean Asylum, in Charlestown, Mass. remarks in the twenty-third annual report of that institution, that "the records of the asylum justify the declaration, *that all cases certainly recent,* that is, whose origin does not either directly or obscurely run back more than a year, *recover under a fair trial. This is the general law :* the *occasional* instances to the contrary, *are the exceptions.*"

It would appear from the opinions above referred to, and from other and various authorized sources, that *first* importance is attached to provision for the curable classes of the insane ; and that ample means should be secured for this end, becomes from every consideration, an imperative obligation ; especially that patients may, in the earliest stages of their malady have the benefit of skilful treatment.

This conducts to the inquiry what present provision has been made in the State for the insane, and is this sufficient for their immediate necessities ? It is known that the asylums at Utica and Bloomingdale, are the only public institutions in the State, and these can by no possibility retain all even of the curable classes, and it is acknowledged that these are adapted in all respects, by architectural arrangements, and by the eminent professional skill of their respective superintendents, for curative hospitals : and we now come to the question what is the provision already made for the now numerous class of incurables ? *The State has made none:* the counties (save those of New-York and Westchester,) *none* that *professional* medical men, or enlightened christians, can sanction as fit for temporary, to say nothing of permanent, use : and by the judgment of those most acquainted with their structure and means of accommodation, and connexion with poor-houses, these must be condemned even for temporary use ; being chiefly *close, unventilated rooms ; narrow dark cells ; cheerless dungeons, cold and damp ;* with accompanying trappings of *iron balls, collars, manacles, fetters and chains ;* and it must be added, the *heavy* blow to *quicken obedience ;* and the *stinging lash* to *enforce silence ;* but these last not always, not oftenest ;—yet if at all, if in but one, rather than what is true, in many cases ; or if but the probability exists that such cruelties *may be, what is the duty of the public, of the whole public ?* I reply, and do not all reply, that *large, entire* provision must be made for these the most-to-be-compassionated of human beings. But why should the State make such provision ? I answer first, because the *expense* of minor establishments, *that are* in *every* way adapted to the necessities of the insane, forbids the idea that they can become the charge of the counties respectively, if attempted, they would at no distant time degenerate into mere receptacles, where neglects would multiply and abuses crowd in. The vigilant and successful superintendent of your State Asylum has observed in a work on insanity, and its modes of treatment in hospitals, " that too much attention cannot be given to the prevention of abuses in lunatic asylums." " *Attendants* of the *most unblemished moral character*, and remarkable for *kind dispositions*, for *calmness* and *intelligence should be procured*, and *well instructed* in their *responsible duties ;* and be induced by proper compensation to *devote themselves* perpetually to the care of the insane." These opinions are corroborated by all who have given consideration to the subject. But it is believed that no elaborate arguments need be advanced to show why county asylums, (and private families with very few exceptions,) are unsuitable for the insane, and should never receive general sanction.

It is remarked by a writer who has become distinguished for efforts to lessen the privations of the afflicted, and to secure protection for suffering humanity, that " with regard to paupers at least, the duty of the State is clear and imperative, and this should be the duty of every Christian government, to provide the best *means for the cure of the curable*, and to *take kind care* of the incurable." The duty of society, besides being urged by every consideration of humanity, will be seen to be more imperative, if we consider that insanity is, in many cases, the result of imperfect or vicious social institutions and observances. We have not space to allude to all these ; but among them are revolutions, party strife, unwise and capricious legislation, causing commercial speculations and disasters ; false standards of worth and rank, undue encouragement of the propensities and passions, social rivalry, social intemperance ; some fashions and conventional usages ; religious and political excitement. These, and many other causes for which society is in fault, are productive of a large proportion of the cases of insanity which exist in its bosom. But if to these we add the still larger number which arise from ignorance of the natural laws, which ignorance society should enlighten, we can fairly lay at its door almost all the cases of insanity which occur. I have advanced the claim of the insane to be received as *wards of the State*, and have shown that this State, by liberal appropriations at various periods to the two public asylums, have acknowledged the justice of this claim ; but I have not, I trust, failed to represent the insufficiency of these appropriations to meet the wants of the *largest* portion of this class : my earnest, my importunate intercession, then, is in behalf of the *incurable insane*, who, lost for life to the exercise of a sound understanding, exposed to suffering and degradation, to neglect and abuse, and often abandoned of friends, are at once the most dependent and most unfortunate of human beings. The basest criminal, who distorts by vile crimes the harmony of social life, who is shut out by just decrees from intercourse with his fellow men in the open walks of life, is still protected by the laws which he has outraged, and his prison opens to admit the minister of religion bearing the holy word of life, the humane instructor and frequent visitor, whose counsels may inspire repentance towards God, and purposes of amended practice ; but the poor wretch whom broken capacities and darkened understanding disqualify for self-care and moral accountability—who, as a young feeble infant, is helpless and unconscious—he is unprotected, unprovided for, *forsaken* of friends, forsaken of all ! He is forsaken—but this will not last ; civil and social organization are advancing to higher stations—reaching after greater perfectness.

I refer again to that valuable State document from which I have already quoted, and respectfully remind you that " it should not be forgotten, that what the State has now done, in the erection of the Asylum at Utica, *forms but the smallest and most insignificant link of a mighty chain of* " *merciful measures which must lengthen with our increased acquaintance with the laws of the human mind, and with the privations of that mind, and can only terminate when the insane are unknown in the land.*"

I will not consume time by suggesting plans in detail for the best accomplishment of what is so much needed to meet these important claims. Establishing the State Asylum at Utica, together with that at Bloomingdale as the curative institutions, may I be permitted to suggest that four or six asylums in convenient sections of the State, established upon a *cheaper plan*, which, while it *assures every needed comfort* and most *careful attendance*, will not need the many extra provisions absolutely essential to a curative institution. These should be built in convenient situations, where abundant supplies of water and of fuel could be had without extra cost; and where extensive grounds for *exercise* and *cultivation* might serve at once to maintain health of body, and a degree of mental tranquility, and to contribute to self-support in some measure. Fire proof buildings well ventilated, two stories high, to spare labor and numerous attendants, these and other accommodaons should be prudently studied. Cottages might be adjacent to a main building, for the most tranquil male patients, somewhat on the plan of the celebrated and successful establishment of *Ghiel*, connected with the hospital at Antwerp. Every Asylum should at all times be subject to the vigilant inspection of qualified and authorized persons, who should never *assume* the administration to be well conducted, but *be assured* of the absolute fact that it is so ; this rigid supervision would imply no distrust of superintending physicians, or of subordinate officers and attendants ; on the contrary, it would confirm and sanction public confidence, and stimulate diligent care into conscientious fidelity.

But whatever deliberation this subject may receive, whatever conclusions may be reached, I will indulge the hope that these will embrace a permanent mode of relief. The great seal of your State, which bears that somewhat aspiring device, the *rising Sun*, the *Heaven-*

bright sky, the *lofty mountain*, the *flowing river*, the *fertile plain*, and a motto that should not have been assumed but by minds stayed to highest purposes; nor retained, but by those whose lofty principles sanction its use,—your State seal is to me the pledge that you will not delay to remedy those corroding moral evils, to which I have asked your attention; that you will not be satisfied with having commenced a good and noble work, but that you will go forward to complete and perfect your system. I solicit your action *now*, on the various ground of expediency, of justice, of humanity, of duty to yourselves, of duty to your families, of duty to your neighbor, and your fellow citizens, of your duty to the Most High God, who, in ordaining that the "poor should never cease out of the land," at the same time ordained that nations, not less than individuals, should find sanctification in the exercise of the higher charities, and the ennobling acts of life.

I am told that the world is selfish, that men seek only outward aggrandizement and temporal prosperity. I assuredly see much of this, but society would cease to exist if liberality and enlarged principles of action did not more prevail. I discover that negligence and folly, vice and crime, sweep widely and fearfully; but I cannot be blind to the fact that there must be a greater amount of care and reflection, of purity and integrity, else the fabric of social life would fall in ruins, and the intellectual become subservient to animal life.

In view, then, of the ascendency of the more elevated principles of humanity, I renewedly solicit your action now upon the subject under consideration. I might recommend this on the low ground of expediency, and prove by numerical calculations that present complete and efficient plans would at no distant time be the cheapest. But while a fit and wise economy ought to be studied, I cannot suppose that you will, in consulting the mere saving of dollars and cents to your State treasury, lose sight of that justice and humanity which most ennoble human nature, and which should be your governing motives; these involve also the highest responsibilities. God, in giving to you understanding above the brute creation, and immortal capacities, has revealed that there is a treasury whose wealth does not fail, where riches may be garnered for the harvest of eternity.

Provide asylums which shall meet the whole necessities of your State; give to your sister States an example yet wanting, of complete

and sufficient institutions for each of these afflicted classes of the insane, and pause only till degradation and suffering are guarded against,
so far as human care and human kindness may prevent the one or diminish the other.   It will be said that much already has been done for
these poor miserables.   I know it, and that is why I expect still larger
benefits to reach them.   It is *because* men have begun, not only to discover evils but to apply remedies; it is because there is a clearer comprehension upon these subjects, that I appeal to you untroubled by distrust.
It has now been learned by experience how much of human suffering
may be diminished, how many ills may be obliterated, how much that
has been deficient may be supplied, how much that has been wrong
may be redressed.   No, I will not believe that it is in New-York I am
to find statesmen and legislators, who will return to their constituents
and say to them that their decisions have stayed the sacred cause of
humanity, and checked the work of justice and mercy.   Am I importunate?   Go, look on such scenes as I have witnessed in your State
these last three months ; you will forget all in zealously devising plans
to heal these great distresses.   Am I importunate?   Importunity finds
justification in acquaintance with the diverse and unfailing resources of
this vast State, which open to energetic and vigorous enterprize the way
to unprecedented prosperity.   Except perverse in the extremest sense,
except blinded by the most sullen self-will, except disqualified by the
rashest movements, New-York cannot but be the Empire State in
that wealth which is computed by ample treasures of gold and
silver, as well as from its permanent advantages from natural position.
It is hardly possible that prosperity should here suffer more than temporary interruption—a mote crossing the disc of your rising sun—a
feeble striving upon a little surface, of your deep flowing river—a passing cloud, shutting out for a moment your sky-reaching mountain.
Look around you, is it not true what I say?   Look abroad, is not that
real which I show?   And if true, if real, if you are, in the adoption
of your State-seal ambitious, without being vain-glorious; if you are
great, without conceit ; if you are just, without speciousness ; if your
noble motto is not a bitter satire upon your acts, then am I more
than justified in the confidence, transcending hope, which inspires me
while urging the claims of the most dependent, and most miserable
portions of the community.   Now, amidst the many acts, the various
deliberations which consume time in your stately Capitol, consecrate a
portion to the highest, most enduring interests—to perpetuating the

bility, and a just appreciation of the claims of humanity, which can find neither justification nor apology. In past ages, it was believed that insanity was a *disease of the mind*, of the mind peculiarly, and distinct from the physical condition. Most of the ancient nations received the idea, that insanity was produced by supernatural agencies; that it was a just judgment from Heaven, directly visited upon the individual, or his parents and family : in short, that it was a judicial infliction from the Supreme Being—hence tortures, chains, and incarceration in gloomy dungeons; and hence derision and degradation, loathing and contumely. And so men argued, 'shall those who receive no mercy from the Just One, not also be cast out; and shall we cherish those abandoned ones whom the Almighty has forsaken?' This terrible error gradually gave place to more humane views, and in the middle ages we recognize the first slow advances in the cause of these poor sufferers. St. Vincent de Paul, that pious, self-sacrificing Apostle, became "*the providence* of God," to soften the hearts of European nations towards the oppressed maniac, and the neglected idiot. With an unquenchable zeal, he traversed vast regions, sustained by a holy charity, teaching men, that to be humane, was to be allied to Deity. He rescued thousands from terrible tortures, and kindled sympathies for the miserable, which, transmitted with increase, from generation to generation, to our own times, have wrought the salvation of thousands and tens of thousands. The monks, to whom for a long period, in Italy and other Catholic countries, the insane were consigned, both for medical and spiritual treatment, through much error, finally attained to a more rational treatment of this fearful malady. Lashes, at one period daily inflicted to subdue paroxysms, were in some places superseded by less severe discipline. But it remained for France to exhibit the first effectual systematic efforts in behalf of the insane. It was in France, first, that thousands of maniacs were brought under control by the influence of *firmness* and *kindness ;* and manacles and fetters, and the blood-imbrued lash, were banished from hospitals and asylums, where they so long had been the rule of government.

It is to Pinel, the great and good Pinel, a physician attending at the hospital of the Bicetre, two miles south of Paris, that we owe this first great triumph of humanity and skill, over ferocity and ignorance.— For the history of this glorious achievement, I briefly translate and abridge a passage from a memoir, read by the son of Pinel before the Royal Academy of Arts and Sciences.

" Near the close of the year 1792, M. Pinel, having repeatedly importuned the government to issue a decree permitting him to unchain the maniacs at the Bicetre, went in person to solicit what had been refused to his written representations. With courage and resolution he urged the removal of this cruel abuse. At length, M. Couthon, member of the commune, yielded to the importunate arguments of Pinel, and consented to meet him at the hospital, to witness these first experiments, as well as to assure himself that this was not a stratagem to give liberty to political offenders. Couthon proceeded, himself, to question the patients, but received only abuse and execrations, accompanied by terrible cries and the clanking of chains. Retreating from the damp and filthy cells, he exclaimed to Pinel, 'Do as you will; but you will be sacrificed to this false sentiment of mercy.' Pinel delayed no longer: he selected fifty, who he believed might be released from their chains without danger to others. The fetters were removed, first, from twelve, using the precaution of having prepared strong jackets, closing behind, with long sleeves, which could be used if necessary.

" The experiments commenced with an English captain, whose history was unknown: *he had been in chains forty years!* As he was thought to be one of the most dangerous, having killed, at one time, an attendant with a blow from his manacles, the keepers approached him with caution ; but first Pinel entered his cell unattended. 'Ah, well captain, I will cause your chains to be taken off; you shall have liberty to walk in the court, if you will promise to behave like a gentleman, and offer no assault to those you will meet.' 'I would promise,' said the maniac; 'but you deride me, you are amusing yourself at my expense ; you all fear me, once free.' 'I have six men,' replied Pinel, 'ready to obey my orders: believe me, therefore, I will set you free from this duresse, if you will put on this jacket.' The captain assented ; the chains were removed, and the jacket laced ;—the keepers withdrew, without closing the door. He raised himself, but fell : this effort was repeated again and again ; the use of his limbs, so long constrained, nearly failed : at length, trembling, and with tottering steps, he emerged from his dark dungeon. *His first look was at the sky!* 'Ah,' cried he, 'how beautiful !' The remainder of the day he was constantly moving to and fro, uttering continually exclamations of pleasure;—he heeded no one: *the flowers, the trees, above all the sky,* engrossed him. At night he voluntarily returned to his cell, which had been cleansed, and furnished with a better bed: his sleep was tranquil and profound. For the two remaining years which he spent in the hospital, he had no recurrence of violent paroxysms, and often rendered good service to the keepers, in conducting the affairs of the establishment.

" The patient released next after the captain, was Chevinge, a soldier of the French Guards, who had been chained ten years, and had been peculiarly difficult of control. Pinel, entering his cell, announced, that if he would obey his injunctions he should be chained no longer. He promised, and following every movement of his liberator, executed his directions with alacrity and address. Never, in the history of the human mind, was exhibited a more sudden and complete revolution; he executed every order with exactness; and this patient whose best years had been sacrificed in a gloomy cell, in chains and misery, soon showed himself capable of being one of the most useful persons about the establishment. He repeatedly during the horrors of the revolution saved the life of his benefactor. On one occasion, he encountered a band of ' *sans culottes*' who were bearing Pinel to ' the Lanterne,' owing to his having been an elector in 1789. With bold and determined purpose he rescued his beloved master, and caused that life to be spared which had been so great a blessing to the insane in France.

" In the third cell were three Prussian soldiers, who had been for many years in chains, *but how or for what they had been committed none knew;* they were not dangerous, and seemed capable of enjoying the indulgence of living together. They were terrified at the preparations for their release, fearing new severities awaited them. Sunk into dementia, they were indifferent to the freedom offered.

" An aged priest came next; he fancied himself to be the Messiah. Taunted once with the exclamation, that if in truth he was Christ, he could break his chains, he answered with solemnity, " *Frustra tentas Dominum tuum!*" Religious exaltation had characterized his life. On foot he had made pilgrimages to Rome and Cologne; he had made a voyage to the western world to convert savage tribes. This ruling idea passed into mania, and returning to France, he declared that he was Christ, the Saviour. He was arrested on the charge of blasphemy, and taken before the archbishop of Paris, by whose decree he was consigned to the Bicetre, as either a blasphemer or a madman. Loaded with heavy chains, he for twelve years bore patiently sarcasm and cruel sufferings. Pinel had the happiness to witness *his recovery in less than a year*, and to discharge him from the hospital quite cured.

"In the short period of a few days, Pinel released from their chains more than fifty maniacs, men of various ranks and conditions, merchants, lawyers, priests, soldiers, labourers—thus rendering the furious tractable, and creating peace and contentment, to a wonderful degree, where long the most hideous scenes of tumult and disorder had reigned."

But the efforts of Pinel for the relief of the insane were not limited to the Bicetre ; at La Salpetriere, a ward bears his name, continually reminding the visitor of what France and the insane owe to this great philanthropist.

The improved method of treating the insane, soon extended to England. Reforms were projected, investigations instituted, and the work advanced, if not rapidly, surely. The Retreat at York, distinguished for its humane influences, was founded by the Society of Friends, who, rich in good works, have always been prompt to sustain humane institutions, and advance enterprises for ameliorating the sufferings which beset humanity. The Hanwell Asylum obtained a celebrity, under Sir William C. Ellis, which has been advanced and sustained by Dr. Connolly.

In Germany, the principles and discipline of Pinel, and his coadjutor, Esquirol, have been established by Heinroth, who has recently died, leaving an example of humanity and fidelity which his pupils and successors hasten to imitate. The asylum at Seigburg, on the Rhine, under Jacobi, whose law and practice was "kindness and firmness," ranks among the best in the European world. The asylums for the insane in Italy have attained a high reputation, contrasted with those of former years.

The rapid diffusion of correct principles and improved modes of treating the insane in the United States, within the last twenty years, is too well known to render any historical detail of our asylums necessary here. New hospitals are annually founded, and old establishments remodelled, and made to keep pace with the rapid improvements of the age. They are superintended by skilful physicians of intelligent minds, and most of them distinguished in their profession, who spend the strength of their best years in advancing the cause of humanity. They "spend and are spent" in the noble effort to heal or mitigate those diseases which derange the healthful functions of the brain, and thus disturb the reasoning faculties and perceptions. The very onerous duties of the superintending physician of a hospital for the insane, and, indeed, of all official persons connected with these institutions, can be appreciated only by those who are very familiar with the routine of their daily duties. We may, with a just pride, rejoice that we have hospitals which will bear a close, and very favorable comparison with any in the old world, and these directed by men whose abilities give distinction to the institutions over which they preside.

I have confidence in hospital care for the insane, and in no other care, which, under the most favorable circumstances even, can be brought to surround the patient. Insanity is a malady which requires treatment appropriate to its peculiar and varied forms ; the most skilful physicians in general practice, are among the first to recommend their patients to hospital treatment, and however painful it may be to friends to yield up the sufferer to the care of strangers, natural tenderness and sensibilities never should stand in the way of ultimate benefit to the patient. And if this care is needed for the rich, for those whose homes abound in every luxury which wealth can purchase, and refined habits covet, how much more is it needed for those who are brought low by poverty, and are destitute of friends ? for those who find refuge under this calamitous disease only in jails and poor-houses, or perchance, in the cells of a State Penitentiary ?

But suppose the jail to afford comfortable apartments, decently furnished, and to be directed by an intelligent and humane keeper—advantages not frequently brought together ; what then ? is not a jail built to detain *criminals*, bad persons, who willingly and wilfully transgressing the civil and social laws, are for these offences, for a time imprisoned ? where is the propriety, where the justice, of bringing under the same condemnation, conscious offenders, and persons *not* guilty of crime, *but labouring under disease?* There is as much justice in conveying to our prisons a man lingering in a consumption, or pining under a consuming fever, as in taking there one who has lesion of the brain, or organic malconstruction. It is more than time

3

this unchristian abuse should cease. In this respect, New York offers an example it would be honourable for this and other states to adopt : insane persons and idiots are not to be found in the jails of that state.

The law there, prohibits the incarceration of the insane in the jails, but does not reach the unfortunate madmen in the penitentiaries at Auburn and Sing-Sing. In Massachusetts, a bill has passed making provision for the insane in the state prison ; but it abandons them to the gracious hospitalities and tender mercies of the county jails. Many are dangerous to society when at large, others are troublesome or "in the way," and may be found herded with the thief and the felon. Nor is this the only injustice—the keepers of jails in Massachusetts, and many other of the states, have shown me how much the sufferings of these afflicted creatures, are enhanced by the perverse dispositions of the prisoners, whose vicious amusement is often found in teasing and tormenting them. In one county jail it was a favorite pastime of the prisoners, to place strips of board upon rollers, and compel the insane and the idiots to jump upon them, when the rollers would be put in motion, and the subjects of this inhuman sport, were thrown upon the stone floor, often with so much violence, as to produce contusions, and in all cases injuries, either moral or physical.

The disposition to annoy and distress insane and imbecile persons, is not confined to our jails ; it is exhibited in the poor-houses, and often witnessed, sometimes accompanied by fatal consequences, on the streets and highways.

If prisons are unfit for the insane, under ordinary circumstances, poor-houses are certainly not less so. Overseers of the poor, the superintendents of the poor-houses, and the poor themselves, are all perplexed and disturbed by the difficulties, the inconvenience, and the impropriety of such a residence for the insane.

Poor-houses, which have for their object the comfort of the aged, the helpless, and the invalid poor, are often so complex in their arrangements and objects, that the purpose of their establishment is lost sight of. Seldom planned with a view to the proper separation and classification of the inmates, order and morality are with difficulty maintained. When to the care of providing for a large and miscellaneous family, is joined the charge of a farm, on the part of the master, and the most various and burthensome duties on that of the mistress of the house, it is not surprising that the difficult task of managing the insane and the idiots, should soonest be neglected, and soonest produce troubles which few have the patience and skill to sustain. Beside, it should be remembered, that while many are capable of judiciously directing an extensive poor-house establishment, very few have either the tact or experience requisite for rightly managing the insane. While in all the northern states, and some of the middle and southern, that is to say, in all the states I have yet visited, I have found almost every form and variety of misery, produced by what many would term abuse, and outrage, and the grossest neglects, I can say, with sincerity, that most of the sufferings and neglects to which I have found the insane exposed, have been not (so much) the result of hard-hearted brutality, as of ignorance, and want of qualification for discharging those duties, and absolute perplexity as to the mode of rendering the objects of their cares, either tranquil or comfortable. Many have truly believed, that an insane man or woman was no better than a mere brute, and less easy to take care of; they have not supposed them susceptible of emotions of pain or pleasure, capable of being controlled through kind influences, or of being restored through any cares they could bestow. It is very frequent, I have found it so, especially in the county-houses of this state, and many in Pennsylvania, that almost the only objections which could be advanced against them, under the present general system, were to be found in the truly deplorable condition of the insane and idiotic inmates. We repeat of poor-houses what we have asserted of prisons—the insane *cannot* be suitably cared for in any such establishments.

Perhaps one cause for the unwillingness felt by some, to promote the establishment of hospitals for the insane, is a doubt of the curability of the malady, or of the superior advantage of hospital treatment over private practice. Such doubts are fast passing from the public mind. Thirty years since, in our country, they might have had plausibility, sustained by want of an experience of benefits resulting from judicious management. A new era has dawned on this department of medical science, and we daily witness the most gratifying results, in the large number of patients restored to their friends, confirmed in bodily and mental health. The twenty-third annual report of the M'Lean Asylum, at Sommerville, near Charlestown, Massachusetts, by Dr. Bell, shows that "the records of the asylum justify the declaration, that *all cases certainly recent*, that is, whose origin does not directly or obscurely run back more than a year, *recover under a fair trial. This is the general* law, the *occasional* instances to the contrary are the *exceptions.*" In this opinion Dr. Ray, of the Maine State Hospital, concurs.

The directors of the Ohio Lunatic Asylum remark, in their third report, "that the importance of remedial means in the *first* stages of insanity, cannot be too strongly impressed upon the public mind."

Dr. Chandler, superintendent of the New Hampshire Asylum, says, in the report for 1843, that "it is *well established* that the earlier patients are placed under curative treatment, in hospitals, *the more speedy and sure is the recovery.*"

Dr. Brigham, superintendent of the New York State Asylum, writes as follows, in his first report of that institution: "Few things relating to the management and treatment of the insane, are so *well established* as the necessity of their *early* treatment, and their removal from home, in order to effect recovery. There are exceptions, no doubt. By examining the records of well conducted lunatic asylums, it appears that more than eight out of ten of the recent cases recover, *while not more than one in six* of the old cases are cured."

Dr. Rockwell, of the Vermont State Asylum, says, in his report for 1841: "It will be seen that a far greater proportion of recent cases recover, than of those which are of long standing. It is very desirable that the insane should be placed under curative treatment in the early stages of the disease."

In Dr. Awl's fifth annual report, I find the following remarks: "We exceedingly rejoice that it is now a settled policy with the citizens of Ohio, to make abundant provision for the reception of *every* insane patient, whether male or female, rich or poor, curable or incurable. *Public safety, equity,* and *economy,* alike require that this should be so."

"Fearful as is the disease of insanity, the experience of this and other institutions of the United States, have clearly shown, that, with seasonable aid, it is by no means an incurable disease. That under *proper medical and moral treatment, a large proportion do perfectly recover.* And of those who are absolutely incurable, a vast number can always be greatly improved, and made comfortable and useful. *In our judgment it is entirely* wrong to consider a certain class of incurables as harmless, and proper to be discharged from the institution, because it ' does not *seem* dangerous to the peace of the community that they should go at large.' This cannot certainly be known, either in or out of the asylum : neither can a bond afford any proper security to the public, for the peaceable and inoffensive are easily excited; and it is possible for the most imbecile lunatic to take life, or fire a city. It is also certain that they must all receive attention, and have a being somewhere in the land; and a majority of them at the public expense. We therefore unhesitatingly conclude, that the only safe and correct course, either for the insane themselves, or for their friends and socie - ty, is to provide ample accommodations for them, where there will be opportunity for every one to experience comfort and relief."

Dr. Brigham, speaking of the benefit of labor for the insane, especially in the open air, adds, that " incurable cases, instead of being immured in jails, and in town and county houses, without em- ployment, where they are continually losing mind, and becoming worse, should be placed in good asylums, and have employment on the farm or in shops. In this way they would in general be rendered much happier, and some would probably recover." " A broad dis - tinction should be made between the *sane* and the *insane* poor, as regards providing for their comfort. The former may have in a good county poor-house most essential comforts, *provided the insane are not kept in it;* but the insane themselves, unless they have *especial* care in reference to their disordered minds, have little or none."

Quoting again from the report of the physician of the asylum at Columbus, showing the benefits of hospital treatment, we read : "It is now five years since this great enterprise of humanity was opened to the unfortunate and afflicted in the state. During this period *four hundred and seventy-three* insane persons have been committed to the care of the institution. Two hundred and three have recovered the right use of their reason, and returned to their friends ; eighteen were discharged, improved in various degrees of mental and physical health ; and a large proportion of the remainder have been reclaimed from wretchedness and suffering, from filth and nakedness, from vio- lence, which caused apprehension and danger, and from anguish and melancholy, which could only be exhibited in silence and in tears. "

The propriety of providing for *all* those who suffer under the vari- ous forms of mental disease, or, more accurately speaking, of physical disease affecting and disturbing the natural and healthful functions of the brain, is found in the daily experience of society, and confirmed by the opinion of medical men.

Dr. Woodward, in the eleventh report of the Massachusetts State Hospital, remarks, that it is not always safe that even the demented should be at large, neither idiots ; it is often necessary to confine both. Idiots are excluded from some of the institutions, but our experience shows that they are often violent, mischievous, and dangerous. There are no institutions in this country designed particularly for them, so that, if confined at all, it is proper that it should be in hospitals for the insane." Another observer of the condition of the insane, and other classes of patients suffering under mental disease, writes : "We look upon the epileptics with compassion. Many of them exhibit the best traits of human nature during their lucid intervals, but at other times they are perfectly uncontrollable, disregarding alike both friends and foes ; and we know of no class more dangerous to go at large."

Dr. Earle, in the report of the Bloomingdale Asylum for 1844, says :

"It appears to be very satisfactorily proved, that of cases in which there is no eccentricity or constitutional weakness of intellect, and where the proper remedial measures are adopted in the early stages of the disorder, no less than *eighty* of every *one hundred* are cured.— There are but few acute diseases from which so large a per centage of the persons attacked are restored.

" One of the chief obstacles to a more general recovery of the patients admitted into public institutions, and one of the principal causes of the great accumulation of deranged people in the community, is the neglect of removing them to an asylum as soon as possible after the commencement of the disease.

" A belief that they can be treated more effectually among their friends, when all experience goes to prove that they are more easily managed, and far more likely to recover, under the care of strangers ; erroneous ideas in relation to public institutions ; the sanguine hope, cherished from day to day, but cherished only to be daily disappointed, that the afflicted person will soon again regain the use of reason, frequently combine, with other considerations, to retard the admission of the patient, until the period most favorable to recovery is past. Thus, the mistaken kindness of relatives has undoubtedly been the cause of rendering the disease of hundreds of maniacs permanent.

"After the first three months of the existence of intellectual derangement, the probabilities of a cure begin rapidly to diminish ; and at the expiration of a year, it is believed they are not half so great as at first. If continued beyond that time, the diminution progresses, so that of such as have been deranged more than two years, the number that recover is comparatively very small ; supposed, by some physicians, to be but about one in thirty. Yet hope is left, and cures are sometimes effected of those whose disorder has existed five, ten, and even fifteen years. It would seem that every consideration of humanity and of duty requires a greater practical attention to these important truths."

" We advocate the doctrine, that a man being insane, all ordinary considerations should yield to the one important measure of securing his recovery, and that this course should be steadily persisted in until he is cured, or it be proved, beyond a reasonable doubt, that his disease is too firmly seated ever to be eradicated by the usual methods of treatment."

Dr. Ray, in the report of the Maine State Asylum for 1844, refers to the beneficial influence of well directed employment for the insane, as follows:

"Of all the remedies for 'razing out the written troubles of the brain,' none can compare with labor, wherein I include all useful employment. No other moral means is adapted to so large a proportion of the insane, and applicable to so many of the various forms of the disease. The excited and the depressed, the gay and the melancholic, the wild and the calm, the curable and the incurable, may be furnished with some form of labor adapted to their particular case, and calculated to produce a beneficial effect upon their bodily or mental condition. Indeed, the great feature which characterizes the management of modern hospitals for the insane, is the extensive use of labor as a means of moral treatment. And therefore it is that these institutions, instead of being as they once were, merely strong houses for the safe keeping of persons whose enlargement would endanger the welfare of society, abounding with instruments of restraint and coercion, and presenting a melancholy scene of idleness, indolence and depravity, have now become places of refuge for the unfortunate, where a spirit of industry is fostered, and a healthful mental activity maintained by various forms of useful employment.   *   *   *

"Incurables who are able and willing to work, are much more contented and enjoy better health, when employed. Even some of the most demented will be found capable of doing something, and though it may not be very profitable, yet it keeps them out of mischief, and thus contributes to the quiet of the house. In the course of the summer, a party of this class of patients, with just mind enough for the purpose and no more, carried into the cellar and shed, and piled up all our wood, amounting to some three hundred cords.

"There is a limit, however, to the use of labor as a moral means. There are always a few patients to whom it has appeared to be decidedly injurious, by increasing, in some way or other, the mental excitement. This effect is apt to be produced in recent cases, when the patient has been allowed to work too soon after the paroxysm, or began by working too long at a time. Labor will naturally produce increased activity of the circulation, and if there is the least disposition to determination of blood to the head, increase of mental excitement is liable to be the result. I have so often observed this fact, that I have deemed it necessary to be exceedingly cautious how we made use of this means with such as were just recovering from violent excitement, beginning with light in-door exercise, and thence trying, as the next step, hard work in the open air, protected from the sun, half an hour or less at a time, and gradually extending the period."

"During the last spring," writes Dr. Earle, at Bloomingdale, "two farmers, each of whom possessed a good farm, were admitted into the asylum, one about a week after the other. They were laboring under the most abject form of melancholy, and had both attempted suicide. In less than a month, their condition being already somewhat improved, they expressed a willingness, and one of them a strong desire, to work out of doors. Being furnished with implements they daily went out together, unaccompanied by any other person, and worked upon the farm with as much apparent interest as if it belonged to themselves. Under this course they continued rapidly to improve, and both were discharged recovered, one at the end of six weeks, and the other three months from the time of their respective admissions.

"Another man was brought to the asylum early in the spring, laboring under a high degree of active mania. His appetite was poor, and his frame emaciated. He was careless of his personal appearance, restless, turbulent, and almost incessantly talking, in an incoherent manner, upon the delusions attending his disease. When out of doors, he was constantly wandering to and fro, and talking to himself, or digging the earth with his hands, without end or object, and generally having his mouth filled with grass. For some months there was but little change in his condition. At length, having become somewhat less bewildered, his attendant succeeded in inducing him to assist in making beds. Shortly afterwards he was employed with the painters and glaziers upon the green-house, and then went to the carpenters' shop, where he worked regularly for several weeks. Meanwhile his bodily health improved, his mind gradually returned to its former integrity, and he was discharged cured of his mental disorder, and weighing more than at any previous period of his life.

"These cases are fair examples of the utility of a combination of medical and moral treatment, for in all of them, medicine was regularly administered until within a comparatively short period before their departure from the institution. They are presented, also, as cogent arguments in favor of giving to manual labor that pre-eminence which has already been assigned to it." * * * *

"The grounds immediately adjacent to the buildings are handsomely laid out and planted with flowers, shrubs, and the choicest fruit and ornamental trees.

"The farm contains about fifty acres, a large portion of which is under high cultivation, and very productive. A substantial and commodious stone building, erected a few years since, serves the several purposes of barn, stable and carriage-house. A spring-house and ice-house are on the premises, and a spacious and handsome green-house in the garden. The following is a schedule of the productions of the farm and garden the past year:

Hay	-	-	-	-	40 tons.
Oats, cut in the milk	-	-	-	4 "
Milk	-	-	-	-	4700 gallons.
Butter -	-	-	-	-	728 lbs.
Pork -	-	-	-	-	2706 "
Potatoes	-	-	..	-	500 bushels.
Corn -	-	-	-	-	75 "
Sugar beet	-	-	-	-	250 "
Blood beet	-	-	-	-	125 "
Mangel wurtzel	-	-	-	..	50 "
Turnips	..	-	-	..	325 "
Parsnips	-	-	-	-	100 "
Carrots	-	-	-	..	30 "
Onions	-	-	-	..	50 "
Cabbages	⌣	-	-	-	3000 heads.
Leeks -	-	-	-	-	4000 "
Celery	-	-	-	-	2600 "
Salsify	..	-	-	-	1500 "

"Besides these, there was a full supply, for the whole establishment, of peas, beans, squashes, tomatoes, radishes, cucumbers, asparagu. spinach, lettuce, egg-plant and pie-plant, together with a good supply of watermelons and muskmelons.

FRUITS.

Apples, 90 barrels for winter use, besides a supply in the summer and fall ; the whole estimated at - - - 500 bushels.

Pears	-	-	-	estimated	60 "
Peaches	-	-	-	-	18 "
Cherries	-	-	-	estimated	100 "
Grapes	-	-	-	-	800 pounds.
Currants	-	-	-	-	an abundant supply.
Strawberries and raspberries		-			a limited supply."

It is said that the establishment of hospitals involves great expense ; that it is much cheaper to maintain the insane elsewhere : is it also computed at what actual cost these are supported in the State Penitentiary, in county jails, in poor-houses, and in families ? what sums are consumed by their uncontrolled habits of destructiveness, what are lost by their crimes when under frenzied impulses they fire buildings, take human life, and make wreck of all social and domestic peace and happiness ? what sums are uselessly expended in conducting the trials of insane criminals ? what the cost of supporting the large class of incurables, who, if timely treated, would have been restored to society and usefulness, to health and enjoyment ? It may be interesting and useful to examine several tables, copied from a report of the State Hospital in Massachusetts, showing the relative expense of old and recent cases, for a series of years, and also some extracts from several reports of other hospitals. For these, see *Appendix*.

These tables determine conclusively that, on the ground of a discreet economy alone, it is wise to establish a State Hospital in New Jersey. But I will not dishonor you by urging this suit on the money-saving principle. I will not unman and unchristianize you by urging other incentives to prompt and liberal action, than those which humanity presents. I am sure it is not a parsimonious spirit which has delayed this work here. I perceive the liberal appropriation of money to sustain the poor-houses, and to fill the many channels of public and private charity. Evidences of a kindly benevolence reach me continually, in provision for the poor and needy, and in care of the distressed : the insane and idiots alone have been too long insufficiently provided for. I speak advisedly in saying, that were a system carefully projected, having for its single object the perpetuity of insanity, by treatment ensuring the incurability of the patient, one more infallible could not be devised than that which consigns to the State Penitentiary, to jails, and alms-houses, the maniac and the demented ; the idiot and the epileptic.

In the document which records the proceedings of the House of Assembly, March, 1839, I find the following eloquent and impressive resolutions called up by Mr. Cattell, "relative to lunatics and a lunatic asylum."

"*Resolved*, 1st. That the confinement of insane persons in jails with criminals, is subversive of all distinction between calamity and guilt, and punishes the misfortune which it is the duty of society to relieve.

"2d. That as experience has shown that recent insanity, in most cases, is readily cured, it is highly expedient that the state should provide a suitable institution for the comfort and relief of the insane poor, and remove them from prisons and poor-houses.

"3d. That an asylum should be erected at the expense of the state, at some proper point, upon such plan as may be best adapted for the purpose of such an institution, *as soon as the finances of the state will warrant a sufficient appropriation.*"

"Which was read and agreed to."

"*Ordered*, That the clerk inform Council, that the House of Assembly have adopted said resolutions, and request their concurrence."

"IN COUNCIL, *March 12th*, 1839.

"Council have agreed to the concurrent resolution from the House of Assembly, in relation to lunatics in jails, &c."

"Without amendment."

Gentlemen, it is believed that the time has arrived for *action* upon the above resolutions. "*The finances of the state will warrant* a sufficient appropriation" for the establishment of a State Hospital for the Insane and Idiots of New Jersey.

Permit me, in conclusion, to urge that the delay to provide suitable asylums for the insane, produces miseries to individuals, and evils to society, inappreciable in their utmost influence, except by those who have given time to the examination of the subject, and who have witnessed the appalling degradation of these wretched sufferers in the poorhouses, and jails, and penitentiaries of our land.

Shall New Jersey be last of "the Thirteen Sisters" to respond to the claims of humanity, and to acknowledge the demands of justice?

Respectfully submitted,

D. L. DIX.

TRENTON, *January 23d,* 1845

APPENDIX.

TABLE *showing the comparative expense of supporting old and re-cent cases of insanity, from which we learn the economy of placing patients in institutions in the early periods of disease; from the report of the Massachusetts State Hospital, for 1843.*

No. of old cases.	Present age.	Time insane, in years.	Total expense, at $100 a year, before entering the hospital, & $132 a year since; last year $120.	Number of recent cases discharged.	Present age.	Time insane, in weeks.	Cost of support, at $2.30 per week.
2	69	28	$3,212 00	1,622	30	7	$16 10
7	48	17	2,004 00	1,624	34	20	46 00
8	60	21	2,504 00	1,625	51	32	73 60
12	47	25	2,894 00	1,635	23	28	64 40
18	71	34	3,794 00	1,642	42	40	92 00
19	59	18	2,204 00	1,643	55	14	32 20
21	39	16	1,993 00	1,645	63	36	82 80
27	47	16	1,994 00	1,649	22	40	92 00
44	56	26	2,982 00	1,650	36	28	64 40
45	60	25	2,835 00	1,658	36	14	32 20
102	53	25	2,833 00	1,660	21	16	36 80
133	44	13	1,431 00	1,661	19	27	62 10
176	55	20	2,486 00	1,672	40	11	25 70
209	39	16	1,964 00	1,676	23	23	52 90
223	50	20	2,364 00	1,688	23	11	25 70
260	47	16	2,112 00	1,690	23	27	62 10
278	49	10	1,424 00	1,691	37	20	46 00
319	53	10	1,247 00	1,699	30	28	64 40
347	58	14	1,644 00	1,705	24	17	39 10
367	40	12	1,444 00	1,706	55	10	23 00
400	43	14	1,644 00	1,709	17	10	23 00
425	48	13	2,112 00	1,715	19	40	92 00
431	36	13	1,412 00	1,716	35	48	110 40
435	55	15	1,712 00	1,728	52	55	126 50
488	37	17	1,912 00	1,737	30	33	75 90
		454	$54,157 00			635	$1,461 30

From Dr. Awl's reports of the Ohio Institution, we extract the following tables :

In the report of 1840, the number of years that the twenty-five old cases had been insane, was 413 ; the whole expense of their support during that time, $47,590 ; the average, $1,903 60. The time that the twenty-five recent cases had been confined, was 556 weeks ; the expense, $1,400; the average $56.

In 1841, whole cost of twenty-five old cases, -	$49,248 00
Average, - - - - - -	1,969 00
Whole cost of twenty-five recent cases, - -	1,330 50
Average, - - - - - -	52 22
In 1842, whole expense of twenty-five old cases, --	$50,611 00
Average, - - - - - -	2,020 00
Whole expense of twenty-five recent cases, - -	1,130 00
Average, - - - - - -	45 20
In this institution, in 1843, twenty old cases had cost,	$44,782 00
Average cost of old cases, - - - -	2,239 10
Whole expense of twenty recent cases, till recovered,	1,308 30
Average cost of recent cases, - - -	65 41
In the Massachusetts State Lunatic Asylum, in 1843, twenty-five old cases had cost, - - -	$54,157 00
Average expense of old cases, - - -	2,166 20
Whole expense of twenty-five recent cases, till recovered,	1,461 30
Average expense of recent cases, - - -	58 45
In the Ohio Lunatic Asylum, in 1844, twenty-five old cases had cost, - - - - -	$35,464 00
Average expense of old cases, - - -	1,418 56
Whole expense of twenty-five recent cases, -	1,608 00
Average expense of recent cases, - - -	64 32
In the Maine Lunatic Hospital, in 1842, twelve old cases had cost, - -- - - - -	$25,300 00
Average expense of old cases, - - -	2,108 33
Whole expense of twelve recent cases, - -	426 00
Average expense of recent cases, - - -	35 50
In the Hospital at Staunton, Va., twenty old cases had cost, - - - - - -	$41,633 00
Average expense of old cases, - - -	2,081 65
Whole expense of twenty recent cases, - -	1,265 00
Average expense of recent cases, - - -	63 25

The results of this table are striking, and show conclusively the importance of early admission to the insane hospitals. Other institutions have instituted the same inquiry with similar results.

MEMORIAL

PENNSYLVANIA

1845

MEMORIAL

SOLICITING A

STATE HOSPITAL FOR THE INSANE,

SUBMITTED TO THE

LEGISLATURE OF PENNSYLVANIA,

FEBRUARY 3, 1845.

Printed by order of the Legislature of Penn'a, February 3, 1845.

HARRISBURG:

J. M. G. LESCURE, PRINTER TO THE STATE.
....
1845.

MEMORIAL.

---

*To the Honorable, the Senate and the House of Representatives of the Commonwealth
of Pennsylvania:*

GENTLEMEN :

I come to represent to you the condition of a numerous and unhappy class of sufferers, who fill the cells and dungeons of the poor houses, and the prisons of your state.
I refer to the pauper and indigent insane, epileptics, and idiots of Pennsylvania.   I
come to urge their *claims* upon the commonwealth for protection and support, such
protection and support as is only to be found in a well conducted Lunatic Asylum.

I do not solicit you to be generous ; this is an occasion rather for the dispensation of
justice.   These most unfortunate beings have claims, those *claims* which bitter misery
and adversity creates, and which it is your solemn obligation as citizens and legislators
to cancel.   To this end, as the advocate of those who are disqualified by a terrible
malady, from pleading their own cause, I ask you to provide for the immediate establishment of a State Hospital for the Insane.

If this shall appear to some of you an untimely demand on the State Treasury ; and
a too hastily, too importunately urged suit, I must ask all such to go forth, as I have
done, and traversing the state in its length and breadth, examine with patient care the
condition of this suffering, dependent multitude, which are gathered to your alms-houses
and your *prisons,* and scattered under adverse circumstances in indigent families; *weigh
the iron chains, and shackles, and balls, and ring-bolts, and bars, and manacles; breathe
the foul atmosphere of those cells and dens, which too slowly poisons the springs of
life ; examine the furniture of these dreary abodes ; some for a bed have the luxury of
a truss of straw; and some have the cheaper couch, which the hard, rough plank supplies!   Examine their apparel.   The air of heaven is their only vesture.   Are you
disquieted and pained to learn these facts?   There are worse realities yet to be
revealed under your vigilant investigations.   The revolting exposure of men ; the
infinitely more revolting and shocking exposure of women ; with combinations of
miseries and horrors that will not bear recital.   Do you start and shrink from the
grossness of this recital? what then is it to witness the appalling reality?* Do your
startled perceptions refuse to admit these truths?   They exist still ; the proof and the
condition* alike ; *neither have passed away.*   The idiot mother ; the naked women in
the packing boxes:* but yet for these last, perhaps, the legal measures resorted to for

---

* See history of counties.

their relief have been availing. Perhaps both judge and jury have interposed for those, some merciful change. This relief may be but temporary, and may disappear with the first indignant excitement which procured it; for the effectual, permanent remedy and alleviation of all these troubles and miseries, this appeal is now made to the Legislature of Pennsylvania; and, gentlemen, you perceive that it is *just, not generous action,* I ask at your hands.

It cannot be forgotten that, successively in the years of 1838 and 1840, earnest efforts were made by benevolent citizens of the state, to procure for the pauper and indigent insane, the benefits of curative treatment and hospital protection. The gentlemen who engaged in this object, I have learned, spared neither time nor labor to accomplish what was justly deemed so important a work. An association of residents in Philadelphia, of which Thomas P. Cope, Esq., was chairman, published and circulated a pamphlet, written with ability, which was designed to give much valuable information on the treatment of insanity, &c. This was received with the consideration the subject merited; and Mr. Konigmacher, of Ephrata, was appointed chairman of a committee, in the House of Representatives, to report upon the subject. This was done with eloquence and precision, in a document of considerable length, which was read in the House, March 11th, 1839. Mr. Konigmacher accompanied his report with a bill, which passed the House of Representatives with but little opposition, and the Senate unanimously; but on account of financial embarrassments, was not sanctioned by the Executive. In 1840, a second appeal from the association of gentlemen before referred to, was printed and circulated at their expense. This pamphlet embodied a mass of statistical information, calculated to throw much additional light upon the subject. The result was, an appropriation by the Legislature, and the appointment of commissioners to carry forward and complete the establishment of a state institution. The work was shortly interdicted through the influence of circumstances which it is unnecessary to explain here.

Meanwhile, the evil for which the wise and benevolent sought a remedy, has gone on to increase. Sufferings have been multiplied with additional cases of the malady. Many who might have been restored by timely treatment, have become, either through the violence of disease, or unavoidable mismanagement, hopelessly insane. Many others are fast verging to the same pitiable condition; and new cases of almost daily occurrence, remind the beholder that a similar destiny awaits these, if no asylum opens its friendly shelter, and renders remedial care in season to avert the impending calamity.

You are not solicited to commence a work of doubtful value, capable of producing uncertain benefits. The age of experiment has passed by : the experience of those of your sister states, who have preceded you in this enterprise of mercy, assures you that thousands, through the skilful care received in hospitals for the insane, have been restored to society and to usefulness, to reason and to happiness.

Beside recent and curable cases, there is yet another class, the very extremity and certainty of whose condition appeals most strongly and affectingly to your humane sensibilities. I mean those from whom, in all probability, the light of reason is forever veiled : dependent, irresponsible, often much suffering beings, they seem from the very entireness and certain duration of their dependence, to demand a peculiar consideration. Abandon not these of your fellow-citizens to any miseries which you can cause to be relieved or mitigated.

This subject comes home to all, to every one : on this ground all alike may suffer ; the rich and the poor, the learned and the uneducated, the young, the mature, and the aged ; from this malady none are sure of exemption ; and the often reverses of fortune teach, that none are so prosperous that they may not need to share the asylum which is solicited now to shelter others.

Through the bond of our common humanity, we may become as they now are. Let imagination for a moment place you in their stead, or rather let it so place those you love, those you cherish, those who are dearer to you than is your own life, and then declare, if you could abandon them to the horrid noisome cell ; and to ignorant pauper attendants ; uninterested, unpaid, and reluctant nurses ; or could you yield them to the strong holds of the jails and prisons, there to be companions of the felon, and the thief, and the abased vicious drunkard : there to be abandoned to their caprices, and subject to their daily taunts, and heartless jeers. I am not suggesting unreal, impossible conditions ; you can witness these scenes as I have done, and learn too; corroboration of these hardships and sufferings from the unwilling keepers of these unfortunate men and women, who, dangerous to the community, through property-destroying or homicidal propensities, must endure this bondage till a state asylum open its doors to receive them. There are some, but the number is not large, who, bound down to low views of the mutual obligations of man to man, and to imperfect perceptions of the sublime truths of the moral law, will argue, that many, very many of those who are found in wretched circumstances in alms-houses and in prisons, have, by their own follies and vices brought on themselves the calamity, which henceforth casts them out from the accustomed walks of life. No doubt this is true ; but why should society visit upon the transgressor who becomes insane, a so much harsher retribution, than upon the transgressor who retains his senses ? It is very well known, that by far the largest portion of those who become wholly dependent on public charity, have been brought to that condition either by their own indiscretion or misdemeanors ; yet these find the sympathy they seek, and the aid they solicit ; for them an appropriate home is often provided, and their necessities are bountifully administered to. There is yet another view of this subject.

Suppose the insane in many cases to have wrought their own ruin, shall man be more just than God? Does not he send his sun to shine upon the evil and unthankful, as upon the obedient and the good ? Again, is it not to the habits, the customs, the temptations of civilized life and society, that we owe most of these calamities? Should not society, then, make the compensation which alone can be made for these disastrous fruits of its social organization? Concede this, and I do not know how it is to be evaded; and your course of action is made plain by a duty not to be mistaken. Economy, justice, humanity, and mercy, that attribute of the Deity, combine to direct your deliberations, and determine your judgment.

Of the *fifty-eight* counties in this State, *twenty-one* contain poor-house establishments ; and the remaining *thirty-seven* sustain their paupers by annual distribution in families, who receive them at "the lowest rate for which they are bidden." I think it may be conceded, that in the majority of cases, defective as is the poor-house supervision for the insane, they are more comfortable, or rather, often less borne down by the accumulation of their sufferings in these institutions, than in private families, where every arrangement is interfered with, and from which all quiet is banished. Few have skill to control the furious, or to manage the refractory; and not many have that patient endurance which is tested to the utmost in the care of excited insane persons.

Next after private families and poor-houses, the insane will be found in the jails and penitentiaries. On this subject, the opinion of some of your jurists has been so explicitly declared, that I feel it but justice to the cause to give this expression of their sentiments place here—justifying the sentences of insane convicts to prisons, on the undeniable ground of necessity, "inasmuch as there is no State Hospital."

"PHILADELPHIA, *March* 5, 1839.

"The want of an asylum for the insane poor, often occasions painful embarrassments to the courts, when the defence in a criminal charge is insanity fully sustained in proof. Although the jury may certify that their acquittal is on that ground, and thus empower the court to order the prisoner into close custody, *yet that custody can be in no other place than the common prisons*, places illy qualified for such a subject of incarceration. We cannot doubt that the ends of justice would be greatly promoted, if such an asylum as the petitioners contemplate were established, with proper regulations, and the courts were authorized to commit to it persons acquitted of crimes on the plea of insanity."

(Signed,)

EDWARD KING,
ARCHIBALD RANDALL,
J. RICHTER JONES,
Judges of the Court of Quarter Sessions.

JAMES TODD,
J. BOUVIER,
R. T. CONRAD,
Judges of the Criminal Sessions.

I fully concur in the above representation.

CALVIN BLYTHE,
Judge of the Twelfth Judicial District.

It is believed that all the judges of the courts of the commonwealth of Pennsylvania, having criminal jurisdiction, would coincide in the above opinion. From many I have the most direct personal assurance to that effect.

Passing from the prisons, &c., we perceive that in the state, are at present two established hospitals or asylums for the insane—not including that populous department of the Philadelphia Alms-house, which is called the Alms-house Hospital for the Insane. The asylum at Frankford, about six miles north of the city, and established by the Society of Friends, in May 1817, and which can receive about fifty patients, and the Pennsylvania Hospital for the Insane, west of the Schuylkill, nearly two miles from the city, have been severally established by the humanity and munificence of private individuals, chiefly citizens of Philadelphia. These two institutions are almost constantly filled to their utmost capacity; or when vacancies occur by the recovery and removal of patients, they are shortly filled by others, whose distressed friends seek for them the benefits which these institutions are so well calculated to secure. The latter asylum, which is under the superintendence of Dr. Kirkbride, can receive but about two hundred patients with their attendants, so that we find a very large number whose recent attack, or the violence of the malady, make peculiarly the subjects of judicious hospital treatment, altogether without the means of relief. The only provision, therefore, and this made by individual benefactions, for the insane of the large state of Pennsylvania, is found in the immediate vicinity of the commercial capital. Far and wide, over an extent of hundreds of miles, from east to west, and north to south, are large numbers of your citizens *declining into irrecoverable insanity* through the want of an institution, which it now depends upon the Legislature of Pennsylvania to establish on a broad and secure foundation.

It is not expected, it is not asked, that at this time you should make ample provision for all the insane of the state. If at this period you build a hospital to receive *recent cases*, and such as may still be judged capable of restoration; if you will take from your prisons such as are there most unrighteously imprisoned, you will accomplish an amount of good, which exceeds computation; a good that will reach to and bless, succeeding generations; and at some more prosperous period in your financial concerns, you may be able to complete, what now you commence upon a moderate and limited plan, that is to say, you may establish as many institutions as the wants of a populous country, and the consequent dependence and maladies of a portion of the community require and will demand.

The *importance of timely remedial treatment* is obvious. The opinion of all the intelligent medical men in Pennsylvania, and throughout the Union, supports this view. An illustration of the advantage of seasonable care, considered merely in reference to economy, is exhibited in the appendix, by tables drawn from the returns of some of the hospitals in our own country. This question, so clearly demonstrated by these, needs no additional argument, yet it may be gratifying to read several brief extracts from the annual reports of several of the hospitals for the insane in the United States.

"The importance of early treatment," says Dr. Awl, "cannot be too strongly urged."

Dr. Ray, of the Maine State Asylum, repeats this in his annual reports with strong emphasis, and his opinion must have weight wherever his name is known.

Dr. Butler, of the Hartford Retreat for the Insane, writes in his report for 1844, "The results of the early commitment of the cases of insanity to the curative appliances of this and similar institutions, present a most convincing evidence of its good policy as well as of its humanity. They justify us in expecting, that of cases where the duration of disease *has been less than one year*, from eighty to ninety per cent. will recover; where it has existed from one to five years, from twenty to thirty per cent.; from five to ten years, about twelve per cent.; and when of longer duration, not more than five per cent. *Delay* in applying the appropriate treatment, rapidly diminishes the chances of recovery."

Dr. Kirkbride, of the Pennsylvania Hospital for the Insane, writing of the importance of *early* treatment for this class of patients, says, in his report for 1842: "Not a month elapses that we do not have to regret that some individual is placed under our care *after* the best period for restorative treatment has passed. The general proposition that truly recent cases of insanity are commonly very curable, and that chronic ones are only occasionally so, may be considered as fully established, and *ought at this day to be every where understood:*" and again in another year's report, the same truth is still urged. "It cannot be too earnestly impressed upon those whose friends are afflicted with insanity, that *all experience* goes to prove, that in its earliest stages it is generally curable, *and that every week it is left without treatment, goes to diminish the prospect of restoration.*"

Dr. Luther V. Bell, whose professional experience and high intellectual ability give authority to his opinions, writes as follows in his report for 1843–44 :—"In regard to the curability of insanity in its different manifestations, there *can be no general rule better established than that this is directly in the ratio of the duration of the symptoms.*"

In the twenty-third annual report of that branch of the Massachusetts General Hospital, known as the M'Lean Asylum for the Insane, near Charlestown, Mass., Dr. Bell again refers with clearness and precision to this subject. "The records of the asylum justify the declaration, that *all cases certainly recent*, that is, whose origin does not directly or obscurely run back more than a year, *recover under a fair trial. This is the general* law, the *occasional* instances to the contrary are the *exceptions.*" In this opinion, Dr. Ray, of the Maine Hospital concurs.

The directors of the Ohio Lunatic Asylum remark, in their third report, that " the importance of remedial means in the *first* stages of insanity, cannot be too strongly impressed upon the public mind."

Dr. Chandler, superintendent of the New Hampshire Asylum, says, in the report for 1843, that "it is *well established* that the earlier patients are placed under curative treatment, in hospitals, *the more speedy and sure is the recovery.*"

Dr. Brigham, superintendent of the New York State Asylum, writes as follows, in his first report of that institution : " Few things relating to the management and treatment of the insane, are so *well established* as the necessity of their *early* treatment, and of their removal from home, in order to effect recovery. There are exceptions, no doubt. By examining the records of well conducted lunatic asylums, it appears that more than eight out of ten of the recent cases recover, *while not more than one in six* of the old cases are cured."

Dr. Rockwell, of the Vermont State Asylum, says, in his report for 1841, " It will be seen that a far greater proportion of recent cases recover, than of those which are of long standing. It is very desirable that the insane should be placed under curative treatment in the early stages of the disease."

In Dr. Awl's fifth annual report, I find the following remarks : " We exceedingly rejoice that it is now a settled policy with the citizens of Ohio, to make abundant provision for the reception of *every* insane patient, whether male or female, rich or poor, curable or incurable. *Public safety, equity,* and *economy,* alike require that this should be so."

" Fearful as is the disease of insanity, the experience of this and other institutions of the United States, has clearly shown that, with seasonable aid, it is by no means an incurable disease. That under *proper medical and moral treatment, a large proportion do perfectly recover.* And of those who are absolutely incurable, a vast number can always be greatly improved, and made comfortable and useful. *In our judgment, it is entirely* wrong to consider a certain class of incurables as harmless, and proper to be discharged from the institution, because it "does not *seem* dangerous to the peace of the community that they should go at large." This cannot certainly be known, either in or out of the asylum : neither can a bond afford any proper security to the public, for the peaceable and inoffensive are easily excited ; and it is possible for the most imbecile lunatic to take life or fire a city. It is also certain that they must all receive attention, and have a being somewhere in the land; and a majority of them at the public expense. We therefore unhesitatingly conclude, that the only safe and correct course, either for the insane themselves, or for their friends and society, is to provide ample accommodations for them, when there will be opportunity for every one to experience comfort and relief."

Dr. Brigham, speaking of the benefit of labor for the insane, especially in the open air, adds, that "incurable cases, instead of being immured in jails and in the town and county-houses without employment, where they are continually loosing mind, and becoming worse, should be placed in good asylums, and have employment on the farm or in shops. In this way they would in general be rendered much happier, and some would probably recover." "A broad distinction should be made between the *sane* and the *insane* poor, as regards providing for their comfort. The former may have in a good county poor-house most essential comforts, *provided the insane are not kept in it ;* but the insane themselves, unless they have *especial* care in reference to their disordered minds, have little or none."

Quoting again from the report of the physician of the asylum at Columbus, showing the benefits of hospital treatment, we read : "It is now five years since this great enterprise of humanity was opened to the unfortunate and afflicted in the state. During this period *four hundred and seventy-three* insane persons have been committed to the care of the institution. Two hundred and three have recovered the right use of their reason, and returned to their friends ; eighteen were discharged, improved in various degrees of mental and physical health, and a large proportion of the remainder have been reclaimed from wretchedness and suffering, from filth and nakedness, from violence, which caused apprehension and danger, and from anguish and melancholy, which could only be exhibited in silence and in tears."

Dr. Kirkbride remarks, in his report upon the Pennsylvania Insane Hospital for 1842, the great importance of bringing patients under early curative treatment, and first, in regard to its economy :

"The economy of subjecting cases of mental derangement to proper treatment, immediately upon the occurrence of an attack, has not been generally understood, *or no state* would have neglected to make adequate provision for the early care of all who were thus afflicted. There can be no question, but that every community, not having within itself the proper means, would save largely by sending their recent cases to some well conducted insane hospital, and retaining them there, as long as there was a prospect for their restoration. If this was done, a large proportion of them would in a few months, be restored to society, instead of continuing as is now too apt to be the case, a charge to their friends or the public. during the remainder of their lives.

"This is not merely conjecture; by referring to the register of this institution, I find that the actual average cost of supporting the first twenty successive cases that were discharged cured—from the time of their admission till their return home, was only *fifty-two dollars and fifty cents* each—while in the first twenty incurable cases that were received in this house, at the same rate of expense, from the time of the commencement of the disease till 1841, the average cost of each, to their friends, was *three thousand and forty-five dollars*. And in the published reports of the Massachusetts State Hospital, it is shown from positive data, that the actual cost to the public of maintaining twenty-five consecutive cases of recent insanity till their restoration, was only *fifty-six dollars* each, while the cost in the same number of chronic ones, already averaged *nineteen hundred and three dollars* and *sixty cents* each.

"The expense in the one instance, is only for a few months, when the individual returns to the care of his family, or business; in the other, it is a support for life, often a long one, and not unfrequently if the individual be the head of a family,—the support of a family in addition."

From allusions made on the first pages of this memorial, to the inappropriate, unjust, and *sometimes* barbarous, treatment of the insane poor, it will be expected that I shall sustain assertion by evidence. I have therefore prepared, from my note book, some account of the condition in which I have found the poor-houses, jails, and prisons of this commonwealth, during more than four months laborious journeyings, devoted to inquiry and investigation. I describe those establishments *as I found them.* The sane paupers in the poor-houses, almost without exception, are well and liberally provided for. The insane, almost without exception, are inappropriately and injudiciously situated. This is not so much the fault of these establishments, as their misfortune. Poor-houses never can be made suitable places for the reception of, and treatment of, the insane. Of the six well directed county prisons in the United States, Pennsylvania has the honorable distinction of containing three, and these I consider established on the best system; but not suitable in any respect as asylums for mad-men and mad-women. Your state penitentiaries, of which I shall shortly take occasion to write more at length, are conducted as they are established, upon the best system human wisdom, and justice, and humanity, has yet devised. But the penitentiaries were not planned and built as hospitals, where the physical maladies of the insane should find remedial and appropriate treatment; nor can they with due regard to the discipline and regulations to which they are subject, be thus occupied. One does not know how to employ mild terms in touching upon the shameful injustice of *sending maniacs, who for years have been known to labor under this distressing malady, to prison.* "To do justly and love mercy is better than sacrifice;" and, gentlemen, to redress these many grievances may be your beneficent and noble work.

In Mr. Konigmacher's report for 1839, the number of idiots and insane in this commonwealth, is represented as *" at least twenty-three hundred."* Of these, it was supposed, *"* that at least *one thousand* were in *county prisons and poor-houses,* the residue being supported on their own resources or upon private charity.*"*

The results of my direct personal enquiry show, that there are large numbers who are not in prisons or poor-houses, whose condition is yet more deplorable : I mean those who are supported *by the towns and counties,* scattered in families who consent to receive them at the lowest rates. But the result of my investigations, generally, is shown in the notes on the counties. I will only add, that a portion of the whole number of insane and idiots are beyond the reach, unhappily, of medical treatment. For them, a comfortable care is all that can be asked, or that can be availing.

The LANCASTER COUNTY JAIL is a substantial and somewhat extensive structure, built of limestone, but the plan is very defective, affording small opportunity for classifying or separating the prisoners. Of the thirty-one prisoners seen there in July and the first of August, three were insane, and four were females. Some of the jail rooms were nineteen feet by twenty, and ten high, often insufficiently ventilated by opening the windows. The area of the exercise yard covers two-thirds of an acre. The allowance of food is *one pound* of bread per day, with as much water as they choose. If they can afford to purchase other articles of provisions it is permitted; but these they work for themselves in the jail. I saw no beds; three blankets are allowed to each man. The punishments are fetters and collar; no solitary cells except the dungeons below, which are damp, and I believe disused altogether. Here I was informed the prisoners are sometimes detained, for months, waiting trial, without employment; left to idleness, that nurse of crime, and to evil communications, which corrupt the juvenile offender, and plunge yet deeper into ignominious habits, the old transgressor. If it were the deliberate purpose of society to establish criminals in all that is evil, and to root out the last remains of virtuous inclination, this purpose could not be more effectually accomplished than by incarceration in the county jails, as they are with few exceptions, constructed and governed. What can be expected of a system, which not only condemns criminals to companionship, but to the most absolute idleness. Neither work nor books, neither counsels nor cautions, find place in the jails of our country. The state penitentiaries are for the most part carefully disciplined, and there are some appliances to heal the moral diseases which corrode the soul and debase the man; but society, with a strange inconsistency, first *establishes* the disease, first inflicts the wound, first imbues the whole heart and mind with evil—and *then,* with christian zeal, hurries with the spiritual physician to the sin-sick victim, and finally marvels that so few cures of the disease crown these benevolent efforts! as if bad habits confirmed, and pollution become familiar, were now to be eradicated and purified by a few months, or even years, of care and restraint. It is respectfully suggested to those interested in this subject, to visit successively the Moyamensing Prison, in Philadelphia; the County Jail of Chester county, at West Chester; and the Dauphin County Jail at Harrisburg; and then, the Allegheny County Jail at Pittsburg; the Erie County Jail at Erie; and the Lancaster County Jail at Lancaster; and they can make a fair and full comparison between a good system and a bad system; between wholesome regulations and vicious influences; between institutions which are an honor to the morals and intellect of a community, and establishments which are a disgrace to both. In two or three particulars it would be unjust and untrue to rank Lancaster jail with the jails at Pittsburg and Erie, as I saw them all; the former was *clean*, a term which in no possible mode or manner could apply to the latter. The officers of the former were sensible of the great defects of the system, and of the demoralizing influences, especially upon young offenders; those of the latter, apparently, cared nothing at all about the matter. In the former, religious teaching sometimes broke in upon the corrupting conversations of the prisoners; in the latter never. The jailor of the Lancaster Prison was very desirous that employment should be introduced as a part of the prison system, and was ready to promote such a change. He also remarked that while he took such care of the insane, as the system and the bad architectural arrangements of the prison permitted, yet it was not possible to render them comfortable or to protect them from the other prisoners, who were disposed to make sport of them, to teaze and irritate them to the utmost, and, if possible, to promote quarrels and fighting. For the insane in prisons, is no State Hospital needed?

LANCASTER COUNTY POOR-HOUSE, founded in 1799, and since increased by the addition of a hospital, is well-built, and well-situated, with an excellent and well-conducted farm attached, and a hospital, constructed of brick, for the invalids, the sick, and the insane. Beside these, are numerous out-buildings commodiously planned, and adapted to the convenience of carrying forward the household labor—as a bake-house, smoke-house, milk-house, wash-house, &c. &c. The recorded number of poor maintained here during the year, from May, 1843, to 1844, has afforded a constant average of two hundred and fifty-four paupers per month, exclusive of three hundred and seventeen way-faring persons who received supper, lodging and breakfast during the year—seventy-eight cases of out-door relief are recorded, at a cost of eight hundred and thirty-four dollars. The salary of the steward is four hundred dollars; that of the clerk two hundred and seventy-five; and that of the matron, or hospital nurse, who has the sole charge of that department, which, at the time of my visit, contained one hundred and fifteen, being more than half the paupers of the establishment, and *forty-six* of these insane, is *ninety* dollars. The salary of the steward is sufficient; that of the clerk *ample;* that of the matron altogether below the half of what would be a just compensation for the various very responsible and difficult duties required of her.— Her cares are never diminished or intermitted, and as she gives all her time and strength faithfully to the work, if some deficiencies are apparent, she cannot be censured. By means of pipes, from a never-failing source, ample supplies of water are conveyed into both the hospital and main building. Both these establishments are extremely neat, and well-conducted, excepting only the lunatic department, and that the defective architecture of the building prevents in no small measure.

The estimated number of insane in Lancaster county, five years since, was rather more than *one hundred.* I have not been able to arrive at any certain result by which the present number can be estimated, but intelligent physicians, whose practice extends over a considerable territory, believe there are not fewer than one hundred and fifty. So little benefit has been derived from the gathering of the insane into the poor-house hospital, which, in this county, has some uncommon advantages, that according to the estimate of a skilful physician, there were but five recoveries in ten years, or but one recovery in every eighty-two patients. About half the patients last August, had the liberty of the premises; others were confined in their cells or to the wards, and a few were ranging a small enclosure, called the exercise yard. This miserable place was utterly comfortless, exposed and inconvenient. The hot sun beat down upon the unconscious or half conscious patients. With bare head exposed to the direct and burning rays, they strayed round the small area, or lay extended upon the ground. Not a tree even shaded the place, and one almost felt that it was but an additional evil, that they were permitted to be abroad, exposing them to the sun or the tempest, the drought, the heat, or the cold, according to the season. Here were no competent "care-takers," except the matron: her assistance and authority were necessary in all cases, directing and superintending the feeble and the recovering paupers. These, who were employed as attendants and nurses, unskilled in the management of the insane, "did what they could," but not what was needed. "I do most earnestly desire the establishment of a State Hospital," said the excellent and benevolent physician—"the insane cannot be fitly treated, either morally or physically, in a poor-house." And again one writes, "the establishment of a State Hospital will be one of the noblest monuments to the humanity of our state, and to the justice and philanthropy of the Legislature who move in it. I hope all hearts and heads will unite in promoting this good and christian work."

The forty-four cells for the insane in the hospital, are four feet by seven, and twelve high; though something better than those occupied a few years since, and intended to have been much better, they are so amazingly defective, that at the first survey, one is forced to exclaim at the attempt to occupy them at all. They are very small, mere closets; some are not ventilated, some not lighted, and very ill-arranged indeed. Several of the very violently excited patients were in apartments below, which should rarely if ever be used for such purposes. "Chains and hobbles" were in constant use here, and though I know it has been the benevolent design of official persons to improve the condition of the insane poor, by a considerable recent addition to the hospital, it is a lamentable failure; and the error of judgment, apparent in the plan and execution of the work, is much to be regretted. In fine, here, as in most poor-houses, is much expense accompanied, so far as the insane are considered, by very unsatisfactory results. This is not said in a censorious spirit, but to prove that the true want is not yet supplied.

YORK COUNTY JAIL, at *York*, was clean. There is attached, a spacious exercise yard, surrounded like most of the prison yards, throughout the state, with a lofty wall. The usual results of prison companionship were apparent here. I found the prisoners *promiscuously* associated, men and women—some in the yard, others in the apartments; none employed, except, as I think, a female prisoner. There was one insane man who had been, that very day, sentenced for horse stealing, to the Eastern Penitentiary. Of this man, Dr. Haller, whose name is a voucher for this history, wrote to the warden of the prison, as follows: "Of his insanity, there can be no doubt. I have had him as an insane patient, in our county hospital, nine years since. You may rest fully assured, that there is no disposition, on his part, to play the crazy man. When much excited, he is rather dangerous. Your physician will find him a fair subject of the insane wards of your institution."

York County Alms-house and Hospital, with the contiguous buildings, make a handsome appearance. The farm is one of the best in the county, and contains one hundred and forty-three acres of cultivated land, and two hundred and twenty-one of woodland. The whole establishment can accommodate three hundred. August 3d, 1844, there were one hundred and one men, women and children ; of these, there were twenty-five idiotic and insane males and females. There is a school for the children, and religious services every Sabbath. Order and good management, were apparent throughout the establishment. As at Lancaster, the apartments were clean, and furnished with excellent beds and bedding. They were also remarkably well ventilated. The buildings are of brick—the main house was erected in 1805 ; the hospital in 1828. It is two stories high, commodious, with spacious rooms and lofty ceilings. These last are especially important in poor-houses and hospitals, where the apartments often become crowded at the approach of winter ; and thus, through want of pure air, much sickness is induced. The cells for the insane, are in the basement of the hospital. They are fourteen by ten, and ten feet high. The windows are grated, three by four and a half. Grating over the doors, three by one and a half feet. The passage is seven feet wide. In winter, warmed by a stove, and pipes conducting near all the cells. The entire length of the hospital, is ninety feet. The breadth, forty. Supply of water, ample. Provisions, wholesome and sufficient. Comfortable as are the insane here, by comparison with most of this class in poor-houses, though some wear *chains and hobbles*, the physician writes of them as follows :

" They receive all the medical attendance that can possibly be rendered to their situation, but in consequence of the want of sufficient apparatus, and the superintendence of prudent and judicious persons, the recoveries are few ; not more than two or three per annum, and those confined to recent cases, where the exciting cause can be plainly understood from those who accompany the patient to the institution." " The establishment of a state asylum would be a matter of economy to all the counties, whether they have poor-houses, hospitals, or not. *It would be the means of restoring thousands of honest poor citizens to their senses*, and their families, who otherwise might have lingered out a horrible existence in filthy cells, or in chains and misery." Such is the opinion of not only the physician of York county-house, but of all intelligent medical men in the state. Estimated number of insane and idiots in York county, about one hundred.

I found the Jail in Adams County in a miserable condition. It is an old, ill-constructed, stone building, a good deal out of repair, and I should think in winter, could hardly be made comfortable. The prisoners sleep upon the floor, on straw beds, and are allowed as many blankets as they need, according to the season. The county allows twenty cents per day for their board, but for the insane twenty-five cents. They have three meals, which are cooked for them; meat usually three times a day. Their washing is done by the family. The students from the Theological Seminary give religious instruction on Sundays, both at the jail and poor-house. I was there in August, and found several prisoners, some about the premises, others in the large exercise-yard. Here also was an insane man—or one whose mental faculties had been defective from birth—yet he had been capable of various employments at his father's house, and reached manhood without giving any alarm so serious as to make his removal a prudential measure. He was subject to paroxysms, and often difficult of control. One day, without any apparent motive, he entered the house with an axe, and deliberately approached one of the farming men, who was sitting with his back towards the door, and at one blow split his head open. This shocking murder inspired the family with the utmost apprehension. He was removed to the jail as dangerous to be at large, about four years since, and there I found him loaded with chains ; a ring about the ankle, was connected by a sort of hinge, to a long, stout iron bar, reaching above the hips, and to this the iron wrist-lets were attached. In the jail, his condition was pitiable; but if at large, neither life nor property would be secure. The only fit place for such, is in a well regulated hospital. The marvel is, that he was not, as *scores of other crazy men have been*, consigned to a state prison ! A young girl, very insane, had not long been removed from the jail, where she was loaded with heavy chains, and endured all the exposures and sufferings incident to a situation in all respects so unsuitable. At times she was very violent. Estimated number of insane and idiotic in the county, from forty to fifty.

The COUNTY POOR-HOUSE at *Gettysburg*, is about a mile from the centre of the town. Early in August, I found it not in good repair. There were from ninety to a hundred inmates, chiefly foreigners. The farm contains one hundred and fifty acres, is well stocked, and well cultivated. There is an ample supply of water ; the health of the family is generally good ; the physician attends two or three times weekly, and oftener if necessary. There is a school for the children, and preaching every Sabbath. Bibles, testaments, and some other books, are liberally supplied. The keeper appeared competent to the performance of his difficult duties ; and interested, so far as he had knowledge, in the good condition of the establishment. The hospital is not so well constructed or arranged as the main building. There were eleven crazy and idiotic patients. In the basement are three "crazy rooms," very fitly named, *eight* by *eight*, *and eight high.* There are also two cells, *four* by *nine,* and *six* by *nine, in the cellar.* They are unventilated and damp, the floors are wood, and they are lighted by an aperture one and a half by one, and barred with wood. These dens can be partially warmed. The insane are very improperly situated, though two of the females, apart from the rest, were in more comfortable rooms. There was no *wilful* neglect, and no means for promoting cure. *Chains and hobbles used from necessity,* to prevent mischief and straying, as in all the poor-houses, with one or two rare exceptions. In well conducted asylums, these are never employed; neither such instruments of terrible torture as the ill-devised "restraining," or, as it is greatly miscalled, *"tranquilizing chair."* I have seen this actually in use only in the Philadelphia Alms-house. They are to be found in the Frankford Asylum, but it is believed, and hoped, have fallen into deserved disuse and condemnation.

FRANKLIN COUNTY JAIL is a large brick structure, covering a considerable extent of ground, including both wings and the exercise enclosures. The cost of this prison was thirty thousand dollars. The occupied apartments, I found clean and exceedingly well ventilated. The prisoners have no employment, except to cook their own meals and wash their clothes. They receive an allowance of one and a quarter pounds of bread per day, and a pound of meat. There were seven prisoners early in August. As usual, all ages, colours, and degrees of offenders are associated ; but the women in this jail, are in a separate portion of the building. Here is no religious instruction ; but the sheriff sometimes lends books and newspapers to those who can read. The jail yard is surrounded by a wall about twenty feet high, built of stone. A pump of excellent water affords the means of thorough cleanliness. The cook room is about sixteen feet square. The prisoners sleep, as is common in a majority of the jails, *on the floor*, a custom which, for cleanliness-sake, should be speedily done away. Each is furnished with a straw bed and blanket. It is a singular fact, that one of these prisoners was born in the county jail. The ill-disposed mother either educated him to vice and misdeeds, or left him exposed to associates, whose example he was quick to imitate. He has but little sensibility to crime or its consequences. Imprisonment has no terrors or hardships for such as he. In jail, he rejoins familiar companions, whose tastes and habits are like his own. Here, supported without labor, and engaged in re-hearsing to each other the exploits of which it is their delight to boast ; they delineate, in glowing colors, every unruly and desperate enterprize. These, together with games within, or athletic sports in the yard, constitute a life not burthened with trials, and under the feeble restraints of which, they qualify themselves anew for evil deeds. In this wise are educated, at the public cost, in county jails, the lawless depredators upon society !

The FRANKLIN COUNTY POOR-HOUSE, near *Chambersburg*, contains on an average, about one hundred paupers. There were eighty the first week in August. There is no school, and *no provision* made for the instruction of the children. There is preaching every other Sunday. The farm, contains one hundred and eighty-eight acres, and is productive. The out-buildings are numerous and commodious. The sup-ply of water from springs and running streams, is ample and unfailing. Such of the inmates as are able, assist at the farm and household labor ; but it was evident that here more competent help was needed, especially within doors. The mistress had alto-gether too much care. The main-building is ninety feet by fifty. It is divided into rooms of good size, pretty well ventilated, clean and in order. All are comfortably furnished, especially with beds and bed-clothing ; but this is a creditable distinction of nearly every poor-house in Pennsylvania, including also general cleanliness. A rough-cast building across the yard, of good and convenient size, is appropriated to the colored people. The hospital, on the opposite side of the main building, is seventy-five feet by thirty-two. The rooms are about nine feet square. The arrangements here are incomplete and not convenient. The only exercise-ground for such of the insane as are not allowed to range the premises, is a small yard, about thirty-five feet by thirty-four, surrounded with a high stone wall. Here is no description of shade or shelter. Nothing worse could be conceived or planned, if the idea of increasing the comfort of these poor creatures was embraced in it.

Beside idiots and epileptics, there were fourteen insane, who require constant care, and under the arrangements which exist here, this is a most arduous task. I found one man chained, for his own safety and that of others, in one of the rooms of the hospital. He was not at that time much excited, but liable to furious paroxysms.— The history was a sad one, but has many parallels. One insane woman was chained near a fire-place, into which she has a fondness for creeping, and there remains much of the time. There was straw in a box near by, where she could sleep !

Some cells, formerly appropriated for the insane, and in every respect unfit to be occupied, are now chiefly disused. I could not learn with any probable accuracy, the number of insane and epileptics in the county; but the poor-house contains more than enough of this class of sufferers to afford substantial reasons for providing speedily a more appropriate asylum !

Bedford County Jail at *Bedford*, is a brick building, containing five rooms of good size, which need white-washing ; there is a good exercise-yard, surrounded by a brick wall, twenty feet high. *through* which the prisoners, at some *leisure times*, have once or twice escaped. The law requires the jailor to furnish one pound of bread per day, and as much water as they want; but the present officer gives them three meals per day, and meat at two of them—the family doing the cooking and also the washing. No moral or religious instruction is given at the jail; but the sheriff lends bibles and books of his own. At the time of my visit there were no prisoners, the last having taken the keys, which were inadvertently hung within their reach, and set themselves at liberty.

Bedford County Poor-house has been established less than three years; it has a farm of six hundred and sixty-six acres, only a small part of which is under cultivation. The superintendent's house is built of brick, and is comfortable and commodious. In it is the kitchen and eating-room for the paupers, who live in a house some hundred yards distant. This very inconvenient and bad arrangement ought to be changed without loss of time. The poor-house proper, is a rough-cast building, two stories high, sixty-five feet by twenty-eight—it is not well planned, and secures neither separation nor classification. There were thirty-three inmates, one idiotic, some sick, and no person residing in the house to superintend or nurse them. There is no provision for the insane, though one woman had been kept here for a time. The experiment was very unsatisfactory to all parties, and the husband concluded to take home the mother of his children, "and try to get along by managing somehow." Of the insane in the county at large, I could learn but little, and nothing certain in regard to numbers. Probably there are not more than thirty who are insane and idiotic.

The poor-house was not clean, and not well furnished. It is not good economy to purchase second-hand furniture for poor-house establishments, even if it was best on other accounts. Much allowance must be made for what is defective in this institution, from the fact of its recent establishment, and the consequent inexperience of those who are concerned in directing and conducting it; time and care may remedy these defects. The house is not visited for imparting religious instruction; no school at present is needed ; the medical attendance is good.

Somerset County Jail, at *Somerset*, is an old stone building; I found it clean, and the prisoners decently clothed. Here were three insane men; all were in the exercise-yard; one was heavily chained. One had been in the jail six years, another one year, and the third eleven months. The mother of one had sent him by the stage driver, some fruit; this he appeared to care less for than to go to his mother. "I must go, I must go," he continually repeated. "I can't stay, I must go, I must go." In justice to the jailor and his wife, I must say that these insane men were taken

2

care of kindly, and, as far as they knew how, and had the means, faithfully. The difficult and often hazardous task was not neglected at the expense of the sufferers. But here was no form of treatment to advance recovery and mitigate paroxysms. The jail rooms were all open, affording access to the exercise-ground. In one apartment I found a man and woman; they had been tried for adultery, were found guilty, and sentenced to the county jail—one for six months, the other period I do not recollect. What moral benefit was derived by either the prisoners or the community by this, neither separate nor solitary confinement, I leave others to determine; but I think that a law prohibiting indiscriminate association of the male and female prisoners cannot be too soon promulgated and enforced.

There is no poor-house in Somerset county, but those who are incapable of self-support, are distributed in the towns, amongst those persons who agree to take them at the lowest rate. In some instances, I learned that they fared well; in many others, neglects and suffering, especially with the aged and helpless, were of frequent occurrence. Humanity and economy unite to recommend the establishment of well-planned and well-regulated poor-houses, generally. Except in a densely populous county, county-houses are much to be preferred to town-houses.

I learned from the commissioners' office in Somerset, that in 1840, the estimated number of idiots, epileptics, and insane, in this county, was seventy-six. I heard of a good many recent cases, and was told that it was probable the present number was not less than one hundred. After all, this is somewhat conjectural. A portion of these are supported by the towns, but the largest part by their friends, and often under circumstances of great trial and affliction. Some are met wandering about the country, owing their subsistence to the charity of those at whose houses they casually stop. The needed meal is cheerfully bestowed, and the torn and tattered garment of the poor wayfarer is often replaced by one that is whole and clean. I am persuaded that no observing person can travel over this state, throughout its length and breadth, and not be inspired with increasing respect for the social virtues of the people. I could detail numerous touching examples which have fallen immediately under my own notice, of a kindly care for the sick and suffering; for poor persons removing from one place to seek, perhaps, a more advantageous situation for work; of wandering, neglected, crazy men and women—the last no uncommon sight—and of little orphan children, received and cherished with a liberal and kind spirit:—not always do the inhabitants give of their abundance, but of their penury, they share with those who have less.

Near Stoystown may be found a young woman violently, I fear irrecoverably, insane. The case is not of recent origin. The parents are poor—and under most painful circumstances, amidst many difficulties, they manage to take care of her at home. For a time, worn out by her violence and destructive propensities, they allowed her to range the county. Often she was exposed, without clothes, and pinched with hunger. Those who found her thus, would bestow a garment, and give necessary food for that day; but the poor demented creature might be seen the next, unclothed and hungry. At this time the father receives aid from the town; but it is for such cases as this poor girl exemplifies, that hospitals are peculiarly needed. How can a family of children, as in this case, be properly managed, when continually witnessing the vagaries and improprieties of the insane girl ; and what is yet worse, of listening to demoralizing language. Many citizens in Somerset county expressed, very earnestly, their desire for the speedy establishment of a State Hospital.

WESTMORELAND COUNTY JAIL, at *Greensburg*, is built of stone, and is tolerably commodious, but very insecure, the safe keeping of the prisoners depending more on the vigilance of the jailor, than the strength of the prison. The rooms were clean, could be well ventilated, and were furnished with cot-bedsteads, clean blankets, and decent benches or chairs. At the time of my visit there were but two prisoners, one, an insane man, very difficult of control, and very dangerous and violent at times. He was altogether unmanageable at home, and public and private safety made it a duty, in default of a hospital, to place him in the jail.

WESTMORELAND COUNTY has no poor-house; the poor are distributed where they can be most cheaply supported. The number of the insane could not be satisfactorily ascertained. I heard of various suffering cases of crazy persons, and of idiots and epileptics, through medical practitioners. I encountered one on my way from Greensburg, who was diligently employed in destroying a hay-stack. There were only females about the house, and as these could not control him, he was necessarily suffered to finish his mischievous work.

I regret that I cannot refer to the JAIL OF FAYETTE COUNTY, in *Uniontown*, in other than terms of unqualified censure. The building is old, ill-constructed, and out of repair. This, comparatively, is of little consequence. It was dirty, ill-kept, and neglected. A wall, nearly twenty-five feet high, plastered within, surrounded the exercise-yard. There were no criminal prisoners : the only occupants of the jail apartments, when I was there in August, were two madmen, in chains; if the rats, of which I heard some intimation, are not included in the category. The men were chained and in separate rooms, or one in a passage and the other in a room, apart for their mutual safety. I did not see their food, and know nothing of its quantity or quality. I saw no bedstead, nor any furniture. The man in the outer room, or passage, was somewhat cleaner than the other, but I must be excused from entering upon special details; the other was covered with soot, and coal-dust, and dirt, and was extended upon the floor, clanking his chains, and beating his head, shouting and singing. Here fell no ray of comfort, hope, or consolation. One of these men is decidedly homicidal, and, with the exception of a short interval, has been, I was informed, in prison *fifteen* years. On one occasion; becoming violently excited at seeing an intoxicated man put into his room, and possibly provoked by him, for no one knows how it was, he fell upon and murdered him in the most shocking manner. When the keeper came to visit his prisoners, a horrible spectacle presented itself—the murdered drunkard, mangled and lifeless : the madman exulting in the deed and covered with the blood of his victim ! He also when at large burned a building.

The other man has been insane about seven years. Both are dangerous, and are subject to paroxysms of fury. Every person must comprehend something of the difficulties of taking care of the insane ; but all know, likewise, that humane efforts can spare them much degradation and suffering, even in a prison.

The POOR-HOUSE OF FAYETTE COUNTY is a mile or two from *Uniontown*. I learned that much improvement had been made in the domestic arrangements within a few years. The superintendent and his family appeared much interested, and desirous of performing their duty; but the building is not well planned, and prevents such classification and suitable separation as the comfort of the inmates and propriety require. The house is too small for the numbers it receives. In August there were seventy-two inmates, and of these rather more than one-eighth were foreigners. The number of men and women were nearly equal; there were but four children, of course no school. Of late no religious services, and rarely visited for the purpose of moral influence. Here were two deaf and dumb, four blind, and an uncommonly large proportion of the inmates of infirm mind, simple, idiotic, and epileptic. Four were violently insane, requiring chains. No suitable apartment in the establishment for these, even allowing the poor-house to be a suitable place. Something should be done at once to enable the superintendent to carry out more properly the objects of the institution. A large, well-ventilated, well-furnished building seems imperatively necessary for a hospital for the sick, and the most infirm of the old people. At all events. such additions should be made that it may not be regarded as necessary to place numbers of aged, sick, men and women together in confined, crowded lodging-rooms! Considering all the difficulties of managing such an establishment, the wonder is that it appeared so well, and this could have been only through a very diligent care on the part of the mistress of the house.

GREENE COUNTY JAIL, at *Waynesburg*, is constructed of stone, and is very strongly built; it is small, but larger than the wants of the county make necessary. It is entirely unenclosed, the doors were all open; there were no prisoners; and I made my way towards it through a rank growth of stramonium and tall weeds, which sufficiently indicated the infrequent use of the building. The path was quite obliterated.

In this county is no poor-house—the poor are placed with those who will take them at the lowest cost. The ascertained number of idiots, epileptics, and insane in the county, is from fifty-five to sixty, of which the largest part are idiots and imbeciles. Two cases of cruel abuse of an insane man and an epileptic youth were related to me by a practising physician. Some time since, an insane man was committed to the jail on a criminal charge. Another is often made intoxicated at the taverns, to afford sport to the idle and vicious. Another, still, who has been insane six years, the physician assured me he believed would have been perfectly cured if he could have had the benefit of hospital treatment. And so it is, that for want of a liberal, well-conducted institution, every year increases the class of incurables, and deprives the state of useful citizens, and families of comfort and the means of support.

WASHINGTON COUNTY JAIL, at *Washington*, is a large stone building, enclosed by a high stone wall, including an exercise-yard, in which I found congregated the old and the young, black and white, men and women, and babies. And beside these, charged with petty and with criminal offences, an insane man, whose fate it was to be associated with thieves and felons, "for he was crazy and not safe to be at large." He had property, the interest of which paid his expenses here, but was insufficient to meet hospital charges. The construction of this jail is not such as to permit much classification. The sheriff appeared quite sensible of the disadvantages to which the place was subject, and said " that having but one exercise-ground, of course, they must all be together, *in the cells and out,* till lock-up hours." The grand jury, in 1842, called public attention to this subject, representing "the propriety of so remodelling the jail-yard, and the jail, that the female prisoners may be kept entirely separate from the males." This, which was meeting but half the evil, was again adverted to in 1843, but it was added, that " having visited the jail, they found the prisoners well-cared for, and the rooms furnished with bibles, in accordance with recommendation." We fear the bibles have been studied to little profit, while so many adverse circumstances were allowed to warp the mind, and tempt to misconduct. The last presentation of the jury on this abuse, was in August, 1844, and still nothing was said upon the subject of classification and employment. I found the jail cleanly swept and aired, and some of the rooms very clean. The prisoners were amusing themselves with games, talking, story-telling, and such like modes of passing time and cultivating the morals.

The COUNTY ALMS-HOUSE is several miles from *Washington.* It is a large brick building, founded about twelve years since. Attached, is a valuable farm, of nearly one hundred and seventy five acres. This, I understand, was managed to the entire satisfaction of the county officers. The house is not planned conveniently for the classification of the occupants. A thorough cleansing was in progress, and such of the inmates as were able, were variously and industriously employed. There were seventy paupers, eight of which were children. *Seven* were insane. A considerable number idiotic, and others epileptic and imbecile. There is no school, and preaching is heard about once a month. The physician is rarely called ; it having been decided that " except in violent cases," the master of the house, who is an excellent farmer and blacksmith, should add to his various duties and professions, that of medical practitioner. There were four insane females, in close confinement, in August. One in a small building, remote from the house, in a field. She was placed there on account of being " exceedingly noisy, screaming and shouting, so that nobody could rest !" A lame man, who I understood to be her husband, had it in charge to take her food to her. The room she was in, was clean; she was also cleanly and comfortably dressed, and at this time, also quiet. In the large yard, common to all the inmates of the establishment, was a small building, consisting of a single room, perhaps twelve by fourteen feet. I did not measure it. At one end was a door. At the opposite, a sashed window, containing twelve panes of glass, I think. On one side, were two windows of the same size. It being a hot day, two were opened, fronting the most frequented part of the house and yard. I looked in, as requested, and saw first, a young woman apparently demented, standing upon a sack of straw. At first, I thought there was no other occupant ; but a little to the right, somewhat concealed from view, as I was at first placed, I discovered a woman of middle age, seated on some straw in a packing-box—and in a state of entire nudity. On the opposite side of the room, stood a similar box, which at first, I supposed to be empty ; but the sound of voices, roused a female. She lay coiled up. I cannot imagine how she could have contracted herself into so small a space. Some straw, too, was in this box, and excepting that, she had neither clothing nor covering of any sort or description. Nor was there any in the room of any kind. Wholly unconscious of exposure, these shamefully neglected maniacs roved about the room, seeming to shrink, yet too much lost to comprehend, into what bitter degradation they had fallen, and to what insensible guardians they were consigned. The boxes into which, now and then, they leaped, cowering down amidst the straw, were such as are seen at almost every door of an English goods store. They were of rough board, about three feet long, by two and a half wide, and deep. And this was here, here in Washington county, where, in 1839, it was officially announced, " that the insane of this county *are so well provided for,* that a state hospital would be useless ;" and further, " the county has it in contemplation to fit up a building, already erected, for the crazy poor." The building has been fitted up it appears, and *furnished,* but exactly how long occupied, I considered it of little use to ascertain ; but was told in general terms, that the unfortunate women referred to, had been in no better condition for several years.

That the intolerable grossness and barbarity of this personal exposure, was neither transient nor accidental, I am assured by the concession of persons on the premises, and by gentlemen who had visited the poor-house by chance, before I came to Washington. I am sorry to employ strong expressions ; I am sorry to censure any persons ; but for this monstrous outrage on decency and morals, I can find neither palliation nor apology. What shall we say ? Here are boxes three feet long, indeed,—a handful of straw thrown in. This the retreat, this the bed, without covering of any kind ; not even the fragment of a rag, or a torn blanket, or the very refuse of cast-off pauper garments to gather about the shrinking form—the windows not shaded even, from the view of seventy or a hundred men, women and children, passing and repassing the room continually. Visitors coming and going ; overseers of the poor making official visits ; religious teachers at intervals ; yet not one making it his or her business to bring about a less intolerable state of things. But one must turn from this subject— rather let those ponder on it, on whom depends the establishment of an institution that shall spare such scenes, and rescue from such barbarisms. I have but to add, that the week following my visit, the grand jury made presentment to the court, then in session, that these facts communicated to that official body, were true: "And that we will not urge further reasons than the facts referred to, as in their opinion, they are sufficient to induce every person to come to the same opinion;" "and they do most earnestly recommend," &c. &c. I have not learned if the representations and recommendations made last August, have taken practical effect; nor have I used any pains to learn the numbers or condition of the insane in the county at large. If the directors of the county-house can have neither desired nor executed more salutary plans for the physical and mental treatment of the insane, than those I witnessed, after *twelve* year's trial, I cannot suppose so rapid progress has been made, as to render future hospital-care unneeded, or the public interference and protection uncalled for, or untimely.

ALLEGHENY COUNTY JAIL, at *Pittsburg,* is a handsome and costly structure, built of stone, and stands immediately adjacent to, and connected with, the court-house. Brought into such proximity to the *halls of justice,* it was but reasonable to look for corresponding advantages.

This jail combines all the faults and abuses of the worst county prisons in this state, or in the United States. Hoping to find something redeeming in its earlier discipline and government, I deliberately and patiently entered upon investigation, but the nature of the revelations these inquiries brought to light, obliged me to relinquish the work to those whose more immediate duty it is to bring about a reformation. The prison was built in view of the separate imprisonment, classification, and employment of offenders; instead of which, I found transgressors of all ages, colours, sexes and degrees, promiscuously associated : little boys listening greedily to gray-headed, time and crime-hardened convicts; the youthful transgressor learning new lessons of iniquity, from those whose vices only kept pace with their crimes; here the sick were unattend-ed, the ignorant untaught, the repentant (if any) unencouraged, and the insane forgotten. The area, stairs, and passages were unscrubbed and unswept; the cells and beds yet worse, uncleansed; and some of them perfectly intolerable through foul air and negli-gence. If it had been the deliberate purpose of the citizens of Allegheny county to establish a school for the inculcation of vice, and obliteration of every virtue, I can-not conceive that any means they could have devised, would more certainly have secured these results, than those I found in full operation in the jail last August. On my second visit, things wore a little better outward aspect, so far as the use of the broom, some clean blankets, and somewhat more decently arranged apparel, were con-sidered. This, the work of an hour, was to last but a day : the visit was prepared for. The ample leisure of the prisoners afforded opportunity for various little works of skill and ingenuity for facilitating oral communication, when by night all, or by day a part, should be locked into the cells. The pastime particularly referred to, was cut-ting the doors in pieces, or rather cutting such apertures through them, as in default of clairvoyance assisted vision and promoted a social feeling, by increasing facilities for conversation. I was somewhat struck with the remark of one of the prisoners, a forger, and a man of some education, though he had failed in the use of its advan-tages—"a man who comes here will lose all respect for the law, and for those who administer it; and all respect for the officers and those who appoint them; and he will go out indifferent to every restraint, and it is a chance if he does not believe him-self as good as those who are instrumental in bringing him here." "You may learn here," said another, "every thing that people outside call bad; and you may look long enough for the good, and not find it at last." At one time, there had been religious teaching by preaching on the Sabbath; but a very respectable pious clergyman told me he had relinquished the work from the conviction, that where evil conduct, through want of a good system of discipline so prevailed, it was wholly unavailing to offer occasional instruction. Dauphin County Jail affords a model upon which the Allegheny County Prison can be reformed and remodelled. I know, some of the most intelligent of the citizens of Pittsburg, are earnest to carry out a change, which, if it be not fruit-ful of great good, shall at least not permit such an increase of positive evil. Attention once directed to these monstrous abuses, reformation will be certain to follow in Alle-heny County Jail.

It is a relief to turn from this to other public institutions of Pittsburg : the Orphans' Asylum situated in Allegheny city, is a charity which rescues many unprotected children from early crime, and saves some from the jail. This institution, so creditable to those who support it, and to the good matron who directs it, is well ordered throughout.

The Poor-house of *Pittsburg*, soon to be replaced by a more commodious establishment, is also in Allegheny city. I found it comfortably arranged, and neat. The two insane of the fifteen inmates, were kindly looked after. The entire number of epileptics, insane and idiotic in this county, was computed to be not less than seventy-five, and might be more.

Allegheny County has no poor-house, but the poor in most of the townships are distributed as is customary in other counties.

Of the Western Penitentiary, I shall speak elsewhere; but I cannot refrain from saying here, that it is one of the most excellently governed prisons I have ever visited. I took sufficient time to see all the prisoners, and to learn the whole state of the institution. It is honorable to the county and the state, and creditable to the warden, Major Beckham, to whose judgment and fidelity, its prosperity is mainly to be ascribed. The moral instructor is greatly interested in his work, and diligent in the discharge of his duties. Here, as is universal in the state prisons, are found the insane and imbecile. Some were so when committed, and in others, the disease has been developed in prison.— They are all kindly treated, so far as a prison affords such influences for that class of prisoners; but these never should be left in a prison, much less sent there while laboring under this malady, as I have proved beyond doubt, has been the case in many instances.

It is to be hoped that the jurisprudence of insanity will receive more effectual, and serious consideration than it has hitherto done in this, and the United States generally ; excepting, latterly in New York, more lately still in Massachusetts, and earlier than either, in Louisiana.

Beaver County Jail, at *Beaver*, is built of stone, and has four rooms, two above, and two below ; there is a small yard protected by a wall twenty feet high. The rooms are about eighteen feet by eighteen, and nine feet high. The prison is out of repair, insecure and inconvenient. The prisoners were all together ; a child, the middle aged, and the man of gray hairs. The boy had been committed on a charge of petty larceny, and probably was guilty. When he is enlarged, he will no doubt come upon the community accomplished in the knowledge of vice and crime. Society gives him this education, *at the free school of the county*, and in acknowledgment of the obligation, he will undoubtedly practice what it has taught. The offender against social and civil law, once committed to a jail, and forced upon the society of other offenders, imbibes a taste for more grave transgressions than he has heretofore contemplated. Here are no restraints that check the influence of "corrupt communications;" here is no employment either for the hands or the mind, helping to strengthen better habits and confirm better resolutions ; here is no moral or religious teacher, kindly and seriously, impressing "line upon line, and precept upon precept;" here is no partition, separating the hardy and mature criminal, from him who has but newly yielded to temptation; here, in short, society seems deliberately to abandon its victim, giving him over to every evil work. I believe no better work can be done in our country than those may accomplish who undertake the establishment of a new, and more just jail system. I am not aware that there are above six disciplined *jails* in the United States ; and I do know that most of them have trained many a convict for the penitentiaries. Whether is it better to prevent disease, or leave it to be not only sure in its attacks, but deadly in its consequences?

BEAVER COUNTY has no poor-house. The poor are supported by the several towns, in families where they can be boarded at the lowest cost. Many sad accounts of the neglects and privations to which this system gives rise, reached me from undoubted sources. Many of the more reflecting and benevolent citizens in Beaver county, are earnest to bring about an effectual change, by establishing a county-house. The question has been discussed for some time, but in August no results had been reached of a definite character.

The intelligent medical men are all in favor of it; this follows of course, as their profession makes them acquainted with injuries and aggressions, which often fail to reach the ear of those whose duty it would be to prevent their repetition. A carefully planned, well-managed county poor-house, produces great benefits; while the want of one often greatly aggravates the misfortunes and miseries of the poor and the infirm.

BUTLER COUNTY JAIL, at *Butler*, is old and out of repair, but well-ordered. The rooms were decently furnished; the prisoners decently clean, but all associated, and without employment. Here was one insane man, who was often violent and dangerous.

BUTLER COUNTY has no poor-house. The poor are supported as in Beaver: distributed at the lowest rates. I heard of several cases of epileptics and insane, through a medical practitioner; but could not learn with any probable correctness, the whole number in the county.

MERCER COUNTY JAIL is in *Mercer*. It is a well built structure of stone, said to be well kept at present. Here was an insane man, who had been a long time in confinement and chained. "At times he is dreadful noisy, and a sight of trouble," said my informant; "but we manage to get on pretty smoothly sometimes."

MERCER COUNTY has no poor-house. So far as I could ascertain, there are from thirty to forty idiots and insane. This is probably less than the actual number. "Some of these wretches suffer horribly, but who is to help it?" was the expression of a tax-paying citizen, who gave me some information respecting these and the other poor. "We need a poor-house, and a place for the unruly crazy ones, and the mischievous idiots. They don't often get care fit for the brutes, unless they chance to have some humane relation."

CRAWFORD COUNTY JAIL, at *Meadville*, is very strongly built of timber, and though exteriorly not wearing a very finished aspect, was within, in a creditable condition; being clean and decent. The food is good, well prepared, and more than sufficient, and supplied from the table of the family who keep the prison. Here were two prisoners, a woman in a room by herself, and an insane man, whose variable and often violent state, made it dangerous to allow him liberty, unless, as at hospitals, he could be attended by some person understanding how to manage him. He was kept clean, though quite as difficult a case as that of the insane men in Fayette County Jail.

In CRAWFORD COUNTY is no poor-house. The number of paupers is small. I heard of several painful cases of idiocy and epilepsy. The case of an idiot boy was described as claiming commiseration. He was often neglected and abused, pursued and tormented by idle boys, and had more than once suffered personal injury. But such events are of frequent occurrence in many places. The vagrant insane and idiots are oftener teazed by the thoughtless and vicious, than sympathized with. It is but a few weeks since, an insane man, driven to frenzy by his street-tormentors, threw a stone at random, which killed a child.

ERIE COUNTY JAIL, at *Erie*, is an ill-planned brick building, containing a number of cell-rooms, floored with stone. The exercise-yard is of sufficient size, and surrounded by a lofty brick wall; over which, however, the prisoners when not watched, contrive by mutual aid to effect escapes. The prison contained, in September, nine prisoners, in a dirty, disorderly condition, altogether, and entirely disgusting. The beds, walls, floors, windows, passages, one and the whole, appeared capable of being thoroughly purified only by the element of fire. The air was intolerably bad. Notwithstanding the hot weather, a large fire was burning in a stove, as they said, "to dry up the damp." This was well enough, provided the doors and windows had been thrown wide, but closed as they were, it made what was bad yet worse. It is seldom one will find a more discreditable prison. The sick were neglected, and all left to their own devices. Here was no moral or religious instruction; no employment, no books; only uncontrolled pernicious intercourse. One of the prisoners was said to be insane; it was a more than doubtful case. It is hoped some wholesome reforms have changed the jail in Erie, before this time.

ERIE COUNTY POOR-HOUSE, a few miles out of town, is not well situated, nor planned to secure the classification of the inmates; but considering the many difficulties always to be overcome in new establishments, and which experience only can effectually meet, so far as the superintendent may be considered responsible, the house is well directed; but the cares are very arduous, and the rooms too much crowded. The buildings are not large enough for the numbers to be received, and there are no suitable apartments for the sick. I do not doubt these deficiencies will be remedied. A small wooden building in the yard, is divided into six cells for the insane, each measuring nearly five feet by nine, and about eight high. In some was a quantity of straw, and I think, bunks. They were very imperfectly lighted, not ventilated, and I cannot think that they can be either safely or sufficiently warmed in winter. It is to be hoped it will not be found necessary to occupy these poor cells; I am sure they are quite unfit for any permanent use. There were forty-eight poor in this establishment in September, ten of which were children. Here were five insane, four epileptics and four idiots, several of them wholly incapable of self-care, not being able even to feed themselves. Estimated number of insane in the county, about forty. Here is no school for the children, and religious instruction as opportunity permitted. Benevolent persons who have leisure, will find a field for usefulness at the Erie poor-house. The burthensome cares of the superintendents, must make attention to instructing the children impossible.

WARREN COUNTY JAIL, at *Warren*, is built of stone, is clean and in thorough repair; it is creditable to those who have charge of it. There was no prisoner in September, but I understand that an insane woman has since been committed for safe-keeping.

Provisions are supplied from the table of the keeper, when there are prisoners. The exercise-yard is securely enclosed.

WARREN COUNTY has no poor-house, and not many poor entirely dependent on the public care; yet these sometimes are subject to neglect in sickness, and a sad sense of homelessness, as year by year, they are transferred from place to place, received on such terms as at the very outset almost assures much discomfort and privation. I heard of not many insane in this county. One female leads a life of exposure, often escaping from those who have taken the responsibility of caring for her. For weeks she frequents a desolate, deserted log house on the mountain, and when urged by the cravings of hunger, wanders to some farm house, where her appetite is appeased, and then disappears, returning only when driven by the same necessity. "She suffers a sight in this way," said my informant; "people hate to have her live so, but some are afraid of her, and some don't care."

VENANGO COUNTY JAIL, at *Franklin*, is constructed of stone, and large enough for county purposes, and ill-contrived enough, to include every inconvenience in occupying it. There were no prisoners in September. The rooms had been swept the day I was there; they needed repairs and whitewashing, and if ever used some decent description of straw-beds and blankets; the remnants of what time and service had destroyed, were scattered about. It was expected, that a man in a state of violent insanity, would be sent there in a day or two, for safe-keeping. It was not easy to conceive that he would be comfortable, especially, if not easily managed. An insane person, in the vicinity, lately committed suicide. It was thought, if the patient could have had early remedial treatment, a cure would have followed. I heard of several interesting cases, through the physicians, whose practice often brings them acquainted with those maladies, and who hold but one opinion respecting the insane—the great importance of placing them in hospitals.

FRANKLIN COUNTY has no poor-house; the poor are placed out at the lowest rates, in families who are willing to receive them for a trifling compensation. This county has but few paupers.

CLARION COUNTY JAIL, at *Clarion*, is a large new building, not well planned or securely constructed. There was, in September, but one prisoner, and he was under sentence to the Western Penitentiary, for a second offence of petty larceny. The keeper here, understood remarkably, the duties of his office, and one could not but wish that his abilities might have a wider sphere of action. In short, that he might have the conduct of some one of the ill-ordered prisons which have been referred to.

In CLARION COUNTY is no poor-house; but few paupers, and few insane.

JEFFERSON COUNTY JAIL, at *Brookville*, is poorly built of stone, and on an inconvenient plan. There were two prisoners in September, charged with murder in the first degree, of which, they were found guilty, but the sheriff held them in such regard, that they frequently, if not always took their meals at his own table. It was allowed to be "a misfortune they had come to, but he thought a heap of them." There is no poor-house in this county, and but few paupers, and few insane. These, so far as I could learn, were kindly cared for.

ARMSTRONG COUNTY JAIL, at *Kittanning*, is not in a very good condition. I saw there, four prisoners in September. One insane, comfortable in apparel and general condition. Food for the prisoners was sufficient, and of good quality.

There is no poor-house in this county, and but few paupers, idiots, and insane.

INDIANA COUNTY JAIL, at *Indiana*, is built of stone, is inconvenient and ill-finished. There were no prisoners in September. It was clean; and when occupied, well attended to, so far as the food and clothing of the prisoners was concerned. Here is no county poor-house. The paupers, of all conditions, are "placed out to those who bid for them lowest." There are thirty ascertained cases of insanity and idiocy. These receive no special medical care or supervision. Several are capable of being employed; but those who have charge of them, are unskilful in directing their labor according to their strength and ability. A case was lately related to me by a medical man, of an insane person who had been very highly excited, and was chained and kept in a cell. After a time, the paroxysm subsided; but the rigid confinement, want of air, and a constrained position, had essentially weakened the muscular fibre. In short, he was pale, emaciated, and feeble, but eager to be let out. The keeper promised this, if he would work; and eager for enlargement, he readily promised to do so. He was accordingly removed from the cell, and directed to load a team with stone. He went to work with alacrity, but soon was exhausted and asked to rest. This was refused, and the command of "work or back to your cell," proved a sufficient incentive and terror, to urge him to the utmost through the day. One day more in feebleness, and with blistered and lacerated hands, he pursued the unequal task, then his strength altogether failed, and to the cell he was remanded; the master saying to him, he "was lazy and must pay for it." After this, the patient's faculties rapidly gave way, and he who might, with judicious care and prudent direction, have recovered reason and ability for a life of useful labor, is now a confirmed idiot. Employment is highly important and useful for the insane; but it is not less important that this should be assigned with judgment, proportioning the task to the physical strength and mental capacity. I was told in a county poor-house, that they did not wish to have their "crazy people carried to a hospital, for they were useful in performing for infirm and disabled persons, offices that were particularly disagreeable, and which the sane paupers could not be made to do!" "We can cure them well enough ourselves, if they will get well, and we need their labor!"

CAMBRIA COUNTY JAIL, at *Ebensburg*, is a miserable building, insecure, and not clean or comfortable as I saw it, so far as necessary furnishing and convenient arrangements were considered. One room was occupied by those notorious murderers, the Flanagans, and I confess I could not see much to impede their escape whenever it should please them to go. An insane man occupied a room adjacent to, and in rear of theirs, affording another example of the want of a suitable asylum. I do not doubt, that under fit direction, he is fully able to earn his own support.

This county has no poor-house; the poor are "let out" to those who are willing to accept a trifling compensation for their board. I heard of several cases of much suffering and neglect of the insane. One man, some miles from Ebensburg, it was stated, was "shut up in a very small room, rarely made clean, badly fed, and miserable beyond what one would easily credit, who is not accustomed to scenes of suffering."

HUNTINGDON COUNTY JAIL, at *Huntingdon*, needed white-wash, scrubbing, and above all, ventilation. There were two prisoners who occupied the same room, without employment and without moral influences. One was said to be insane; I had reason to doubt this; there might have been a degree of eccentricity, united with moral perversion, but the case was by no means clear.

HUNTINGDON COUNTY has no poor-house; but the poor are boarded with those who name the lowest receivable price. From the best information received, the idiots, epileptics, and insane, in this county, may be estimated at about sixty. The desire for a State Hospital was strongly expressed by intelligent citizens.

I seldom refer to cases existing in private families, and never by name; but there is one in Huntingdon county, so well known, and so publicly exposed, that I feel a description of his condition, as given to me by a citizen, will be in place here, and serve to illustrate the fact that there are terrible sufferings, and miseries which call for speedy relief. On the banks of the canal, near the Juniata, stands a farm house, to which the cooks of the canal boats are accustomed to resort for supplies of milk, butter, &c. Immediately adjacent to the house is a small shanty, constructed of boards placed obliquely against each other. In this wretched hovel is a man, whose blanched hair indicates advancing years; not clad sufficiently for the purposes of decency; "fed like the hogs, and living worse; in filth, and not half covered: the decaying wet straw upon the ground, only increases the offensiveness of the place." In the rains of summer, and the frosts of winter, he is alike exposed to the influence of the elements. There is no fire of course. There is no room for such a luxury as a fireplace or stove! And there you may see him now, affording a spectacle so miserable and revolting, that you are thankful to retreat from a scene you have no authority to amend. It is but a few days since nineteen cases, from sources of unquestionable authority, have been communicated to me: some accompanied with solicitations to interpose in behalf of these poor maniacs, whose sufferings almost transcend belief. These are in private families, chiefly of humble circumstances; and most of all, those who are connected with them utterly perplexed by the trials of their lot, and ignorant how, or in what manner, to manage the refractory and violent mad-men. These all need care and protection in a Lunatic Asylum. They cannot elsewhere be brought into decent conditions, or rendered in any sort as comfortable as the lowest of the brute creation.

MIFFLIN COUNTY JAIL, at *Lewistown*, was ill-arranged; dirty beds on a dirty floor, walls needing white-wash, the rooms, the admission of pure air; and the prisoners, of which there were several, the free application of soap and water.

This county has no poor-house. The poor are distributed as cheapness and convenience determine. For the insane, idiots, and epileptics, there is no appropriate provision; they have no medical attendance, and 1 heard of no recoveries amongst the poor. Many I did not see; those who described them, concurred in the opinion that "something was needed for their help, and they thought well of a State Hospital."

JUNIATA COUNTY JAIL, at *Mifflintown*, contained no prisoners; most of the rooms were occupied as a saddlery, being converted, "till further demand for the county," into work-shops and store-rooms. Not long since an insane woman was shut up here. She was subject to the most furious and alarming bursts of passion, and the jailor's wife declared it her belief that she "was more ugly than crazy;" but other testimony, from competent judges, settled the fact of her insanity, and of the danger of her being at large. At this time (September) she was wandering "somewhere over the country," having escaped from the restraints of the prison. From the best information I could collect, one may estimate the number of idiots and insane in Juniata county at about thirty-five; most of them are incapable of employment. There is no poor-house in this county; the poor are distributed according to the prevailing usage where there is no county institution.

CENTRE COUNTY JAIL, at *Bellefonte*, contained no prisoners in September. That portion of the building which was occupied by the sheriff's family was in complete order, and well arranged. The jail rooms were much out of repair, and in all respects unfit for use till cleansed in every part. The condition was exceedingly discreditable to whoever had charge to maintain the place in decent order. One room was convert-ed into a pigeon-house, and seemed also to be shared with the rats. Fortunately the county has little use for the jail, and this is yet more fortunate for prisoners. I regret to add, that since I was at Bellefonte, I am informed a young man, recently become insane, is incarcerated and chained in this prison, which, I am sure, could afford no apartment tolerably decent for any living creature. Cases daily are related to me, which seem even more strongly than most I have recorded, to urge the establishment of a Lunatic Asylum and Hospital.

CENTRE COUNTY has no poor-house. Some details of suffering reached me. The number of insane poor is computed at forty, including the idiotic cases. I understand many indigent families receive liberal aid from the more prosperous citizens, especially, near Bellefonte; but, much doubt was expressed respecting the general condition of the aged poor and sick through the county at large.

CLEARFIELD COUNTY JAIL, at *Clearfield*, is remarkably well built, in complete order, and had no prisoners at the season of my visit.

In this county is no poor-house, and but few paupers. So far as ascertained, the idiots and insane are fourteen, these are chiefly with their friends; they have no special attendance. I could hear of no recoveries: the physicians related a number of cases where at one time they tried to induce the friends to adopt a remedial treatment; but, at home they could not carry this out, or thought they could not, and the patients are now considered past cure.

ELK COUNTY, at present has no jail, no poor-house, and but few paupers; could earn nothing of the insane—doubt if there are any.

CLINTON COUNTY JAIL, at *Lock Haven*, is a small building in temporary use for detaining prisoners. The two rooms were in decent order.

In this county, is no poor-house, and not many paupers. Several cases of idiocy and insanity. A physician remarked that every year increased the number of incurables, "through want of seasonable and necessary care."

LYCOMING COUNTY JAIL, at *Williamsport*, is constructed of stone, is well built, and in good order. In this county is no poor-house. The estimated number of insane is above seventy. The paupers are set off yearly to those "who bid cheapest."— "Some are well dealt by, and others suffer great hardships."

TIOGA COUNTY JAIL, at *Wellsborough*, is substantially built, in rear of and beneath the court rooms. The rooms are inconveniently constructed, being more suited for the secure detention of offenders, than most county prisons, but ill-devised in many respects. Here is no enclosed exercise-yard, and, but for special care on the part of the jailor, prisoners subject to long detention, would, from dampness of the cells, suffer in health.

TIOGA COUNTY has no poor-house; but few paupers, few idiots, and few insane. I saw but two of the latter class, who were subjects for hospital care.

BRADFORD COUNTY JAIL, at *Towanda*, is an old, inconvenient building, gone much out of repair. Here were three prisoners in October. My visit was made in the morning before breakfast. I found the prisoners, who had already arranged the apartment, and were themselves clean and neat, reading and talking in a quiet manner. I understood, that the food was well supplied, three times a day, from the kitchen of the keeper. Insane persons have been kept in the jail—there are none at present.

In this county is no poor-house, the old system is still followed for supporting the poor—"Let out at the lowest rates." The estimated number of insane and idiots is nearly twenty; there is no provision for these adapted to their necessities.

One insane female wanders constantly from Troy, in Bradford county, to Elmira, in New York, and south returning to Williamsport. When her garments fail, she shows the ragged gown, and another is given by some kind-hearted person. She asks food only when hunger compels her to enter the way-side dwelling; and is supposed to lodge sometimes in the woods, sometimes in out-buildings. She is harmless and silent.

COLUMBIA COUNTY JAIL, at *Danville*, had but one prisoner early in October. The jail rooms were in order. In this county is no poor-house. The present mode of disposing of those who become a public cost, is the same as in all the northern and most of the interior counties. Physicians informed me, that the insane suffered much for want of suitable care.

UNION COUNTY JAIL, at *New Berlin*, was vacant of prisoners. It is well built, was clean and suitably arranged. In this county is no poor-house. The poor are supported as in Columbia county. The cost of supporting each individual, was variously estimated at from forty to sixty dollars per annum. Of the insane, a considerable number are under the care of relatives. Their condition varies according to the forms the disease manifests, and the dispositions and ability of those who have them in charge. A physician acquainted me at New Berlin, that within the limits of his own practice, there are now six insane persons, proper subjects for an insane hospital, and he writes "to give you some data. I inform you, that beside myself, there are fifteen practitioners of medicine in the county ; all of whom traverse a considerable territory. *We feel the want of a hospital constantly.*" I heard of about thirty cases of idiotic and demented persons in Union county, but this cannot embrace all of the class, though it may exceed the number strictly needing remedial treatment.

LUZERNE COUNTY JAIL, at *Wilkesbarre*, the last week of October, contained two men and two women prisoners. There are four jail rooms ; two above and two below. Those on the first floor are arched. All require whitewash, and are insufficiently ventilated. The building is of stone, and the exercise-yard enclosed by a high wall. The construction of the prison, is such as to subvert discipline. The men and women, at this time, were in separate parts of the building, but could converse at will. The poor of this county are supported in the several townships, in those families who take them on terms most favorable to the public interest. The highest estimate of the insane and idiots, of which, the latter is most numerous, is forty-six.

WYOMING COUNTY JAIL, at *Tunkhannock*, is *solidly* constructed, and it was designed not only to be well built, but upon a good plan. Great mistakes have been made, and if it continues to be occupied, it will be found absolutely necessary to make some alterations for the increased admission of light and air. The cells or dungeons, are almost in total darkness. Of these, there are two, about seven feet high, and nearly ten by fifteen. The interior wall is eighteen inches thick. A small aperture in the door, seven by nine inches, admits so much light and air, as can thus find entrance. The grates in the outer wall are nearly two feet by two. The entrance door which communicates with the kitchen has a small aperture opening from the area, and at this, I found the two prisoners amusing themselves with a member of the family. The supply of food is ample ; and it must be owned that the prisoners appeared in high health. But then they were not locked into the dungeons.

In this county is no poor-house, and but few who are wholly dependent on the public for their support. I heard of but two insane.

SUSQUEHANNA COUNTY JAIL, at *Montrose*, is not a very good building. It was tolerably clean, and the food of the prisoners wholesome and sufficient. There were but two prisoners the last of October ; one a boy, who was imprisoned for assault. He was passionate, and had been irritated unreasonably, as he believed. He certainly needed some moral influences here ; some instruction which should help him in future to rule his temper.

In this county is no poor-house. The estimated number of the insane, is about thirty-five ; some of these are supported by their friends, others at the public cost, at the lowest prices. I heard of several very painful examples of severe usage. One, of a man, who, from no brutal impulse, but conviction that it was "the only way to tranquilize crazy people," most severely beat his own wife—whose violent conduct and language created the utmost domestic confusion. We need a State Hospital surely, for such as these.

WAYNE COUNTY JAIL, is at *Honesdale;* it is well built of stone, and contains four centre cells. These cell-rooms are strongly finished, but defectively ventilated, and are not altogether convenient. The prisoners are well fed. There was but one in October. I heard of but few insane in the county. There are no poor-houses, but the poor are distributed through their respective townships.

PIKE COUNTY JAIL, at *Milford,* is out of repair, and not very well constructed. The prisoners were supplied liberally at their meals, when there were any in detention. I found the prison vacant. There is no poor-house in this county, but the poor are supported as in Wayne. The ascertained number of insane is small.

MONROE COUNTY JAIL, at *Stroudsburg,* was out of repair. There was but one prisoner, and he seemed imbecile; they called him "foolish," where he was known. In this county, the poor are supported in the several townships, as in Wayne and Pike. I heard from a physician of extensive practice, that there were several cases of insanity requiring remedial treatment.

CARBON COUNTY JAIL, at *Mauch Chunk,* was entirely unoccupied the last of October. It is not conveniently constructed in any respect, but I understand that hitherto there has not been much occasion to use the prison-rooms.

In this county is no poor-house, but many poor persons. The benevolent inhabitants use much exertion to alleviate the sufferings of the sick and helpless. I heard of several cases of insanity and idiocy in the county, but could not ascertain that these were in particularly suffering conditions, though some were negligently exposed.

NORTHAMPTON COUNTY JAIL, at *Easton,* was vacant of prisoners the first week in November. The apartments are clean, though the prison is not constructed upon a good plan. At present, I have understood, it is well kept; though being subject to the same system as nearly all the jails in the state, it is liable to like abuses and immoralities.

THE COUNTY POOR-HOUSE, near *Nazareth,* and the numerous buildings connected with it, are in a condition highly creditable to the *town and the state;* so, indeed, with rarest exceptions, are all the Pennsylvania German poor-house establishments: well built and liberally supported.

The main building at Nazareth, consists of a large stone house, forty feet by ninety, and three stories high with the basement. Adjacent to this, is a hospital for the sick and the insane, constructed with brick, thirty feet by eighty, and also three stories high, including a thoroughly finished basement. There are various out-buildings, workshops, farm-buildings, as barns, sheds, &c. The farm contains two hundred and fifty-five acres, all cleared except about five. The land is productive, and the whole well managed, and under good cultivation. Early in November, I found here one hundred and thirty-seven paupers—eighty-one males, and fifty-six females; of these thirty-five were children under fourteen years of age, and sixteen were insane.

The master and mistress of this establishment, deserve high praise for their vigilance and discreet management. Such of the inmates as were able, were employed according to the measure of their strength and capacity.

3

A number of the idiotic and insane were in the main building, others occupied rooms in a large wooden house, partly used for work-shops, on the lower side of the court-yard ; others again were on the first floor of the hospital ; and the violent and ungovernable, were in very comfortable, well finished rooms, of sufficient size, in the basement. To these were attached small exercise-yards, enclosed by a high brick wall. The deficiency was found in the want of skilful nurses, acquainted with the care of the insane. As a receptacle, this affords comforts not often found in connection with an alms-house ; but it cannot be made a curative establishment : neither those medical nor moral influences can be brought together here, which the wants that are peculiar to insanity demand.

One defect may be remarked of this, as of all the hospital establishments connected with the alms-houses, and many of which have been built almost without regard to cost as this ; that at Reading, Berks county, and those at York and Lancaster. It is in constructing the apartments for the sick and infirm, and those for the insane, in such proximity, as almost to ensure the disturbance of those who most require quiet and repose. There are times when this does not seem to be a serious evil, but one can have no assurance that these seasons of calm may not be followed by long and distressing disturbances : cries and shrieks, which banish sleep and distract the mind enfeebled by illness.

The arguments are very strong and conclusive, which advocate the separation of insane patients from the poor-houses. They are fitly established only in asylums solely appropriated to their use, adapted to their wants, and directed by persons whose only business is to guide and govern the affairs of the institution.

One cannot but respect the motives which have prompted the county hospital provision for the insane ; and not the less, that it is not all which the good of the patients require. A State Hospital is needed to supply what these *cannot* procure—a more complete remedial treatment.

LEHIGH COUNTY JAIL, at *Allentown*, is a large stone building, containing numerous rooms, but none in very good order in November. This jail is not so securely built, or carefully kept as to prevent escapes. The latest occurred the night before my visit, when the only prisoner remaining had effected his freedom by descending from the second story above the basement, through an opening made by a former convict into the room below, thence into the passage, and so on through the entries past the family-rooms, by the front door upon the street ! He was under sentence for a larceny, but the imprisonment did not seem to have wrought a very salutary influence. For he was charged with not having left the prison empty-handed. I understood that the food for prisoners in this jail, and at Easton, was supplied from the table of the keeper.

LEHIGH COUNTY, at present, has no poor-house ; measures have been adopted to establish one. The citizens very justly concluding that it is both more humane, and more economical to build a county-house, than to support as heretofore, the poor of the county, by letting them out to families willing indeed to take them at the lowest rates, but not securing or giving needful care.

The condition of the insane poor was represented as deplorable. I saw none in this county, but intelligent medical men concurred, as elsewhere, in the opinion that a hospital would be an inestimable blessing to the citizens of Pennsylvania.

SCHUYLKILL COUNTY JAIL, is at *Orwigsburg;* in October it contained seventeen prisoners, twelve men and five women. The latter were in apartments by themselves and occupied two rooms, over-heated, not ventilated, tolerably clean, and sufficiently furnished. There were beds and bedsteads. They go below to receive their food, which is passed from the men's yard, on which side is the kitchen, through an aperture in the gate-door, which connects the two exercise-yards. Conversation is not prevented. The men's rooms were quite decent; the size twenty-five by eighteen, and twenty by fourteen. Some of the prisoners were ironed for security. They receive three meals per day; the provisions sufficient in quantity and of good quality. No books, (except a few loaned by the keeper,) no employment, no moral or religious instruction; ample time and opportunity for conversation, and corrupting companionship.

SCHUYLKILL COUNTY ALMS-HOUSE, is well situated a short distance from *Schuylkill Haven;* the apartments of the main building are commodious, well-furnished, and kept in clean and neat order, but insufficiently ventilated in the cold season. Improvements have been making here in the general internal arrangements for several years. The various out-buildings are in repair, and the large new hospital for the sick and insane, chiefly for the latter, indicates that the citizens of Schuylkill county desire to do, what can be effected in a county establishment, in procuring a degree of comfort and humane management for the insane. Of this class there are here about twenty-five, ten of which were in the hospital; these, both men and women, were in charge of a person called the steward, who is, or was, one of the paupers. I had no reason to doubt his fidelity so far as his knowledge and ability should conduct him; he appeared attentive so far as I had an opportunity of observing, but his qualifications could not be such by education, as to make him a competent and responsible "care-taker" of the insane, farther than the mechanical labor is concerned. I understood a woman was sent daily from the main-building to assist in the early arrangements connected with the female apartments. I should think a better plan would be to appoint a competent female superintendent to take care of the women and to lodge at the hospital; she might also assist in watching the sick, and attending to the invalids. The hospital apartments here, I think, are about seven by nine, and ten feet high, the windows were of good size, and the cells could be ventilated, and warmed perhaps sufficiently with care. Several of the patients were exceedingly ungovernable, and most of them I fear not likely to recover the use of their faculties.

The farm connected with this county-house is large and valuable; it is said to be very well managed. Here is no school for children, and religious services rarely; but places of public worship in the neighborhood, afford opportunity for those of the inmates to attend who are able, and inclined to go.

NORTHUMBERLAND COUNTY JAIL, in *Sunbury,* was in decent order. I found no prisoners, but learned that this prison was subject to all the objections which apply to the majority of county prisons. The prisoners were well supplied at their meals from the keeper's table, as I was told.

This county has no poor-house; the poor are distributed in the several townships as convenience and economy determine. I learned from a medical practitioner, and others, that there were in the county many cases of insanity, urgently claiming appropriate care; but the entire number of idiots, epileptics, and insane, I could not learn. Many suffer from absolute neglect, and some become, it is feared, incurable through want of remedial treatment.

I cannot conclude this very brief notice of Northumberland county, without referring to a "son of the soil," whose best energies are now successfully devoted in a siste[r] state to conducting an institution for the insane : I refer to Dr. Awl, of Ohio, a name known there, and repeated with affectionate gratitude by many, whom, in the providence of God, he has been instrumental in restoring to health, and to the blessings of family and social life. His annual reports urge constantly a timely care for insane patients, and humane provision for all, whether recoverable, or beyond the reach of human skill to cure.

PERRY COUNTY JAIL, at *Bloomfield*, was in order, and clean. There was but one prisoner; a young man charged with murder. His habits and character have earned for him no right to look for lively sympathy in his present jeopardy; but his case was judged of very leniently by some of the citizens—"He had only killed a poor old man who was half intoxicated, and who did nothing when he was alive."

PERRY COUNTY POOR-HOUSE, near *Landisburg*, is a respectable establishment, having some good buildings, and a productive farm. The inmates, who in October numbered about forty, and were chiefly aged and infirm persons, appeared tolerably comfortable, and the rooms were arranged with reference to convenience and general order. A somewhat more immediate supervision might be better. The family who have the direction of the establishment, reside in an adjacent dwelling. Here is no school; religious meetings, I understood, occasionally.

The rooms or cells for the insane, were in a small wooden building; these were above ground—*very small*—lighted somewhat, but very defectively ventilated, and badly constructed, the barred partitions exposing the patients to observation. There were three of the insane altogether incapable of being at large, or associated with the other inmates of the place. The day I was there, though fires were necessary throughout the establishment, the clearness of the weather permitted them to be taken into the small enclosures, near the cells. I found them sitting upon the damp ground, in slight apparel, and exposed, of course, to colds and rheumatic attacks. I think in the winter some difficulties, if not danger, would be encountered in supplying the cells with sufficient warmth. The charge of keeping these poor creatures in any degree decent or comfortable, could not be easy, and would require a high sense of duty for its faithful performance. I have reason to apprehend they experience much suffering.

The number of insane and idiots in this county, I should judge was small, but I could not rely on certain information.

CUMBERLAND COUNTY JAIL, at *Carlisle*, was pretty clean, and for a prison so ill-built and ill-planned, pretty well arranged. The supply of food for the prisoners, appeared to me not sufficient. The allowance is *one pound of bread per day*, and *three* pounds of meat per week, with nothing in addition—water as much as desired—they cook for themselves in one of the apartments of the jail. There is a large enclosed yard common to the family and the prisoners. There were seven in confinement in October, on various charges; no means of improvement from abroad or within; no instruction, and no employment; and no impediment to evil communications. The jailor, on his part, did all the county required.

CUMBERLAND COUNTY POOR-HOUSE is remarkably well situated, and has a well-managed, productive farm. The establishment is expensive to the county. In October there were one hundred paupers, seven of which were insane, not including some who were idiotic and of feeble minds. At that time none were constantly in close confinement. An *idiot* girl has been the mother of four children; two of these were born and died before she was placed in the poor-house. Alms-houses, unless there is a well arranged classification of the inmates, are surely not fit places for the insane and idiots. The "crazy cells" in the basement, I consider unfit for use in all respects. The insane and idiots in the county is said to exceed one hundred. *Chains and hobbles are in use.*

DAUPHIN COUNTY JAIL, at *Harrisburg*, is undoubtedly one of the best conducted county-prisons in the United States. Like the jail in Chester county, it adopts the separate system with employment, and such instruction and advantages, as prisons constructed on this plan, secure to morals and habits. The provisions are excellent, and the food well prepared, and supplied in sufficient quantities. As a system, it is subject in common with the Philadelphia County Prison, and that of Chester, to an objection in retaining criminals, whose offences render them subject to the State Penitentiaries, and to terms of imprisonment exceeding a year in duration. This mistake will, it is believed, be remedied both by justice, and a necessity which a little longer experience will make plain. The discipline and moral training of the Eastern and Western Penitentiaries, adapt them to effect the objects of prison detention for extended sentences more surely, than it is possible to secure in county prisons, where there are no teachers qualified and expressly appointed, to give appropriate instruction.

Religious service is held in the Dauphin County Jail on every Sabbath afternoon, by the clergy of Harrisburg, who have volunteered their services, and so fulfil the law of Christ, preaching repentance and the forgiveness of sins, "unto the poor and the prison-bound." This instruction needs to be followed up by additional lessons. Many cannot read; they should be taught. Many are profoundly ignorant upon the plainest principles of morals, so far as teaching and example have reached them. They need help in these things; more aid than the inspectors or warden can have leisure to give; and these official persons are both vigilant and interested to benefit and reclaim the prisoner.

A well chosen library for the prison is much needed; and it is hoped that the benevolent citizens of Harrisburg will make it *their* work and duty, to supply such books as are suited to the moral and mental wants of the convicts.

Repeated visits to the Dauphin County Jail, have satisfied me of the kind and just discipline which prevails. Punishment is infrequent, and when imposed, is of no greater severity or duration, than is absolutely necessary for securing compliance with the mild and necessary regulations of the institution.

The dimensions of the cells are eight feet by fifteen, and ten high ; lighted at one end near the ceiling. Pure water is introduced through iron pipes, and the cells are maintained warm and dry by means of hot water thrown through small iron pipes in each cell. The bunks are furnished with a straw bed, replaced as often as necessary ; and a sufficient quantity of clean bed-clothing. The apparel of the prisoners is comfortable and adapted to the season. I have found the prisoners in health and as good condition, physically, as the same number of persons following like employments and of steady habits abroad. There is no hospital room.

On the 1st of January, 1844, say the inspectors, in their report of the prison, there were *twenty-three* prisoners—fourteen of which were sentenced to labor ; four to imprisonment, (" who might have employment if they wished,") and five, also, conditionably employed, were waiting trial. During the year 1844, there were received *one hundred and sixty-five* prisoners, and during the same period, *one hundred and sixty-nine have been discharged* ; leaving in prison, January 1st, 1845, fourteen. *Died, none.* The health of this prison is indeed remarkable.

The inspectors also remark, " As to the efficacy of the system of separate confinement, *combined with labor*, being the most perfect yet devised for the punishment and reformation of offenders, our experience during the past year, fully confirms all that our remarks expressed in the last annual report—*giving precedence* to the ' Pennsylvania, or separate system.' " The report concludes with a merited commendation of the warden, and other officers, for fidelity in the discharge of their duties. The fidelity extends to the inspectors, and is as commendable as it is rare in county jails.

The DAUPHIN COUNTY POOR-HOUSE, near *Harrisburg*, is a substantial brick building, of three stories with the basement, and one hundred and fifteen feet by forty. It is generally clean, comfortable, and well furnished. I have visited it twice, and the whole condition of the establishment shows creditably for those who superintend it, and gives evidence of the benevolence, and just spirit of the citizens who established and support it. The number of inmates, the third of February, was one hundred and sixteen, of which, twenty-nine were children ; thirteen imbecile and slightly deranged, three epileptics, and four very crazy. One insane woman, has for several years occupied a cell in the basement, which measures fifteen feet by six ; it is lighted, and warmed by a stove set in the partition. She has long refused to go abroad. For those of the insane, who are quite enough to be enlarged, *chains* are employed to restrain them from rambling to a distance. These are as light as is consistent with strength, but yet are a source of great discomfort and evident mortification to the wearers. This class here fall a good deal under the personal direction of the superintendents. The farm consists of two hundred acres, one hundred and forty of which are cultivated ; a grist-mill is on the premises, and is considered a valuable part of the property. The food is ample, and of good quality. The bread, which is of fine wheat flour and mixed with milk, is excellent. The bed-clothing and wearing apparel is comfortable. The children, who are of suitable age, are sent to the district school. Religious services are frequent. Medical attendance as often as required.

LEBANON COUNTY JAIL, at *Lebanon*, is built of stone, and is much on the same plan as other jails constructed thirty or more years since. It was tolerably clean. The only prisoner was a half-crazy imbecile man, who was committed for mischievously "burning the woods." He appeared to me incapable of any responsible act. His room was comfortable, and he was well cared for.

LEBANON COUNTY POOR-HOUSE, near the town, is a finely situated and liberally established institution. All the buildings are in repair, and the whole place respectably arranged, combining much comfort and convenience. This populous house had many infirm and invalid inmates. Several aged females, almost or quite imbecile, were not in so neat a condition as one would wish, but I learned that it was nearly impossible to render them more so. The house is very well furnished; the provision, as usual in the poor-houses, of excellent quality, and amply supplied. Wearing apparel also, as usual, good and sufficient. Beds and bed-clothing of excellent quality. This is an excellence which quite distinguishes Pennsylvania alms-houses, especially those of the Germans. There were no cases of violent insanity here in November, but several idiotic and imbecile men and women.

BERKS COUNTY JAIL, at *Reading*, is an old building, constructed with stone, upon an inconvenient plan, and subject to the objections of the common system of indiscriminate association of prisoners. I understand the plan of a new county prison is under consideration. Several prisoners occupied two of the four jail apartments. Here are no moral or religious influences, and no means for general or special improvement. Idle habits are confirmed, and good habits, if any, weakened or destroyed.

BERKS COUNTY POOR-HOUSE, near *Reading*, is an extensive establishment, providing amply for the necessities and comforts of its numerous inmates. The buildings are large and commodious, constructed of brick, and well finished, and furnished. There were, in the Autumn, two hundred paupers; eighty of which were sick, infirm, and insane, belonging to the hospital department. Of the insane, there were twenty-two. The salary of the matron of the hospital is insufficient. She is a person of uncommon energy and ability for that place. But while every care is taken that a poor-house can give, the insane cannot, for want of the medical and moral treatment which their cases peculiarly require, be often restored. I am satisfied there can be few recoveries here, though the apartments appropriated for this class, are constructed and furnished on the plans most approved in modern hospitals for the insane. I can imagine nothing better. I have seen nothing elsewhere that will compare with the excellence of these arrangements altogether. No cost appears to have been spared to make the inmates comfortable, so far as the building and furnishing are concerned. The deficiencies are want of suitable exercise-grounds, for those who were too much excited to have the range of the premises, and who were incapable of employment; and the want of competent nurses to aid the matron. The whole place was thoroughly neat. It may be offered as a model to all the counties in the state, for poor-house hospitals for the sick, and incurable insane, epileptics, and idiots. Here they are safe and comfortable, as far as their condition permits. The insane and idiots in the county at large, I heard variously computed at from eighty to one hundred.

In the main-building is a school for the children. The supply of well chosen books is altogether deficient. For a time there was very little moral or religious teaching. I understood this was to be resumed at no distant season. In nearly all the poor-houses in Pennsylvania, is found an apartment or chapel, exclusively appropriated to religious services. A knowledge of the language of the people is of course indispensable to useful influence. Few of the inmates understand English, except the most common colloquial phrases, and many of them not even these.

MONTGOMERY COUNTY JAIL, at *Norristown*, is a large stone building, capable of receiving many prisoners. I saw but one in November. The prisoner was not very clean, but neither was there much neglect. The ventilation was imperfect, and usually the rooms over-heated; a very common fault in prisons and poor-houses. I understood the food was sufficient and suitable in quality.

MONTGOMERY COUNTY POOR-HOUSE is several miles north-west from *Norristown*, and is a liberally managed establishment, so far as the furnishing of the various buildings and supply of provisions is regarded. There are three large dwelling houses, beside numerous out-buildings, Two of the former have been long built; but one is new, and was designed to increase the accommodations for the sick and the insane. Attached to the poor-house is a large and productive farm, under good management.

The new hospital, erected at considerable cost, and I doubt not, in the idea of procuring much good for those who should occupy it, is unfortunately not well planned. The principal defects are in the basement, where the insane are placed. The cells for this class in the old building, were condemned by all who saw them, both in their construction, and the wretched condition to which the inmates were abandoned. To remedy some of these acknowledged evils the new cells were made. I confess, except that change of place may have been a benefit, I see nothing gained; nothing can be more defective than the ventilations and mode of warming the whole range of cells. They are offensive, dreary, and comfortless in the extreme. These miseries are augmented by the entire incapacity of those who have the immediate care of this department; the woman I saw employed there had neither tact nor skill for that most responsible and difficult charge. An assistant, a blind man, could not be supposed to render assistance that would avail much. I do not know that there was a disposition to neglect duty, but, ignorance of how to manage, and to meet the peculiar wants of these maniacs, was obvious at every step. I have found nowhere in Pennsylvania, so bad and hopeless a condition of things for the insane, especially, for the excited and troublesome patients. I am sorry to say this, and especially, because I must believe that the overseers of the poor in the county, had meant to reach some better results.— There is a very small confined yard, enclosed by a lofty wall, in which the insane men and women, for they are brought pretty promiscuously together, when out of the cells, may walk. This place is but a few yards square, and so shut in, as to have little the benefit of pure air; it also prevents a free circulation of air from reaching the cells. This admits remedy by knocking down the wall and extending it, so as to enclose *at least half an acre*, but better one or two. The patients were very indecently exposed, and I left this department of the establishment grieved and astonished. The upper stories of the building were well directed, and comfortable altogether, unless the needed repose of the sick and aged was disturbed by the shrieks and vociferations issuing from the insane cells, below the infirmary. This could hardly fail to be the case. At the Berks County Poor-house Hospital, one felt that the miseries of the insane were mitigated; at the Montgomery County-house Hospital, they seemed perpetuated and aggravated. In the one was decency, cleanness, and measured comfort; in the other nakedness, exposure, and filth.

Bucks County Jail, at *Doylestown*, is a well built prison, in good order and repair. The apartments being comfortable and decent. I found here four prisoners, two men and two women, committed for immoralities, all occupying one room by day It would appear that if evil communications are corrupting, they were not likely to leave the prison with amended purposes or repentant minds.

The County Poor-house is in Warwick township, three miles from *Doylestown*. The situation is elevated, pleasant and healthful. The farm is large, productive, and well cultivated. All things pertaining to it, are creditable to the management of the superintendent.

The main dwelling was generally neat and comfortable. There were in November one hundred and fifty paupers, twelve of whom were confined in apartments removed from the main building, and in and adjacent to the hospital. The whole condition of, and arrangement for, the insane, especially for the men, was very bad; very bad, indeed. Eight or nine were crowded into one small over-heated, unventilated room; the discomforts of which, were intolerable. The attendant, a pauper, appeared to do all in his power to maintain some little cleanness, but want of space, and many other wants, rendered these efforts nearly useless. A small lodging room over the apartment, in which I found most of the men, contains their beds, and miserable enough they were; yet here eight or nine are crowded each night, and in one bed two are required to lodge. The rattling of the *chains and hobbles* was the accompanying music, to cries and other most discordant sounds. The history of some of these cases, as related at the poor-house, and as I learned them elsewhere, are very sad. An epileptic, particularly, moved my sympathies. He was at the time I saw him, tolerably rational, and quite conscious of where he was, and how situated; but being liable to fits, at almost any hour, he was shut in with the other patients, who embraced the worst cases on the premises. He had a book, and looking up, as I paused beside him, said: "It's a hard place to be in, but I must bear it." It was hard, indeed; nay, it was more—it was horrible. What an experience of life; what a living death. The breaking down of the mind, under that terrible disease, was almost too much to be borne; yet how was all this aggravated by such companionship. Such loathsome revolting scenes! What contrasts does life not afford!

Delaware County Jail, at *Chester*, is a stone building, old, inconvenient, and very badly planned, but cleanly kept. On my first visit in July, I found three prisoners, two males and a female; two had severally been committed for vicious conduct. I found all of them together. And to my remark on the impropriety of such mis-arrangements, was answered, that it had "*always been the custom* to keep the prisoners together, and they had not thought much about it!"

I re-visited this prison in October, and found ten prisoners ; nine men, and one woman ; the latter at that time employed in the kitchen. The rooms were not very clean ; they were over-heated, the beds as usual on the floor, and the prisoners of all ages and colours, congregated to amuse each other according to their fancy. The allowance of food is one pound of ship-bread to each prisoner, and as much water as they wish. The county, not the sheriff, is responsible for all defects here.

DELAWARE COUNTY POOR-HOUSE, several miles from *Chester*, is a large stone build-ing, clean, well furnished, and well directed. The provisions are good and sufficient, and the food well prepared. Here were eighty-five inmates the third week in October; of these but few are children. From twelve to fifteen are insane and idiotic; were clean, and comfortable, with the exception perhaps, of wearing *chains* and *hobbles*. None were in close confinement; though such cases often occur. A small wooden building, constructed near the main dwelling, contains six cells, cleanly white-washed and scrub-bed, furnished with a small but comfortable bed, but not capable of being warmed at all; accordingly they are disused during the cold season. Each is lighted by a grated window. There are in the basement of the main building four cells, lined with sheet iron, which are used for the violent patients when necessary. There are no recoveries reported in the poor-house through remedial treatment. "The most we expect," said one of the family, "is to do what we can for their comfort; we have no means for curing them." The entire establishment seemed excellently conducted, and but for the difficulty of managing the insane and idiotic, would afford a quiet home for the aged and infirm.

It is estimated that there are in Delaware county about seventy cases of insane and idiotic persons. The poor-house farm is large and productive.

CHESTER COUNTY JAIL, at *West Chester*, is built of stone, upon the plan of separate imprisonment. The cells are of good size, perfectly clean, and well aired. The pro-visions supplied, are of excellent quality. The allowance is three meals daily, and as much as satisfies the appetite. There has been but one death, by disease, in four years, and this was by consumption, developed before admission; and one prisoner was pardoned in consumption, who was also sick when received. I think one man, who was received in a state of intoxication, committed suicide. An accident which has happened to a few lines upon my note-book prevents my stating the whole case. I copy from the warden's report to the board of inspectors, the following facts :

We had in prison on the 1st of May, 1843, - - - - - - -	32
We received, during the year, white males, - - - - - -	41
" " " " females, - - - - - -	3
Coloured males, - - - - - - - - - - -	25
" females, - - - - - - - - - - -	4
Making in all, - - - - - - - - - - -	105
In prison on the 1st of May, 1844, - - - - - - - -	28

" The total number sentenced to labor, during four years, since removed from the old prison, is seventy-nine. Of these, forty-seven could read and write; twenty-four could not read nor write; and eight could read only. Thirty-three of these prisoners were intemperate; twenty-eight of them temperate, and eighteen were moderate drinkers.

"We have manufactured, during the year 1843–44, fourteen thousand three hundred and ninety-four yards of cotton cloth, four thousand three hundred and fifty-seven yards of carpet, and made bags, four hundred and ninety-four. These have met a ready market, and afford a fair profit."

I visited this prison in July, and saw all the prisoners, of which there were twenty-nine. Twenty of these were convicts, and nine were waiting trial. They were in excellent health, often replying to my inquiry in the words, "I am right hearty." They conversed cheerfully, were clean in their persons and apparel, and presented a remarkable contrast to the sixty-eight prisons I have since visited, always excepting the Moyamensing Prison, and that of Dauphin county. Some of the jails referred to were in Maryland, Virginia, and Ohio.

There were two of the prisoners above named, who, though in apparent health, were insane, a German and a Pole; the insanity of the former was produced by irregular life and intemperance. The case of the latter I did not learn. They both were in comfortable rooms, and were carefully attended. The defects at present in this prison are deficient moral instruction, and the want of a sufficient supply of well chosen books; these should be furnished without delay. Those who cannot read should be taught, and to this writing and arithmetic might without disadvantage be added. I saw a letter written by a prisoner, who had served out his time, and settled himself to an honest life. It was addressed to the warden, and shows that he was sensible of the kind influences which had been extended to him in prison.

"*Mr. Robert Irwin:*

"Sir :—I cannot but think from the gentlemanly manner you treated me while I was with you, you will be glad to hear from me; and I do assure you, I shall always feel the most sincere gratitude and affection for you, and the other officers connected with the hall. The kind and manly course pursued by you and all in authority, is calculated to reform any one that has the least spark of honesty left in his heart. I have, by sad experience, found that any but an honest and upright course, will lead to wretchedness and misery."

Perhaps the writer might have arrived at this conclusion if he had spent his two years in idleness, associated with all the corrupt offenders received during that period, but I hold the faith that he was saved by being withdrawn from evil associates, and evil habits, and subject to discipline through kindness, employment, and the use of books.

Chester County Poor-house, near *Marshalton*, has been undergoing a steady improvement for some years, in its discipline and domestic arrangements. It is a large, old building, almost surrounded by smaller buildings and out-houses. There is a valuable farm under good cultivation. Early in July, there were *one hundred and fifty* paupers, from twenty to thirty of which were idiots and insane persons. Forty of the entire number were coloured, (these occupied part of two comfortable houses,) fifty were Irish, and sixty were Americans. About forty-five of the whole number are children. Five of the insane were in close confinement ; ten were often added to this number, but at times were so well as to be allowed at large upon the premises, sometimes restrained by irons; the residue were always at liberty to go about the houses and yards. The health of the place was generally good; very few were seriously ill, but there were a few chronic cases. "About the hardest trial we have here," said the kind-hearted superintendent, "is parting with the children." The little creatures clustered around him like a swarm of bees; it was no "make-believe love," between them : the very babies stretched out the little arms to go with him.

I spent a long time about the buildings ; and from cellar to attic, and attic to cellar, through the whole, all things were clean and in order. The mistress had inspired the people with an ambition rarely found amongst the inmates of a poor-house : an emulation each of the other, in maintaining well-ordered apartments. Not a speck of dirt was to be seen about the wash-boards, the window-sills, or any where ; even the rooms for the craziest men and women, partook the general care. Here one saw that the oldest and least convenient buildings, might be made respectable and healthful, by proper attention to cleanliness and ventilation. All the insane were made as comfortable as their condition in a poor-house permitted. But here are no recoveries—here are no means for procuring essential benefits—what can be done is done, and it is a consolation amidst such inevitable miseries, to witness efforts for alleviating sufferings and evils which do not admit entire remedy. Curable cases should never be received here.

The PHILADELPHIA COUNTY JAIL, at *Philadelphia*, situated in the district of *Moyamensing*, is a massive stone building, in the Gothic style of architecture. From the rear of the front edifice, the extensive halls run back at right angles ; these contain three tiers of cells on either side. The two upper tiers being reached by means of railed corridors and galleries, extending the entire length of the blocks, which are ventilated and lighted from the roof. One block is appropriated to prisoners before trial. The other receives convicts who are sentenced, and who are here furnished with employment, and subject to a wholesome, but not rigid discipline. These blocks are exclusively for the male prisoners. The women's prison, divided by a high wall and intervening garden, is a separate building and establishment, disconnected in all domestic arrangements, from the men's prison. This department is especially well ordered, clean, comfortable, and well managed. The prisoners are supplied with suitable work—with books, and have the benefit of moral and religious teaching, (not at the expense of the city or county,) from the moral instructor, who visits the prison at large, and from an association of pious and devoted women, who spare no pains to reclaim the offenders, and restore the outcast. Their benevolent efforts are not confined to the prisoners during their terms of detention, but they endeavor to extend care and influence beyond the walls of the prison. Their disinterested and faithful exertions, sometimes meet with their highest reward, in the good results which attend upon, and follow these labors. There are many in all prisons, who set at nought counsel, and scorn reproof, but this is no argument whereby a Christian community would find justification in refraining from employing every consistent and reasonable exertion to recover the sin-sick soul—to inspire virtuous sentiments, to raise the fallen, and to strengthen the weak. The moral teacher in this prison, is a missionary employed by a benevolent society. Would it be more than justice demands, since the courts sentence so many convicts to these prisons, for long terms, for the city to appoint and support a chaplain, at its own cost? The many hundred prisoners in the county jail, though a very unpromising class of pupils, certainly not the less on that account, should be faithfully visited and instructed. Is it not a mistake, however, to sentence to the county prison, offenders, whose crimes make them legitimate subjects for the Eastern Penitentiary? Sent there, where sufficient and effective arrangements are made for teaching the ignorant, and nourishing the moral nature, where the regulations are all in all, better adapted for their benefit, than can be those of the county prison; they would be subject, not to a severer discipline, but would receive a stricter justice, whether we consider their rights as men, or their condemnation as criminals.

The cells of Moyamensing Prison, are of good and convenient size, well lighted, and ventilated, and in winter, well warmed. They are maintained clean, and well furnished, and are supplied with pure water, by pipes. The food is of good quality, and of sufficient quantity. It is well prepared, and usually distributed with care. I have visited all the cells in this extensive prison, and conversed with the prisoners, and having spent the largest part of nine days in a diligent examination of their condition, and of the general arrangements and the discipline, I do not hesitate to say, it is conducted in a manner highly creditable to the officers, whose duty it is to govern and direct its affairs. There are some defects, but they may be chiefly remedied with due attention. Well chosen additions to the library are much needed, as also care in the distribution of the books. The prisoners were at liberty to communicate to me, their grievances, if they had any, and to represent their condition without restraint. The only grave complaint, and it was twice repeated, was from a prisoner who desired a greater *variety* of food. Mutton and veal to vary his meals diet, and a larger variety of vegetables! There were three or four insane men, who had been committed on various petty charges, and were not subjects for this prison, or any other.

The EASTERN PENITENTIARY contained in January about three hundred and sixty-two prisoners. Within two years, *twenty-seven well attested* cases of insanity, have been brought to this penitentiary. I do not wish to enter now upon an elaborate discussion of this subject. The gross injustice of sentencing and committing men to prison for crimes committed while governed by the delusions of insanity, appears so obvious, that no person of the least humanity or intelligence will deny the position. Is it not time that the penal code of Pennsylvania should be revised? In this respect especially it demands consideration. The criminal jurisprudence of insanity has engaged much attention during the last thirty or forty years. France has led the way to this just reform, declaring with precision and perspicuity, "that there is no crime nor fault when the party accused was in a state of insanity at the period of the act." The penal code of Louisiana contains an act to the same effect, though less concisely expressed. That of New York lays down the same principle, with distinctness and precision: "No act done by a person in a state of insanity, can be punished as an offence, and no insane person can be tried and sentenced to any punishment, or be punished for any crime or offence committed in the state." These decrees, so philosophically just and humane, are worthy of being copied into every statute book of every nation. Several of the German principalities have long since adopted them. We have been slow in the United States to recognise this duty to a class of sufferers having peculiar and undeniable claims on the considerate and merciful care of every people. The English law on this subject is obscure; and successive acts of Parliament are both perplexing and contradictory. The high judicial authorities have from time to time declared opinions on these points, which, considering the times in which they were expressed, are distinguished only by their errors: and these inexcusable, because, information of undoubted authority, was within reach. The able medical governors of the hospitals and asylums, were both willing and competent to define insanity.

A vast many persons honestly believe, that most offenders for whose defence the plea of insanity is urged in courts of justice, are merely feigning a malady in order to escape the punishment consequent on crime. False pretences may be set up, and such have been, but to sustain these with the means of knowledge society now possesses in the experience of intelligent medical men, who have made this branch of their science a study, is not easy. The truth is, insanity is not a malady to be easily counterfeited, and those who undertake to simulate this disease, must have a very thorough acquaintance with its manifestations. There is no need to apprehend that in these cases either judge or jury may be imposed upon, if information is sought from those competent to determine this very grave and important question.

The insane who have been committed to the Eastern and Western State Penitentiaries, receive in those prisons such care and humane consideration, as the discipline, and general organization of these places permit. But granting for a moment that the insane do not suffer a great injustice in being committed to the state prisons, they inevitably, from the plan and arrangement of these institutions, are severe sufferers by such imprisonment; and one finds a sufficient argument for a State Hospital in the unhappy circumstances of the insane patients in the prisons, and jails, and alms-houses of Pennsylvania; without referring even, to another class, numerous and claiming benevolent consideration: I mean those who are not in affluent circumstances, and who borne down by this domestic calamity, are not able to meet the expenses of removal to, and cost of support in those institutions which are already established, and which have proven so great a blessing to large numbers of your citizens.

Pennsylvania has the high praise of having established a model prison on the separate system, which in its whole plan and government is worthy of being copied, wherever civilized life makes the establishment of prisons necessary, for the security of society. I express this opinion in a full confidence, based on extensive knowledge of prisons and prison systems of discipline; and I am satisfied that no unprejudiced, intelligent mind, can examine deliberately and faithfully, the wards of the Eastern Penitentiary, and not arrive at the same conclusion. The best systems, it is acknowledged, exhibit defects; and the best systems badly administered may produce the worst consequences; but in the prison at Cherry Hill, one witnesses both the good system, and the good administration united; and we wish not to see its harmonious order and just, but mild discipline, disturbed by the strange anomaly of uniting a State

Prison and a State Hospital, criminal wards and lunatic wards. We wish not to see misfortune punished as crime, and crime raised to a level with misfortune.

I have said that within two years, *twenty-seven* insane persons have been committed to the Eastern Penitentiary, charged with various crimes. The history of many of these, I have traced. I have resolved that no labor shall be spared on my part, in bringing facts to light. The testimony of intelligent citizens throughout the state, and the opinion of medical men acquainted with these cases, having had them under their care as patients, settles these points definitively. Men having been known as insane for years, committing recent crimes, still under the influence of insane delusions, are every month tried, and condemned, and sentenced, precisely as if they were in possession of a sound mind, and were responsible for their speech and deeds. The fact of their known insanity, is often recorded on the books of the prison, by the officers who convey them there. One often hears the now somewhat trite assertion, "Since we have no State Hospital, they must go to prison, that the lives and property of the public may not be destroyed!"

To this custom of sending so large numbers of insane men to the penitentiaries, may be referred many of the aspersions and objections which have been adduced against the "Separate System."

All the POOR-HOUSES in the city and county of *Philadelphia*, reveal scenes of suffering through defective provision for the insane, and great mistakes in the care and management of them.

A majority of the paupers in this county are gathered into the poor-houses, that is, if the city and its districts, the Northern Liberties, Southwark, Kensington, Spring Garden, and Penn township are included. Most of the other townships and villages in the county, I am informed, follow the "old custom" of "letting out the poor," or annually placing them in families, who agree to take them at the lowest rate, as in West Philadelphia, a part of Blockley township, &c. &c.

At *Germantown* is a POOR-HOUSE, which I have not visited since June; but I found it at that season, very clean and comfortable. The pleasant weather permitted most of the people to be abroad, including some insane men, who under a degree of restraint, still found pleasure in the air and in exercise. One insane woman remained chiefly in her apartment, which was very comfortable, well situated and neatly arranged. This room she had decorated in a most fantastic manner with flowers, and leaves, and fragments of coloured cloth; she was tranquil and silent. There are many indigent persons in this township who find aid from the more direct charities of the benevolent citizens, and are with that assistance saved from the entire dependence consequent upon resorting to the poor-house.

I think it probable that in winter this establishment must be quite too much crowded for health, or for that degree of comfort and accommodation which should be secured to the aged and infirm inmates.

ROXBOROUGH POOR-HOUSE, which also receives some of the poor from Manayunk, I visited three times early in the summer of 1844. I found a remarkably neat, well regulated establishment; too much crowded indeed, even at that season, and affording no suitable provision for the insane of which there were five, and one idiot; beside these there were seventeen paupers. One, a young girl, in a state of dementia, was at times subject to violent paroxysms and was exceedingly difficult of control. Another, a German woman of middle age, from Manayunk, was highly excited, and for the safety of others, as also for her own security, was closely confined *in the cells in the cellar*. Her strength and violence made it necessary for a man to take charge of her, the women of the house fearing and dreading her attacks. The superintendents of this house expressed much dissatisfaction and uneasiness at being obliged to use these underground apartments for this purpose. They were damp and in some respects unsafe.— So far as the habits of the occupants and the situation of the cells would allow, they were made comfortable; and I think uniformly as the paroxysms subsided the insane were removed for a few hours to the upper part of the dwelling, and in suitable weather, taken into the enclosed yard at one end of the house.

There were no means here for any care of the insane, that could conduct to recovery. The exposures of every sort to which they are subject in alms-houses, should be recollected by those who have the responsibility and power of determining if these shall last, or if by speedy legislation a fit asylum be opened for those who, in ceasing to exercise the reasoning faculties, cease from self-care, and have no more the capacity for governing their actions.

The PHILADELPHIA ALMS-HOUSE, west of the *Schuylkill*, is a vast structure built of stone, and capable of receiving above two thousand paupers. The main buildings alone, arranged in a parallelogram, cover and enclose an area of nearly ten acres. The average number of paupers in 1842, was fifteen hundred and forty-six, the inmates dispersing somewhat in the summer, but thronging again in winter. December 7th, 1844, the number was seventeen hundred, of which six hundred and ninety-nine only, were natives of the United States.

This vast establishment is suitably furnished, and kept in remarkably neat order. Ventilation is complete, and every hall and ward exhibited a uniform attention to that promoter of health—thorough cleanliness. I remarked the want of regular employment for a vast number of the inmates, and learned, with no less surprise than regret, that the original judicious plan of providing work for the paupers, according to the measure of their strength and ability, had been superseded; and further, that the machinery, and other apparatus for carrying out a part of the original system, so necessary to preserve in any degree the morals of the place, was now on sale. I am not acquainted with the motives which have led to this determination on the part of the official governors of the alms-house; but it seems, according to all experience in life and civil economy, a great error of judgment to admit such numbers of able-bodied men and women to the benefits of the institution, and to maintain them either in idleness, or with insufficient occupation. The school was not regularly organized when I was there, and I could not learn that the moral training was such as most persons would determine to be sufficient to form the character, to correct ill-habits, and early to deepen impressions of truth, integrity, and good sentiments. There seemed to me too little education of the conscience. I am sensible that many children brought to this house, are already imbued with pernicious ideas ; that their propensities are often vicious, and their habits corrupt and corrupting. All this but strengthens the argument for their more careful education, that so they may, if possible, be saved from successive grades of demoralization, and from the prisons of the land. I do not impute to those who direct these children, any intentional omissions of duty, believing they perform all the guardians require, but I suggest that perhaps the present system will admit of improvement and reform.

The Blockley Alms-hospital is a very expensive institution, and those aids for sustaining it at less cost to the city, with equal comforts for the inmates, which are adopted in some large establishments of this sort in other states, are not here resorted to ; for example, the large fruit, vegetable and flower gardens, sometimes cultivated and affording an income of some thousand dollars to the poor-houses. are not here made available.

Again, useful employment is afforded, as at the Rochester Alms-house, in New-York, during the season when labor is not practicable on the farm, by cracking stone. for M'Adamizing the streets and roads.

Employment in these institutions, even if not made to yield a considerable income, seems of much importance. The virtuous poor are always willing to work according to the measure of their strength ; while the idle vagrant, compelled to labor in the alms-house, will be more ready to seek work abroad, where he can be paid for it.

Of that department of the alms-house hospital, which is occupied for the insane, I feel great unwillingness to speak ; but I believe I am not the first to suggest that it has great and fatal defects. Attention has been called to the subject, through the journals of the city, and I trust that there will be no long delay in changing the whole order of this department of the institution. In one respect, and it is no little praise to accord, it was unexceptionable ; it was *clean, thoroughly clean.*

The men's department alone for the insane, received from January 1st, 1843, to January 1st, 1844, three hundred and ninety-five patients ; of these, it is painful to record, that two hundred and forty-eight cases were produced by intemperance, and were not strictly hospital patients. The remaining one hundred and forty-seven are recorded under the general head of insanity.

Dr. Jarvis, of Louisville, (Ky.) who visited this hospital in 1837, and has since written a treatise on Insanity and Insane Asylums, thus describes the mode of treating excited patients at the Blockley Alms-house ; being a mode of restraint never at any period practised in our best asylums for the insane, and now, with one exception perhaps, disused altogether throughout the country. "A poor female was confined in a 'restraining chair' made of plank ; one strap confined each arm, another the waist, and another passed over the thighs, and held her down to her narrow prison. This girl was in a state of furious excitement; she was using the greatest struggles to extricate herself; she was kicking her feet endeavoring to strike every one near her; she was boisterous and spat on any one within reach; she was the very image of a raging fury; and we were told that she had been in this excitement for three years, and the same means of straps and chairs had been as long used to calm her."

4

My first visit to this alms-house was in June, 1844. There were many visiters at that time beside myself. I anticipated something like change ; amendment, since 1837. I supposed that in seven years the abominations of the present system, would so have disgusted, not only the official guardians of the house, but the whole public, that with one indignant voice they would have united to demand and enforce a more rational, not to say merciful, organization of the establishment. It was not so.

Entering the men's wing, we found the hall and rooms vacant; except three or four, in which were several excited patients who were necessarily shut up for a time : for how long a time one could not tell—nor who should determine these questions of restraint; here is no one competent, governing director: "care-takers," are selected from the paupers, and of their qualifications in general for such delicate and very difficult duties, others can judge who know somewhat of the wants and dependence of the insane. The patient's rooms were very clean, and sufficiently furnished. We descended to the *exercise-yard*, and directly the men were "driven forward by a keeper," into a small grassed area, where they might sit down, or lie down, or do what they listed. Some were chained, and others muffled, that they might not do mischief. As if their own collective vociferations were not productive of sufficient discord, a fiddler from the other department was brought to increase the confusion. The worst feature here to my thought, was the *indiscriminate association* of all these insane men, without the smallest regard to the degree of insanity, or to the different physical and mental states they might exhibit; those who were conscious of their own malady, who were conscious *where* they were, "in the alms-house crazy-ward," those who did not comprehend this, or comprehending, did not care; the drooping melancholic, the noisy maniac, the drivelling idiot, and the spasm-shaken epileptic, all were here *together*.

From this scene revealing so little of appropriate and remedial care, we turned away, and followed our conductor to the women's department. Here, save a few, who were in their rooms, in states of vehement excitement, we found the patients collected into one large room—the hideous tumult of which beggars description. The recent and the established cases ; the tranquil and the excited ; the conscious and the unconscious; were here in one "great, monstrous, horrid company," to adopt the expressive description of one of them; crying, shouting, laughing, screaming, moaning, complaining, rolling on the floor, moping in the corners, assuming all attitudes, and rousing each other to higher and higher exasperation ; here they were, and here too, was sent the pauper musician, with the sharp, shrill, dissonant fiddle, adding discord to discord, and commingling the war of words, with the war of sounds, in rivalry of Babel ! But this does not complete the picture. In a remote part of this large room, in a "tranquilizing chair," that monstrous invention, which merits a place with the instruments of inquisitorial torment, or the machines of rack and torture employed in the middle ages, by regal despotism, in *a tranquilizing chair*, was fastened a young and beautiful girl, in the highest state of frenzy, yet, now and then, becoming, for a few moments, tranquil. She smiled sweetly, in her woe, and uttered half sentences, that moved many to tears. It was a sad and pitiable sight. Closely bound, hands, feet, and waist, she could only move the head and neck a little. Her beautiful hair fell in waves upon her neck, and there was a charm in her appearance, notwithstanding the wildness of the eye, that attracted all strangers. The "board of guardians," not less than the more infrequent visiters, drew towards her. I asked who she was, and whence she came. No one could tell. She had been found wandering in the outskirts of the city, and was brought there a few days before, raving mad ! I saw her once again, some weeks later ; she was still highly excited, and more unmanageable than before. I was consoled, to learn, subsequently, that her friends had traced her from the upper part of the county, above Frankford, and had removed her home. A merciful change, but how much more merciful, if she could have had the benefit of skilfully directed hospital care.

My second visit to the alms-house, produced new distrusts of the management of the lunatic department, and confirmed first opinions. I found in the men's ward, a poor man in a "tranquilizing chair," whose countenance wore an expression of agonized suffering I can never forget. His limbs were tightly bound, his legs, body, arms, shoulders, all were closely confined, *and his head also*. Feeble efforts to move were broken down by this inexorable machine. Upon the head, sustained by the apparatus, which confined the movements of the neck, was a quantity of broken ice. This, as it gradually melted, flowed over his person, which however, was in some degree protected from the wet by a stiff cape, either of canvass or leather. It was a very hot day, but he was deadly cold, and oh, how suffering! To suffer would have been his lot, perhaps, under any circumstances; but this treatment, "employed *to keep him still*," was a fearful aggravation of inconceivable misery. I asked how long he had been under this restraint. "Four days!" What, day and night? "No, at night we take him off and strap him upon the bed." How long will you keep him so? "Till he is quiet." How long have you ever kept the patients in this condition? "Nine days, I believe, is the longest. ' It does not require much knowledge of the human frame, and of its capabilities to endure suffering, and resist destructive and injurious influences, to know whether such a mode of treating insane persons is remedial and restoring in its effects, or whether it does not seriously endanger life, and lay the foundation of various fatal ailments, in addition to the malady under which they are suffering. I am sure the intelligent and skilful medical men in Philadelphia, will concur in the opinion, that this department of the alms-house calls for speedy and entire reconstruction. This can be accomplished with but little difficulty, and at small additional expense. To doubt the willingness of the citizens of Philadelphia to promote this much needed change, would be to distrust that humanity and liberality which has never been found deficient, when benevolent objects have been presented for their consideration and support. Why the alms-house alone, of the numerous public charities of Philadelphia, should show a condition so adverse to the objects it proposes to accomplish, is a problem I cannot resolve.

If idleness is the nurse of vice and crime, it would seem consistent with the purest political economy, to provide employment for all who are able to labor in the alms-house. If education is important to the youthful mind, especially moral culture, then a more careful attention to the school would be a public as well as individual good. If benevolent institutions for the protection of the friendless, and the recovery of the sick and disabled, to health and usefulness, are recognized as important and necessary in crowded cities, and a densely inhabited country, then it is well that these should be so established as to procure for the recipients of charity, all the benefits which they can be made capable of securing.

The exciting causes of insanity in large cities, are numerous. The poor and indigent are also numerous. If an extensive alms-house is necessary to receive the crowds, the thousands of sane paupers, surely a hospital, on a curative foundation, is also necessary, and to be preferred to a mere receptacle. In the one case, the maniac may be restored to reason and usefulness ; in the other, there is a possibility, but it rests upon slight probability. It may be argued by some, that many who are sent to this hospital, are the victims of their own vices and indiscretions, and are undeserving the special care solicited. Many of them are unworthy; in all probability the majority may have abused their privileges, wasted property, and impaired their health by indulgences and excesses, which must be condemned. But shall not these find mercy, and pity, and succour? You do not abandon the criminal in the jail; the juvenile offender finds a "Refuge;" and the halls of your penitentiary echo to the voices of those who, by earnest counsels and instruction, strive to reclaim the convict from perverse and criminal habits, to rectitude and duty. Let not the erring, perhaps once vicious insane, alone be abandoned.

One of your own citizens has not long since said publicly, what none have attempted to disprove: "That unless means are taken to discover the real condition of the insane in the alms-house hospital, the people of this community will justly incur the infamy of sustaining a moral nuisance, an establishment disgraceful to humanity, and a libel upon the present state of our knowledge of the proper treatment of mental disease."

The city and county of Philadelphia needs its own hospital and asylum for the treatment and protection of the insane ; as the cities of New York and Boston, sensible of the necessity of such provision for this class of their poor, have theirs. All large cities, as witness those just referred to, and not less Philadelphia and Baltimore, need for their own dependent citizens, a well established hospital.

It is but few years since the Alms-house of Suffolk county, Boston, revealed scenes of horror and abomination rarely exhibited, and such as we trust are now, in *the mass* at least, no where to be found in the United States. These mad-men and mad-women were the most hopeless cases, of long standing, and their malady was confirmed by the grossest mismanagement.

The citizens at length were roused to the enormity of these abuses ; to the monstrous injustice of herding these maniacs in a building filled with cages, behind the bars of which, all loathsome and utterly offensive, they howled, and gibbered, and shrieked day and night, like wild beasts raving in their dens. They knew neither decency nor quiet, nor uttered any thing but blasphemous imprecations, foul language, and heart-piercing groans. The most sanguine friends of the hospital plan, hoped no more for these wretched beings than to procure for them greater decency and comfort; recovery of the mental faculties for these was not expected. The new establishment was opened, and organized as a curative hospital. The insane were gradually removed, disencumbered of their chains, and freed from the foul remnants of garments that failed to se-cure decent covering. They were bathed, clothed, and placed in comfortable apartments, under the management of Dr. Butler, now superintendent of the Retreat, at Hartford. In a few months behold the result: recovering health, order. general quiet, and measured employment. Visit the hospital when you please, at "no set time or season," but at any hour of any day, you will find these patients decently clothed, comfortably lodged. and carefully attended. They exercise in companies or singly, in the spacious halls : they may be seen assembled reading the papers of the day; or books loaned from the library ; some labor in the yards and about the grounds ; some busy themselves in the vegetable, and some in the flower-garden; some are employed within doors, in the laundry, in the kitchen, in the ironing-room, in the sewing-room. In every part of the house a portion of the patients find happiness and physical health, by well-chosen, well-directed employment. Care is had that this does not fatigue, that it is not mistimed : and the visiter sees, amidst this company of busy ones, some of the incurables who so long inhabited the cages, and wore away life for years in anguish, encompassed by indescribable horrors. And though, of this once most miserable company, less than one-sixth were restored to the right use of their reasoning faculties, with but few excep-tions, they are capable of receiving pleasure, of engaging in some sort of employment. and of being taken to the chapel for religious services, where they are orderly and seri-ous. Such, to the insane paupers of Suffolk county, Boston, have been, and continue to be, the benefits of the hospital treatment. Than theirs, no condition could be worse before removal from the old building; now none can be better for creatures of broken health and impaired faculties, incompetent to guide and govern themselves, but yielding to gentle influences and watchful care.

Gentlemen, I have endeavored to show you in the preceding pages,—*First*, that the provision for the poor and indigent insane of your state, is inappropriate, insufficient, and unworthy of a civilized and christian people : *Second*, that it is *unjust* and *unjusti-fiable* to convict as criminals and incarcerate those in prisons, who, bereft of reason, are incapable of that self-direction and action, by which a man is made responsible for the deeds he may commit : *Third*, I have, in the description of your alms-houses, adding the opinion of the most intelligent men of your state, shown that these are, in all essential respects, unfit for the insane; and that while they may, with uncommon care and devotedness on the part of the superintendents, and other official persons, be made decent *receptacles*, they cannot be made curative hospitals nor asylums, for affording adequate protection for the insane : *Fourth*, still less can these ends be accomplished in private families, even where pecuniary prosperity affords the means of supplying many wants. But in those where this calamitous malady is united with poverty and pinching want, it is barely within the bounds of probability that the patient should recover. There is then but one alternative—condemn your needy citizens to become the life-long victims of a terrible disease, or provide remedial care in a State Hospital. Let this be established on a comfortable, but strictly economical foundation. Expend not one dollar on tasteful architectural decorations. In this establishment, let nothing be for ornament, but every thing for use. Choose your location where the most good can be accomplished effectually, at the least cost. Let economy only not degenerate into meanness. Every dollar indiscreetly applied, is a robbery of the poor and needy, and adds a darker shade to the vice of extravagance, in misappropriation of the public funds.

Choose a healthful situation where you can command at least one hundred acres, and better if a larger tract, of productive land, mostly capable of cultivation. Let the supply and access to pure water, be ample and convenient : also consider the cost of fuel, which is a large item in the annual expenses. Furnish your establishment by means chiefly of convict labor, from your two state penitentiaries, with mattresses, bed-clothing, chairs, &c. &c. You thus secure a sale for *their* work, and get good articles at reasonable cost for your own use. You will recollect that at some future time other hospitals will be needed and demanded, but let the location of the *first* have reference to sparing as far as possible to the poor at large, the heavy charge of travelling expenses. A substantial brick, or unhewn stone building, not more than three-stories high with the basement, to save labor, and the consequent multiplying of attendants, having the officers' apartments in the centre, and those of the male and female patients in the two wings respectively, will be found most commodious. Numerous minor considerations will, at a suitable time, receive a share of attention. But one thing should not be overlooked in a hospital designed to benefit *the people at large.* In this state it must be recollected that the medical superintendent, the governing, resident physician, who alone can be head of such an institution, and also his assistant, must have *practical acquaintance with both the German and English languages,* which are spoken in this commonwealth. Nearly half the insane of the lower classes, east of the mountains, are Germans, and cannot, in general, utter a sentence of English; and the medical adviser would find no little embarrassment in directing the moral training and treatment of his patients, except he could speak their language fluently, and was familiar, by residence and practice, with some of their peculiarities and local customs. I have perceived the importance and value of this, from being frequently accompanied to the poor-house hospitals by the attending physicians ; and as they have mixed with the inmates, addressing one in one language, one in another, I have seen that in a State Hospital for the Insane in Pennsylvania, it is absolutely necessary to possess these qualifications in order to be really successful.

If the mere outward manifestations of disease were to be studied, and decided on, if no other influence were to reach the patient than a medical prescription for a symptom which could not be mistaken, it would be of little consequence in what language the physician conversed, or whether he possessed at all the gift of speech; but as much beside is to be embraced in intelligent, skilful hospital practice, your physician for the State Asylum must speak readily the two languages of the country, at least. The medical superintendent of a hospital for the insane, needs not only a quick perceptive faculty in detecting the characterizing symptoms of the various forms of this malady, but adding to this an acquaintance with the social habits of both the German and English classes, he should possess energy, promptness of action, and ready determination ; he should have *active* business habits, and devotion to his profession. The very onerous duties which devolve on him will not nourish self-indulgence, or allow leisure for various pursuits: he must consecrate himself to the work, and he must concentrate all his energies, physical and mental, to promote the success and prosperity of the institution; making it so far as human means are concerned, an asylum where the curable may find health, and the incurable alleviation and solace for their sufferings.

Gentlemen, of the Legislature of Pennsylvania, I appeal to your hearts and your understanding; to your moral and to your intellectual perceptions; I appeal to you as legislators and as citizens; I appeal to you as men, and as fathers, sons, and brothers; spare, I pray you, by wise and merciful legislation now, those many, who if you deny the means of curative treatment and recovery to health, will *by your decisions, and on your responsibility*, be condemned to irrecoverable, irremediable insanity: to worse than uselessness and grinding dependence; to pain and misery, and abject, brutalizing conditions, too terrible to contemplate; too horrible to relate!

Grant to the exceeding urgency of their case. what you would rightly refuse to expediency alone. Benevolent citizens of your commonwealth were the first of civilized people to establish a society for alleviating the miseries of prisons; shall Pennsylvanians be last and least in manifesting sensibility to the wants of the poverty-stricken maniac? Is the claim of the Lunatic less than that of the Criminal? Are the spiritual and physical wants of the guilty to be more humanely ministered to, than the bodily and mental necessities of the insane? You pause long, and hesitate to condemn to death the blood-stained murderer; will you less relentingly condemn to a *living-death*, the unoffending victims of a dreadful malady?

The wise and illustrious Founder of Pennsylvania, laid broad the basis of her government in justice and integrity: now—while her sons with recovering strength, are replacing the shaken *Keystone of the* ARCH, may they, as in the beginning, find *their Salvation,—Truth, and their Palladium,—*RIGHTEOUSNESS!

Respectfully submitted,

D. L. DIX.

Harrisburg, February 3, 1845.

APPENDIX.

TABLE *showing the comparative expense of supporting old and recent cases of insanity, from which we learn the economy of placing patients in institutions in the early periods of disease; from the report of the Massachusetts State Hospital.*

No. of old cases.	Present age.	Time insane, in years.	Total expense, at $100 a year, before entering the hospital, & $132 a year since; last year $120.	Number of recent cases discharged.	Present age.	Time insane, in weeks.	Cost of support, at $2.30 per week.
2	69	28	$3,212 00	1,622	30	7	$16 10
7	48	17	2,004 00	1,624	34	20	46 00
8	60	21	2,504 00	1,625	51	32	73 60
12	47	25	2,894 00	1,635	23	28	64 40
18	71	34	3,794 00	1,642	42	40	92 00
19	59	18	2,204 00	1,643	55	14	32 20
21	39	16	1,993 00	1,645	63	36	82 80
27	47	16	1,994 00	1,649	22	40	92 00
44	56	26	2,982 00	1,650	36	28	64 40
45	60	25	2,835 00	1,658	36	14	32 20
102	53	25	2,833 00	1,660	21	16	36 80
133	44	13	1,431 00	1,661	19	27	62 10
176	55	20	2,486 00	1,672	40	11	25 70
209	39	16	1,964 00	1,676	23	23	52 90
223	50	20	2,364 00	1,688	23	11	25 70
260	47	16	2,112 00	1,690	23	27	62 10
278	49	10	1,424 00	1,691	37	20	46 00
319	53	10	1,247 00	1,699	30	28	64 40
347	58	14	1,644 00	1,705	24	17	39 10
367	40	12	1,444 00	1,706	55	10	23 00
400	43	14	1,644 00	1,709	17	10	23 00
425	48	13	2,112 00	1,715	19	40	92 00
431	36	13	1,412 00	1,716	35	48	110 40
435	55	15	1,712 00	1,728	52	55	126 50
488	37	17	1,912 00	1,737	30	33	75 90
		454	$54,157 00			635	$1,461 30

Average expense of old cases, - - - - - $2,166 20
Whole expense of twenty-five old cases, - - - - 54,157 00
Average expense of recent cases, - - - - - 58 45
Whole expense of twenty-five recent cases till recovered, .. - 1,461 30

From Dr. Awl's reports of the Ohio Institution, we extract the following tables :

In the report of 1840, the number of years that the twenty-five old cases had been insane, was 413 ; the whole expense of their support during that time, $47,590 ; the average, $1,903 60. The time that the twenty-five recent cases had been confined, was 556 weeks ; the expense, $1,400 ; the average $56.

In 1841, whole cost of twenty-five old cases, - - -	$49,248 00
Average, - - - - - - - -	1,969 00
Whole cost of twenty-five recent cases, - - - -	1,330 50
Average, - - - - - - -	52 22
In 1842, whole expense of twenty-five old cases, - - -	$50,611 00
Average, - - - - - - - -	2,020 00
Whole expense of twenty-five recent cases, - - - -	1,130 00
Average, - - - - - - - -	45 20
In this institution, in 1843, twenty old cases had cost, - -	$44,782 00
Average cost of old cases, - - - - - -	2,239 10
Whole expense of twenty recent cases, till recovered, - -	1,308 30
Average cost of recent cases, - - - - -	65 41
In the Massachusetts State Lunatic Asylum, in 1843, twenty-five old cases had cost, - - - - - - - -	$54,157 00
Average expense of old cases, - - - - -	2,166 20
Whole expense of twenty-five recent cases, till recovered, - -	1,461 30
Average expense of recent cases, - - - -	58 45
In the Ohio Lunatic Asylum, in 1844, twenty-five old cases had cost,	$35,464 00
Average expense of old cases, - - - - -	1,418 56
Whole expense of twenty-five recent cases, - - -	1,608 00
Average expense of recent cases, - - - - -	64 32
In the Maine Lunatic Hospital, in 1842, twelve old cases had cost, -	$25,300 00
Average expense of old cases, - - - - -	2,108 33
Whole expense of twelve recent cases, - - - -	426 00
Average expense of recent cases, - - - - -	35 50
In the Hospital at Staunton, Va., twenty old cases had cost, -	$41,633 00
Average expense of old cases, - - - - -	2,081 65
Whole expense of twenty recent cases, - - - -	1,265 00
Average expense of recent cases, - - - - -	63 25

The results of this table are so striking, and show so conclusively the importance of early admission to the insane hospitals, that many other institutions have instituted the same inquiry with similar results.

TABLE (*from Dr. Awl's sixth report for* 1844, *of the State Hospital, at Columbus, Ohio,*) *showing the comparative expense of supporting old and recent cases of insanity.*

No. of old cases.	Present age.	Duration, in y'rs, of insanity before admission.	Cost of support before admission, at $2 per week.	Number of recent cases.	Age.	Duration of insanity before admission.	Time, in weeks, spent in the asylum.	Cost of cure, at $3 per week.
1	42	18	$1,872 00	1	29	1 month.	20	$60 00
2	45	11	1,144 00	2	22	6 "	18	54 00
3	35	13	1,352 00	3	35	5 "	15	45 00
4	40	12	1,248 00	4	26	4 "	9	27 00
5	38	15	1,560 00	5	41	8 "	43	129 00
6	38	10	1,040 00	6	37	5 "	16	48 00
7	42	10	1,040 00	7	27	7 "	59	177 00
8	40	15	1,560 00	8	34	4 "	15	45 00
9	40	20	2,080 00	9	31	1 "	18	54 00
10	40	9	936 00	10	22	9 "	13	39 00
11	50	10	1,040 00	11	18	1 week.	11	33 00
12	48	11	1,144 00	12	29	2 months.	52	156 00
13	45	9	936 00	13	23	5 "	25	75 00
14	35	10	1,040 00	14	24	8 "	5	15 00
15	57	27	2,808 00	15	28	2 "	13	39 00
16	57	10	1,040 00	16	45	4 "	14	42 00
17	28	13	1,352 00	17	28	4 "	26	78 00
18	49	21	2,184 00	18	41	1 "	23	69 00
19	43	15	1,560 00	19	24	3 "	15	45 00
20	45	10	1,040 00	20	32	2 "	15	45 00
21	29	14	1,456 00	21	20	5 "	33	99 00
22	33	10	1,040 00	22	20	8 "	29	87 00
23	40	28	2,912 00	23	21	5 "	8	24 00
24	39	10	1,040 00	24	31	5 days.	16	48 00
25	40	10	1,040 00	25	25	10 months.	25	75 00
			$35,464 00					$1,608 00

Average number of years for each case before admission into the asylum, 13⅗.

Average number of weeks spent in the asylum, 21½.

Average cost of each case before admission into the asylum, $1,418 56.

Average cost of each recovery in the asylum, $64 32.

MEMORIAL

KENTUCKY

1846

MEMORIAL

SOLICITING AN

APPROPRIATION FOR THE

STATE HOSPITAL FOR THE INSANE,

AT LEXINGTON;

AND ALSO URGING THE NECESSITY

FOR ESTABLISHING A

NEW HOSPITAL

IN THE GREEN RIVER COUNTRY.

BY D. L. DIX.

FRANKFORT, KY.
A. G. HODGES:::::::::STATE PRINTER.
1846.

MEMORIAL.

To the General Assembly of the Commonwealth of Kentucky :

GENTLEMEN:—I ask the indulgence of placing before you some remarks suggested by repeated and careful inspection of the State Hospital for the Insane, at Lexington ; and also the results of journeys recently made through forty four counties of your State, in view of ascertaining, as far as possible, the numbers and condition of this class of sufferers who have not been brought under remedial hospital care.

I would respectfully and earnestly urge the duty of providing a remedy for prominent defects and deficiencies in the present establishment, and suggest some reasons which appear absolute and consistent, for early additional provision in a southern district of the State for this numerous and increasing class of sufferers. Justice and humanity unite to present these claims, and it may be added, that both present and future *economy* in the administration of the public funds sustain their plea.

I approach you with confidence as the advocate of those who, alas, cannot plead their own cause—of those in whom the light of the understanding is darkened, and who are crushed under the weight of an overwhelming malady—yes, I approach you with confidence, for I am told that the citizens of Kentucky have heretofore been neither slow nor reluctant in responding to the calls of duty, and acknowledging the claims of those, who through privation and disease are made *wards* of the State—legalized dependents on its beneficent and guardian care.

Legislators of Kentucky, I do not now urge the necessities of these afflicted ones, so much in the *hope* of your effective and generous action, as in the *belief* that you will not hesitate to provide amply for those who, in the providence of God, cannot provide for themselves : yes, I *believe* that with united mind and will, you will act wholly upon that sacred rule of universal obligation, which enjoins upon Legislators no less than upon individuals in their social relations, to do for others what they in similar circumstances would have meted to themselves.

Of all the calamities to which humanity is subject, none is so dreadful as insanity. Pinching want, hideous deformity, acute disease, mutilation, deafness, blindness ; all these are distressing in their effects alike upon the sufferer and those with whom he is connected ; but sad as are these distresses they leave to the unfortunate, human sympathies and priceless affections. They admit the assuaging influence of consolation and tender care, *recognizing* through these the love that prompts, and the hand that ministers. Not so is it with those who are smitten with the visitation of *insanity*— that disease which produces utter dependence for the supply of all physical wants, and rends away the noblest attributes of humanity.

The heart grows cold, and no gentle or generous affections flourish there. The brain no longer exercising its functions healthfully, reveals only distorted images of the mind. Healthful, intellectual vigor is prostrated, and man, from bearing affinity with spiritual natures, becomes in an hour, transformed to a mere brute existence, manifesting little beside low animal instincts. This malady, the offspring of civilization, increases annually in our country, and demands not on the solid ground of *humanity*, and the less stable basis of *expediency*, but through the uncompromising law of *necessity*, that its progress be arrested and its controllable causes subdued. The evil and the remedy are both before us. Experience and observation have dispelled that long received error which ascribed to the *mind* the production of insanity, and have demonstrated the physiological fact that the proximate cause of this disease is bodily. The *manifestations* of the mind are distorted through physical disease, or disturbance of that organ through which the reasoning faculties find expression. Insanity in strict definition, has ceased to be called *mental disease;* it is rather mental disability. This fact established, we seek for insanity, as for other bodily ailments, 'those remedies which will *soonest* and *most surely* restore the lost balance of the system. Moral means in various measure, in all diseases, but eminently so in this, comes in aid of medical agents, and it is both conceded and urged by the highest authorities, that *these can be effectually combined only in an establishment specially devoted to the remedial treatment of the various forms of this malady.*

It is a prominent characteristic of insanity, manifested with rare exceptions, in all varieties of this disease, that many of the persons and objects amongst which it is developed, become sources of discomfort, or of serious annoyance and excitement to the patient, thereby nourishing and aggravating irritation and morbid susceptibilities.

Disagreeable thoughts are continually revived by things with which they are associated, as well as by persons whose kindest attentions are construed into proofs of ill-will and ill-design. Thus the mind of the patient is disquieted sufficiently to counteract any curative process the administration of medicine might be preparing. Withdrawal from all outward and familiar disturbing causes counteracts morbid associations, and wholesome influences obtain predominance.

Friends at home rarely possess the means of relief which a violent and sudden exhibition of insanity demands, even if in all cases they can have the advantage of the services of a skilful medical practitioner, familiar with the Protean phases of this disease. The discriminating and watchful *hourly* attention these often, for considerable periods require, can be had only within the walls of a judiciously organized and vigilantly governed Hospital. Here, where mild and gentle, but firm and decided influences are brought to bear, the raving maniac becomes yielding and calm, and the insensible are roused to an interest in the affairs of life, and throw off melancholy and inertia.

Although for a given time a patient may live at greater expense in a hospital than in a poor-house, or in a private family, this is no argument against the former; for granting that expense alone is the consideration, the number of cures wrought through the agency of hospital treatment timely adopted, will in a short period leave the balance-sheet of expense altogether in favor of the latter. But it is not a question of expense which is to be discussed, it is the *rights of suffering humanity ;* in Kentucky it is no longer a question whether the poor and friendless maniac, and the helpless subject of dementia shall be provided for ; and whether the well-established hospital shall open its doors to but a few favored ones, and reject the many ; heretofore it has, I think, been the purpose to provide for *all.* But numbers have now increased vastly beyond the capacity of the present establishment to receive ; and it is well known to all who have inquired into the facts, that the lodging apartments are in many cases, crowded to the great disadvantage and discomfort of the occupants. What was once an *ample* provision is no longer *sufficient.* The increased population of the State, and of course the increased number of patients, call for accommodations in measure with this increase.

The first consideration however seems to be attention to the *comfort* and *safety* of the patients resident in the hospital which is already established, by adding such improvements as will place it in rank with the best institutions for the management of the insane in the United States, and put it in the power of the able and devoted Superintendent to do that justice to his patients, and the cause of humanity, which his judgment and skill as a physician, and his kind and humane dispositions suggest.

Within the last three months, I have repeatedly visited the hospital at Lexington, and have been permitted freely to see every department of the entire establishment. With such ample opportunities for observation, I think I am able to do justice to all who share in the administration of the affairs of the institution. The judicious and watchful attention of the resident physician and his assistant, have commanded my confidence and respect. The Commissioners, as official visitors, are as vigilant as they are disinterested. The Steward and Matron are devoted to their very onerous duties, through a hearty interest in the welfare of those whose daily comforts so much depend on their fidelity. One cannot sufficiently commend the neatness and order which are maintained in this large establishment ; and that these circumstances are preserved under existing inconveniences, must surprise even the most casual observer. This is done at an expense of manual labor and continual oversight, laborious in the extreme.

A transient visitor, passing through the Institution, giving perhaps but a few hours to an examination of its various departments, unacquainted with the details of its domestic economy, and knowing little or nothing of the peculiar and unremitting care which most of those two hundred and twenty patients require ; seeing little of the special labors which the defective construction, and the inconvenient arrangements of the present buildings produce,—such a visitor may come away from the hospital, as many I have known, even within the short period of my acquaintance with the Institution ; and believe that all is as it should be, and that nothing is wanting to make this a complete and effective establishment.

The most obvious defects may be briefly enumerated as follows :—The kitchen is much to small for the variety and amount of labor to be performed in it. It is deficient in *all* arrangements which would facilitate the accomplishment of work in that department. For the want of a well constructed *range*, with boilers and bakers, the cooking is done by a large iron stove, not the least objection to which is the greater quantity of fuel which it consumes than would a properly adjusted fire, and cooking-apparatus. It is estimated that the saving in fuel alone for a year or eighteen months would cover the expense of erecting a well-constructed and commodious kitchen.

The establishment affords but *one dining-room,* and in this long and cheerless hall must be congregated nearly all the patients, both from the men and women's departments, to partake their meals at one and the same time. That these should be disposed with less comfort than is requisite for a large part of the patients is, under existing arrangements inevitable. And here we see congregated all classes of patients, the incurable and the convalescent; the mirthful and the sad; the unconscious and those whose keen sensibilities are quickened to acutest suffering; these all must come together, and on these are wrought healthful, or oftener injurious influences, according to the form of the malady under which the patient labors. It is deemed an imperative necessity in all well-organized hospitals that the patients be classified with reference to their mental condition and physical wants. Here your Superintendent has *no choice*; it cannot be done, so remarkably defective is the internal construction of these buildings.

There are in this whole establishment, neither bathing-rooms nor washing-rooms of any description. In ordinary domestic arrangements these are needful for comfort and refreshment, as well as for their essential hygienic influences; how much more at all seasons, must this be the case in establishments which receive several hundred inmates, and most of these variously diseased. In no class of diseases indeed, is either warm or cold bathing considered so essential to the curative process, as in that of insanity; yet we have here a hospital which should be complete in all remedial appliances, wholly destitute of even the most simple accommodations for water-bathing. How the benefits of personal cleanliness are commanded at all here, is the wonder. First, laboriously, the water must be "packed" from the spring to the kitchen; next heated in small quantities at a time, in a receiver upon the cooking-stove; thirdly, it must be conveyed in buckets over two flights of stairs (if for the women's department, if for the men's, across the yards, &c.,) into one of the *day-rooms,* where, after use, it must again and finally, be borne in buckets over one flight of stairs to some waste-drain on the premises. It cannot be necessary to enlarge upon this subject.

The necessity is urgent for the early introduction of water throughout the State hospital; it is requisite in the culinary department, and in all beside. Here again would be a diminution of expense in the item of labor. The quantity of water required for daily consumption in large institutions is not comparable with that demanded in private households. Of thirteen hospitals, with the internal arrangements of which I am acquainted, there is *daily* consumed in each, for all purposes, from *one hundred and twenty,* to *one hundred and sixty barrels,* and this for purposes only of absolute necessity. At Utica, N. York, when the number of patients as yet did not reach two hundred, the daily consumption of water was nearly *four thousand gallons.* Nor did this, in whole, supply the baths, the house-cleansing, washing, and cooking departments. The water at Utica was forced from a well by means of a pump driven by horse-power, to the attic story of the centre building, and thence distributed through pipes over the entire establishment. One horse will force from forty-five to fifty hogsheads in an hour. Every arrangement is made to guard against a conflagration. The roofs are all fire-proof. An engine, and large number of buckets are always *in order and in place,* for instant use. There is an engine at the State Hospital here, but the distance from the spring to the rear buildings, would render its use of little avail. In fine, the first and greatest necessity is to secure an ample supply of water *in* the buildings, as well for security, as for health and convenience.

The laundry is very defective. The ground floor, occupied for cleansing the apparel, &c., is so imperfectly constructed that the health of those who labor there is seriously exposed. The ironing-room is but half the size necessary for the ready and convenient performance of that branch of labor. There is no drying nor airing room at all. In damp and wet weather, therefore, several days sometimes intervene before the requisite changes of body or of bed-garments can be had. A properly constructed washing-house appears desirable, not less for health than for the reduction of labor, and the great reduction in the expenditure of fuel. There is no infirmary in the hospital, nor are there apartments either in the men, or the women's ward, where, in the event of special sickness from fevers, or other incidental illnesses, patients might be kept quiet, and receive all the cares their condition would claim.

Dr. Luther V. Bell, whose reputation not only in our own country but in Europe, gives authority to his opinions, remarks as follows, upon the treatment of the insane : " The value of properly adapted architectural arrangements ; of a complete classification of patients ; of a well educated, morally elevated, and well paid class of attendants ; of well directed and perseveringly applied employment ; of mechanical and of agricultural labor ; of such amusements of mind and body as experience proves to be best adapted to occupy and direct the diseased intellectual functions and moral susceptibilities; and lastly, such an intercommunication with the sane, in social intercourse, public and private devotional exercises, and in the lighter and gayer re-unions of life, as the peculiarities of each case demand, must be felt and acknowledged, wherever the insane are entrusted to the care of the refined, the well-informed, and the conscientious. Beyond the judicious, energetic, and experienced application of such moral agents as these, and an adequate medical treatment, there is, and can be no mystery in the treatment of the insane."

The State Hospital at Lexington is pleasantly situated, and at convenient distance from the city. There is attached to this institution about thirty acres of land, but it is much to be regretted that it has not the advantage of owning a farm of one or two hundred acres, whereon those of the patients who are able to labor, and who would be benefited thereby, might be employed. All recent experience shows that a tract of land for agricultural purposes is almost, if not quite, indispensable to the interest both of the patients, and to the domestic economy of the hospital. Whatever shall seem to aid remedial measures, and advance recovery to health, seems demanded at the hands of those who, possessed of this priceless blessing, owe as a thank-offering to heaven, every care to such as are smitten with disease.

Dr. Earle, of the Bloomingdale Asylum refers repeatedly in his valuable reports, to the advantage of well-directed employment for the insane, and offers examples illustrative of this opinion, from which I select the following. " During the Spring of 1844, two farmers, each of whom possessed a good farm, were admitted to our Asylum within a week of each other. They were laboring under the most abject form of melancholy, and had both attempted suicide. In less than a month, their condition being somewhat improved, they expressed a willingness, and one of them a strong desire to work out of doors. Being furnished with implements, they daily went out together, and worked upon the farm with as much apparent interest as if it belonged to themselves. Under this course they continued rapidly to improve, and both were discharged recovered, one at the end of six weeks, the other at the expiration of three months from the time of their respective admissions."

"Another man was brought to the Asylum, laboring under a high degree of active mania. His appetite was poor, and his frame emaciated. He was careless of his personal appearance, restless, turbulent, and almost incessantly talking, in an incoherent manner, upon the delusions attending upon his disease. When out of doors, he was constantly wandering to and fro, talking to himself, and digging the earth with his hands, without end or object, and generally having his mouth filled with grass. For some months there was but little change in his condition. At length, having become somewhat less bewildered, his attendant succeeded in inducing him to assist in making beds. Shortly afterwards he was employed with the painters and glaziers upon the green-house; after this, he went into the carpenter's shop, where he worked regularly for several weeks. Meanwhile, his bodily health improved, his mind gradually returned to its former integrity, and he was discharged cured of his mental disorder."

"These cases are fair examples of the utility of a combination of medical and moral treatment, for in all of them medicine was regularly administered until within a comparatively short period before their departure from the institution. They are presented also as cogent arguments in favor of giving to manual labor that preeminence which has already been assigned to it."

The following schedule of the productions from fifty acres of the Bloomingdale farm, cultivated by the patients under the direction of the farmer and gardener, may be read with interest.

Hay,	40 tons.		Mangel Wurtzel,	50 bushels.
Oats cut in the milk,	4 "		Turnips,	325 "
Butter,	728 lbs.		Parsnips,	100 "
Milk,	4700 gallons.		Carrots,	30 "
Pork,	2706 lbs.		Onions,	50 "
Potatoes,	500 bushels.		Cabbages,	3000 heads.
Corn,	75 "		Leeks,	4000 "
Sugar Beets,	250 "		Celery,	2600 "
Blood Beets,	125 "		Salsify,	1500 heads.

Beside these there was a full supply, for the *whole* establishment, of peas, beans, squashes, tomatoes, radishes, cucumbers, asparagus, spinach, lettuce, egg-plant, and turkey-plant, beside a good supply of water-melons and musk-mellons. Of *fruits*, we had

Apples,	500 bushels.		Cherries,	100 bushels.
Pears,	60 "		Grapes,	800 lbs.
Peaches,	18 "			

Beside currants in abundance, strawberries and raspberries.

By the labor of the patients and gardener three years since, I observe from the annual report of the Connecticut Hospital, that the garden, which contains *an acre and a quarter* of land, surrounded by a carriage-road, and a border planted with evergreens, rose-bushes, and other flowering plants, produced as follows:

Lettuce, 1100 large solid heads.	Cucumbers for pickles, 7 barrels.
Cabbages, 1400 do. do.	Beets, 147 bushels.
Radishes, 700 bunches.	Carrots, 24 "
Asparagus, 2800 do.	Parsnips, 25 "
Rhubarb, 300 lbs.	Onions, 120 "
Marrowfat peas, 14 bushels.	Turnips, 80 "
Sweet Corn, 419 dozen ears.	Tomatoes, 40, "
Summer Squash, 715 dozen.	Early potatoes, 35 bushels.
Squash peppers, 48 dozen.	Winter squashes, 7 wagon loads.
Cucumbers, (table) 756 dozen.	Celery, 500 large heads.

These articles, all of the very best and earliest kinds, and valued at market prices in Hartford, would have amounted to more than 625 dollars. The farm was like the garden, well cultivated." I have quoted these examples, which might be greatly multiplied, to show the excellent economy of a judicious cultivation of the lands pertaining to public institutions, and to enforce the double argument for attaching good farming and gardening land to Hospitals for the treatment of the insane.

I have referred at some length to the special wants and deficiencies of the only establishment for the reception of the insane within the bounds of this wide Commonwealth, and have urged perhaps with importunity, that these wants should be supplied, and that these deficiencies should be remedied. I leave this subject with those whose good sense and convictions of justice will, I trust, conduct to such effectual legislation as shall be in harmony with the humane sentiments of the citizens at large, creditable to the Legislators, and honorable to the Commonwealth.

Many States are active in laying broad and deep the foundations of numerous charitable institutions; in enhancing that real greatness which knows no decline or extinction; let not these outstrip Kentucky in moral elevation, and enlightened wisely directed beneficence. Let it not be said here as of old, in Attica: " The Athenians *know* what is right; but the Lacedemonians *practice* it.

I have yet another plea to urge, another boon to crave. It is for *yourselves and your children* that I ask *additional* benefits. More complete and entire provision is needed for the unruly or unconscious idiot, the helpless epileptic, and the raving maniac. Heretofore your appropriations from the State Treasury since the establishment of the Hospital, have appeared to keep pace with the public need, at least it seems to me that this has been the intention. The Report of the Superintendent of the Hospital reveals the facts of an overcrowded institution, and of numerous applications for admission, for which, of course, there is now no provision. Several hundred insane persons according to the most moderate estimate, are now suffering, in various parts of the State, for want of well-directed remedial treatment. As yet, I have visited but forty-four counties ; but from the best sources of information I have been able to consult, it is evident that much suffering exists, and many patients are annually becoming *hopelessly* insane through want of seasonable appropriate care. Friends are often indisposed to place the patient away from home, but if the dispositions were usually favorable to hospital treatment, there at present exists no accommodations for receiving them. In Kentucky alone, of all the States I have traversed, it has not been my painful experience to find the insane poor, filling the cells of poorhouses, or the dungeons of the jails. I have not a single example to offer of an insane person found either in a poor-house or jail, except one patient, whose violent paroxysms and homicidal propensities made it necessary to place him for his own safety, and that of his family, in a county jail, till the session of the court, when the legal measures required for his transfer to the hospital could be adopted. The fact that the *State* assumes the expenses of the pauper insane, explains the entire absence of similar cases of culpable neglect, and dreadful suffering and privation, exposure and distress, which are to this hour frequent in almost, if not quite, every State in the Union.

In Kentucky the affluent and self-supporting classes are the severest sufferers. Just views respecting the healing and kindly influence of hospital care are not so widely diffused as could be wished, and except in the event of sudden and very violent attacks of this fearful malady, the patient is detained by mistaken tenderness within the family circle, till the disease is confirmed, and hope of cure is extinct.

All experience shows that insanity *seasonably treated is as certainly curable as a cold or a fever.* Recovery is the rule; permanent disease the exception.

Dr. Bell, in one of his Reports of the McLean Hospital, at Somerville, states that the records of the institution justify the declaration, that "*all cases certainly recent,* that is, whose origin does not directly or obscurely run back more than a year, *recover under a fair trial.*" In this opinion Dr. Ray, formerly of the Maine State Hospital, now physician elect to the Butler Asylum, R. Island, fully concurs.

The Directors of the Ohio Hospital, at Columbus, observe in their third annual report, " that the importance of remedial means in the *first* stages of insanity, cannot be too strongly impressed upon the public mind."

Dr. Woodward, of the Massachusetts State Hospital, repeats in nearly every report, and renews arguments, for the *seasonable* treatment of the insane.

Dr. Chandler, late of the New Hampshire Hospital, says, in the report of 1843, that " it *is well established,* that the *earlier* patients are placed under curative treatment in hospitals, the *more sure and speedy* is the recovery."

Dr. Brigham, Superintendent of the State Asylum at N. York, states that, "few things relating to the management of the insane are so *well established,* as the necessity of their *early* treatment, and their removal from home in order to effect recovery. By examining the records of well constructed lunatic asylums, it appears that *more than eight in ten recent cases recover,* while *not more than one in six* of the old cases are cured."

Dr. Awl, of Ohio, remarks in his fifth report, " that fearful as is the disease of insanity, the experience of this and other institutions of the United States, have clearly shown, that *with seasonable* aid, it is by no means an incurable disease; that under *proper medical* and *moral treatment,* a large proportion do perfectly recover. And of those who are absolutely incurable, a vast number can always be greatly improved, and made comfortable and useful. We unhesitatingly conclude, that the *only safe* and correct course, either for the insane themselves, or for their friends and society, is to provide ample accommodations for them, where there will be opportunity for every one to experience comfort and relief."

Dr. Earle, of the Bloomingdale Hospital, in the report for 1844, states that " it appears to be very satisfactorily proved, that of cases where there is no eccentricity or constitutional weakness of intellect, and where the proper remedial measures are adopted in the *early* stages of the disorder, no less than eighty of every one hundred are cured. *There are few acute diseases from which so large a per centage* of the persons attacked are restored."

" *One of the chief obstacles* to a more general recovery of the patients admitted into public institutions, and one of the principal causes of the great accumulation of deranged people in the community, *is the neglect* of removing them to an Asylum, as soon *as possible after* the commencement of the disease. The mistaken kindness of friends in detaining the patient at home until the period most favorable to recovery is past, has undoubtedly been the cause of rendering the disease of hundreds of maniacs permanent." "After the first three months of the existence of derangement, the probabilities of cure rapidly diminish, and at the expiration of a year, it is believed that they are not half so great as at first. If continued beyond that time, the diminution progresses, so that of such as have been deranged more than two years, the number that recover is comparatively very small; supposed by some physicians to be about one in thirty; yet hope is left, and cures are sometimes effected of those whose disorder has existed five, ten, and even fifteen years. *It would seem that every consideration of humanity and duty requires a greater practical attention to these important truths.*"

An experienced writer on insanity, says, " It appears to me, that no idea relating to this unfortunate portion of our fellow-beings is more essential to keep before the community, than *the importance of attending to the first indications of insanity, and the immediate adoption of judicious medical and moral treatment.* The records of hospitals establish the fact that insanity is a disease that can be generally cured, if early and properly treated, while it is equally well established, that if the disease is neglected, or suffered to continue for two or three years it is difficult of remedy. That such should be the result is evident from the nature of the disease. Insanity is a disease of the physical system—a disease of the brain, and the *mental disorder is but one of its symptoms.* Insanity never arises till the *brain,* the *organ* of the mind, becomes affected."

Dr. Rockwell, of the Vermont Asylum says, " It is *very important that the insane should be placed under treatment in the early stages of the disease.*"

Dr. Kirkbride expressly urges in his reports of the Pennsylvania Hospital for the Insane, " the exceeding importance under every aspect of the case, of *early, prompt removal* to suitable hospitals; by which large numbers would be restored to health and to society, who now are a burthen to themselves and their friends."

Drs. Allen, Stribbling, Fisher, Butler, Stedman, Galt, and others who conduct the hospitals in the United States, concur in these views, and urge them in all or nearly all the reports which are annually issued from their respective institutions.

In the Ohio State Asylum, 1842, *twenty-five* old cases, suffered to become incurable, had cost to the State and counties $50,600, while *twenty-five recent* cases, brought under seasonable treatment, had cost but $1,130, that is, forty-five dollars twenty cents for each individual.

In the Massachusetts State Hospital, *twenty-five* old cases had cost the State $54,157, while the whole average number of recent cases recovered, cost but *fifty-eight* dollars, *forty-five* cents. Similar facts are exhibited upon the records of other institutions, and we have thus positive demonstration of the usefulness of hospital treatment in the two-fold, but not comparable results of health-restoring, and property-saving advantages.

Surely, if partial deafness, or failing sight, or inflammation upon the lungs assail our friend, we do not rashly defer calling on the physician to aid, by his superior knowledge our own cares, nor do we fail to surround the invalid with all those circumstances which shall seem most likely to control and cure the disease. On the access of fever or pneumonia, we lose no time in applying the most approved remedies, together with the most skilful nursing, yet we venture, with a strange hardihood, to tamper with that delicate organ, the brain, and delay the remedial measures till the case becomes, if not quite hopeless, nearly so. I have paused longer on this topic than I was aware, but its exceeding importance, the influence the decisions of friends and relatives exert on *life and health, and all life's dearest interests,* urge all who have knowledge on this subject, to enforce earnestly and firmly the duty of seasonable attention to appropriate care, and medical treatment for the insane. Numerous and deeply affecting examples of domestic trial, and individual suffering, through ill-judging and ill-judged management of the insane, exist in many private families in Kentucky. These cases not being a *public* charge, and not under official control, I do not feel at liberty to record ; but sure I am, that there will be few readers of these pages who will not be able to furnish, through their own recollection, examples which will sustain my position,—examples powerfully appealing to every just and humane sentiment in the community.

Are there not many who will read this page, who, like myself, can recal the lone husband and father wearing out a woful life in the dreary block-house, almost within the shadow of his own roof; ' without clothes, for if he was furnished, he would rend them in pieces ; without bed, for if that was supplied, it would be destroyed; without bathing or shaving, till he resembles the beasts of the forest; without fire, for with it he would burn the building ; in a cheerless block-house, for if a less solid structure, he would break through it !'

Are there none who remember the dull victim of melancholy delusions, harrassed by unreflecting neighbors, hurrying away to find refuge from their thoughtless persecutions, beneath the waters of the nigh flowing river? Are there none who recollect the son and brother, swinging his clanking chain within a slight and comfortless cabin, clamoring and hooting at the passers by, vociferous, dangerous, and destitute of all appropriate care ; dangerous when at large, and wretched under the weary bondage of his chains ? Will none have heard of the delirious epileptic girl, whose troublesome habits and mischievous propensities bring upon her the cutting lash, and who, driven by this merciless discipline, to wilder freaks, and more frequent paroxysms, is an object of deepest pity. These scenes, these hapless conditions of the insane are terrible, but these, and others not dissimilar, are not unusually the result, so much of barbarious dispositions on the part of kindred, (the last case excepted,) as the consequence of ignorance upon the right treatment demanded for the insane, and a failure to *realize* the great sufferings which ill-directed management create and aggravate. Let all, and each, throughout our country, learn the benefits of hospital treatment, and unite to secure these benefits to all the insane, of whatever rank or condition.

The dread of severe measures, in the treatment of the insane in hospitals is passing away from the minds of all who seek information concerning them. In these *the rule of right, and the law of kindness* are known to prevail. Severity and harsh measures of coersion are long since abandoned. Gentleness and persuasion unite with a mild decision, to control the wayward and the perverse, and to quiet the raving maniac.

The good and truly noble St. Vincent de Paul, was the first apostle in this holy work to turn men's thoughts in Europe, to more humane and more rational modes of treatment. With a devotion which no hardships could subdue, he traversed vast regions, and taught men the sublime lesson, that to be humane, was to be allied to Deity. Pinel, in France, carried to this blessed reform the manly tenderness and clear reasonings of his noble heart and intellect; thousands owe to his determined exertions their salvation from a bondage more terrible than death; their recovery of the lapsed powers of the mind; their restoration to reason, to usefulness, and to happiness. England and the United States are far advanced in this humane work; but, all is not done; too much remains to be done; let none supinely rest while such loud calls are raised through the land for the succour of these afflicted beings.

Gentlemen of the Legislature, I ask of you such an appropriation from the State Treasury for the hospital at Lexington, as shall place that, your first and most liberally established institution for the insane, upon a suitable foundation. As this, when completed, will be altogether inadequate to the necessities of your citizens, I ask for the establishment of a new hospital in the Southern, or Green River Country; and to this end, solicit the early adoption of such preliminary measures as shall enable you the next year, rapidly to carry forward and complete that work. The evils of delay are incalculable; they must be obvious; they should not be allowed to increase. I ask, that in the choice of a site for a new hospital, the very important appropriation of a tract of land of sufficient extent to furnish labor for the patients, and supplies for the institution, may be a first consideration. This should be chosen in a healthful district, command cheerful views, be accessible to and from a shire-town, be of convenient access by good stage-routes and water conveyances from different portions of the State; it should have an ample and unfailing supply of pure water; be so situated as to command fuel at moderate rates; and abundant stores of provisions at reasonable cost. It is worthy of consideration to embrace in this view the advantage of vicinity to a stone-quarry, or to clay strata suitable for the manufacture of brick. I respectfully suggest the appointment of an efficient Board of Commissioners to carry these objects into effect.

Legislators of Kentucky, from the discussions arising out of conflicting interests, and diverse opinions, questions of various weight, and some, possibly, of doubtful advantage; before you shall dissolve this session, consecrate one hour, uninfluenced by selfish aims, local prejudices, or political differences, to the solemn and sacred interests of suffering humanity. United by an exalted motive, be the instruments of a wide spreading happiness, and the creators of enduring benefits. The heart of many a child of misfortune, released from pangs of deep distress, through your just legislation, shall upbear you daily to the gates of heaven in prayers of gratitude. To use the language of one of our high-souled citizens, " the truest tokens of grandeur in a State are, the diffusion of the greatest happiness among the greatest number; and that God-like Justice which controls the relations of the State to all the people who are committed to its charge." Let your hospitals and your asylums rival your schools and your colleges; so multiply the "links in that golden chain by which Humanity shall connect itself with the throne of God!"

The clarion note of "Kentucky, old Kentucky"!—rings through the land. She claims eminence in her political station amidst the Star-crowned Sisters; she exults in the far told history of her military renown; but there is a moral eminence far transcending political distinctions; and a more glorious renown than is sounded from the trumpet of victorious battles:—bid her to a place in the firmament of heaven; there enthroned by her holy deeds of charity and love, inscribe her name on that scroll of history borne by angels—and sealed by arch-angels for the archives of eternity!

Respectfully submitted,

D. L. DIX.

Frankfort, February, 1846.

APPENDIX.

TABLE *showing the comparative expense of supporting old and recent cases of insanity, from which we learn the economy of placing patients in institutions in the early periods of disease ; from the report of the Massachusetts State Hospital, for 1843.*

No. of old cases.	Present age.	Time insane, in years.	Total expense, at $100 a year, before entering the hospital, and $132 a year since; last year $120.	Number of recent cases discharged.	Present age.	Time insane, in weeks.	Cost of support, at $2 30 per week.
2	60	28	$3,212 00	1,622	30	7	$16 10
7	48	17	2,004 00	1,624	34	20	46 00
8	60	21	2,504 00	1,625	51	32	73 60
12	47	25	2,894 00	1,635	23	28	64 40
18	71	34	3,794 00	1,642	42	40	92 00
19	59	18	2,204 00	1,643	55	14	32 20
21	39	16	1,993 00	1,645	63	36	82 80
27	47	16	1,994 00	1,649	22	40	92 00
44	56	26	2,982 00	1,650	36	28	64 40
45	60	25	2,835 00	1,658	36	14	32 20
102	53	25	2,833 00	1,660	21	16	36 80
133	44	13	1,431 00	1,661	19	27	62 10
176	55	20	2,486 00	1,672	40	11	25 70
200	39	16	1,964 00	1,676	23	23	52 90
223	50	20	2,364 00	1,688	23	11	25 70
260	47	16	2,112 00	1,690	23	27	62 10
278	49	10	1,424 00	1,691	37	20	46 00
319	53	10	1,247 00	1,699	30	28	64 40
347	58	14	1,644 00	1,705	24	17	39 10
367	40	12	1,444 00	1,706	55	10	23 00
400	43	14	1,644 00	1,709	17	10	23 00
425	48	13	2,112 00	1,715	19	40	92 00
431	36	13	1,412 00	1,716	35	48	110 40
435	55	15	1,712 00	1,723	52	55	126 50
488	37	17	1,912 00	1,737	30	33	75 90
		454	$54,157 00			635	$1,461 30

From Dr. Awl's reports of the Ohio Institution, we extract the following tables:

In 1841, whole cost of twenty-five old cases, - - - - - - - $49,248 00
Average, - - - - - - - - - - - - - - 1,969 00
Whole cost of twenty-five recent cases, - - - - - - - 1,330 50
Average, - - - - - - - - - - - - - 52 22

In 1842, whole expense of twenty-five old cases, - - - - - - - $50,611 00
Average, - - - - - - - - - - - - - - 2,020 00
Whole expense of twenty-five recent cases, - - - - - - - 1,130 00
Average, - - - - - - - - - - - - - 45 20

In this institution, in 1843, twenty old cases had cost, - - - - - $44,782 00
Average cost of old cases, - - - - - - - - - - 2,239 10
Whole expense of twenty recent cases, till recovered, - - - - - 1,308 30
Average cost of recent cases, - - - - - - - - - - 65 41

In the Ohio Lunatic Asylum, in 1844, twenty-five old cases had cost, - - $35,464 00
Average expense of old cases, - - - - - - - - - 1,418 56
Whole expense of twenty-five recent cases, - - - - - - - 1,608 00
Average expense of recent cases, - - - - - - - - 64 32

In the Massachusetts State Lunatic Asylum, in 1843, twenty-five old cases had cost, $54,157 00
Average expense of old cases, - - - - - - - - - - 2,166 20
Whole expense of twenty-five recent cases, till recovered, - - - - - 1,461 30
Average expense of recent cases, - - - - - - - - 58 45

In the Maine Lunatic Hospital, in 1842, twelve old cases had cost, - - - $25,300 00
Average expense of old cases - - - - - - - - - - 2,108 33
Whole expense of twelve recent cases, - - - - - - - 426 00
Average expense of recent cases, - - - - - - - - 35 50

In the Hospital at Staunton, Va., twenty old cases had cost, - - - - $41,633 00
Average expense of old cases, - - - - - - - - - 2,081 65
Whole expense of twenty recent cases, - - - - - - - - 1,265 00
Average expense of recent cases, - - - - - - - - 63 25

The results of this table are striking, and show conclusively the importance of early admission to the insane hospitals. Other institutions have instituted the same inquiries with similar results.

REVIEW

KENTUCKY

1846

A REVIEW

OF THE

PRESENT CONDITION OF THE

STATE PENITENTIARY OF KENTUCKY,

WITH BRIEF NOTICES AND REMARKS UPON THE

JAILS AND POOR-HOUSES

IN SOME OF THE

MOST POPULOUS COUNTIES.

WRITTEN BY REQUEST.

PRINTED BY ORDER OF THE LEGISLATURE.

BY D. L. DIX.

FRANKFORT:
A. G. HODGES:::::::::STATE PRINTER.
1846.

REVIEW.

To my Readers, respectfully :—

I have very cheerfully complied with the request of several members of the Legislature, and many citizens in counties I have visited, to furnish the result of observations upon the present condition of the Penitentiary at Frankfort, and some extracts from my note-book relating to the Jails, and to the modes of supporting the poor in this State, so far as observation has extended. In regard to the insane poor, I here say but little, and furnish no illustrative facts, for *in the jails and poor-houses of Kentucky there are no insane.* The spirit of humanity and sense of justice has prevailed here, and provision for kind oversight and hospital treatment for a large part of this class, has been made at Lexington. This provision is insufficient for all the insane of the State,—those in moderate and affluent circumstances cannot, without additions to the present Institution, and the establishment of another, share these great benefits; but they have, as was right, first been supplied to the most necessitous. I have discussed this subject elsewhere, and pass to others which claim consideration.

The hope is indulged that the perusal of these pages may lead to a more careful attention to the construction of jails, and to a reformation and alteration of many already built, as well as direct the thoughts to the expediency of establishing in some of the most populous districts, work-houses, or *houses of correction.* These are greatly needed, especially for women-offenders. It is apparent, that for a series of years, even if it were ever a *proper* arrangement to unite prisons for men and women convicts, that it must be attended with great expense, to conduct decently, under a system that the people will tolerate, a prison for women, under the same administration as the State Penitentiary. A county-house of correction might receive for a long time all the women-convicts who are likely to be sentenced to imprisonment and labor.

A very benevolent feeling towards the poor prevails in this State; and many families, by judicious assistance, added to their own labors, are saved from becoming paupers. So far as a condition of entire dependence can be guarded against, great good is thus secured for the individual, as well as good to society in general. Nothing sinks a person's self-respect, and creates the " don't care feeling," like suspending exertion for self-support. We see daily the effect of this influence in large towns and cities.

The system adopted in Kentucky for the support of pauper idiots, is peculiar to this State, and combines both evils and advantages. Indiscriminate association of idiots in families with other children, has often been observed to have injurious influences : on the contrary, these unfortunates are more carefully and kindly looked after by parents than by strangers. But I think there can arise no question as to the greater fitness of gathering these often helpless creatures into an Asylum in which they may be surrounded with every needed care. The sum now annually paid out by the State for the maintenance of indigent idiots, would, in two years, suffice to build a spacious and comfortable Hospital, or rather Asylum, into which all might be gathered, and to support them therein, and after that time, the cost would be, it is computed, much less. In 1845, the sum of $17,500 62 cents was paid out of the Treasury for this class, that is, for 450 individuals. The allowance is not to exceed $50 to any one beneficiary; but in cases where parents or friends afford partial support, it is proportionably less. The increased number of idiots during seventeen years seems to have exceeded the proportion usually computed, allowing for the increase of population. I ascribe this in part, and in large part, to the intemperance of parents. The fact that habits of intoxication induces partial or entire imbecility in children, in frequent instances, is too well established to require proof here. This result is often apparent in infancy and childhood, and is also developed at later periods in active insanity, which passes rapidly into dementia, and is followed by permanent idiocy.

Idiots are not here placed in poor-houses, and this is right. They never should be; they are, in Kentucky, either boarded in private families, having a guardian, who receives the appropriation of the State, or in their own families, who receive the pension from the State, and in some cases, if dangerous to go at large, they are removed to the State Hospital.

The following table shows the amount of the annual State appropriation for this class during the past seventeen years:

A Statement showing the amount paid out of the Treasury of the Commonwealth of Kentucky, for the support of Idiots, from the year 1829, to the year 1845, inclusive, viz:

For the year 1829,	$ 8,640 47
For the year 1830,	10,049 72
For the year 1831,	11,746 65
For the year 1832,	12,974 19
For the year 1833,	11,949 17
For the year 1834,	12,765 82
For the year 1835,	12,563 62
For the year 1836,	15,227 28
For the year 1837,	14,966 94
For the year 1838,	16,797 87
For the year 1839,	16,876 75
For the year 1840,	17,358 41
For the year 1841,	13,568 59
For the year 1842,	15,536 13
For the year 1843,	14,880 33
For the year 1844,	16,468 87
For the year 1845,	17,500 62
Total,	$239,871 43

I have spent much less time in the several counties through which I have journied, in Kentucky, than is my usage, when visiting prisons and poor-houses; but there has been no necessity for more. I have found invariably, from the records of the county Clerks, and from an examination of the jails, that there are fewer paupers, and fewer prisoners in detention, than I have found in any other State. While I most heartily and decidedly condemn the construction of the prisons, a few excepted, and while I see no urgent call for the establishment of poor-houses, except in large towns and in cities, and have felt deeply convinced of the absolute need of additional provisions for the insane of *all* classes, in Kentucky, I have perceived an awakening and earnest spirit upon many great questions involving social happiness, and public prosperity. More interest is felt in the cause of common school education, and greater attention is given to secure competent teachers in all institutions of learning.

I have every where been, stranger as I am, and traveling alone, received courteously and respectfully, and my objects promoted with ready good-will, and often with a zeal and kindness which has greatly lessened the weariness and difficulties of my journeys. On a deliberate review of the past, I find that no four months, during the last five years have offered to my observation as little of human privation, misery, and suffering in any form, and under any circumstances, and *all* circumstances, and an equal amount of ease, and enjoyment of the common comforts of life, amongst the largest numbers, and so wide a diffusion of general cheerfulness and contentment, as in the forty-four counties through which I have passed, in Kentucky.

I should prefer to see the benefits of moral and mental culture more widely diffused, more careful habits of self-discipline, a more just estimate of social advantages, and of civil rights, but without question, *progress, advancement*, and rectitude, are in the ascendant; the aspects of society vary : much is to be done, but the " life of man is in him," and however one might, from glancing hastily on the surface of society, at times fasten the gaze more steadily and anxiously upon the shadows, rather than upon the lights of the picture, the conviction is kindled into full belief, that the shadows are dispersing, and the lights breaking into fuller radiance. All States and people seem at times to be merged in a moral eclipse; so it has been from the beginning, and so will it continue to be. But God's spirit strives with man, and the Created own the influence of the Creator.

The principal defects of the county prisons herein described, with but two or three exceptions, are as follows :

They are badly planned, dangerous often for the keeper, if he has in custody desperate prisoners; inconvenient of access; often insecure, and exposing the prisoners to communication with persons outside, or, they are so extremely close as seriously to impair health, and often endanger life. They are chiefly *unfurnished, unventilated, damp, imperfectly lighted ; not warmed, and not cleansed* when occupied; not sufficiently supplied with water, and deficient in some of the most important arrangements for daily cleanliness and health. The prisoners are without employment for mind or hands; occasionally a few books are loaned by the keeper. The jails are seldom so built as to afford the means of separating or classing the prisoners. But I need not multiply examples of defect in the construction of county prisons. I know of but one point where there is not disadvantage or suffering, and that is controlled by the jailer : the prisoners, with rare exceptions, are amply supplied with food of good quality.

As a man, till he is by court and jury found and proved guilty, is, in the just eye of the law supposed to be innocent, as he is as yet not legally condemned nor sentenced, it seems to me to be illegal, as well as inhuman, to surround him for weeks and months with painful circumstances, affecting him both mentally and physically—impairing, or at least wasting the mind, and confirming, if not originating idle and injurious habits. Man is made for action; if not furnished with the means of doing well, he will surely do ill; he will be hourly growing worse; he will continually recede farther and farther from virtue, and sink lower and lower in the scale of humanity. The county jails of our country, with few exceptions, are seats of misery, and *schools* of *vice*. In these, every better sentiment is effaced ; and whether the prisoners are ultimately acquitted and discharged, or found guilty and sentenced to the Penitentiary, they quit the county jails worse, more corrupt, more degraded, than when they were first arrested. These results are beginning to be viewed in their true light, and communities are wakening to the facts of the inconsistency and injustice of holding culprits in prisons under such circumstances as to *ensure* their moral degradation, and destroy in them the traces of good which crime, and folly, and sin, heretofore had spared. Not till county prisons are differently constructed, and differently administered, need we look for reformations in the penitentiaries, or improvement upon the restoration of convicts to society?

On this subject I need not here expatiate, for I find a just sense awakened upon the condition of the county prisons in all but three or four counties. The most enlightened of the citizens, and the most humane of all classes, speak strongly on these subjects; and none with greater emphasis than the Judges of the Courts, and members of the bar generally. Even in Lincoln, Fayette, Clinton, and Jessamine counties, strong expressions of disapprobation and of disgust and indignation respecting either the construction or the management of their jails reached me. It cannot be long that defects in the construction, or misapplication of the use of the county prisons, will be tolerated.

STATE PENITENTIARY OF KENTUCKY, AT FRANKFORT.

This Institution, established in 1798, and partly rebuilt and remodeled since 1840, has from time to time had great difficulties to contend with, from various causes, but from none more serious and depressing to its financial concerns, than during the past year and a half, consequent upon the disastrous fire which consumed the work-shops, tools, stock, &c., throwing at once the affairs of the prison into the utmost confusion, and creating inconveniences which to this hour affect the prosperity of its condition ; and which must still for a considerable period, continue to be experienced, from delays in restoring the buildings.

In examining and commenting upon the prison as it now is, justice demands that these adverse circumstances should be kept in mind.

This Penitentiary is not a model, by comparison ; it is not excellent, for the objects proposed, viz : *correction*, and more for *reformation*. In short, it exhibits some great defects. But there are in connection with it two very encouraging circumstances: first, that the public mind is every year becoming more alive to the importance of improving the government and discipline of prisons, and more sensible of the obligation the virtuous portion of the community owe, to exert a reforming, enlightening influence over criminals, and all transgressors. The best interests of society, and of our country, no less than the high duties of Christianity urge this; but secondly, an encouraging view is afforded in regarding this prison, from what, after much inquiry and examination seems to be the fact, that whatever are the faults now observable in its discipline and administration, it is certainly in many respects, in a better condition, so far as the prisoners are considered, than it has ever been before. This opinion is based on conviction, and expressed from the belief that it is due to the present lessee and keeper of the State Penitentiary. Whether it depends upon this officer, upon the Executive, or upon the Legislature, or upon all these influences combined, to procure a speedy and effectual remedy for defects to be stated, it is believed that no delay need intervene, and that none will be allowed to intervene, if the *utility* of changes and improvements can be demonstrated. These will be referred to in course of a brief description of the above named Institution.

The prison and its appendages are enclosed within a stone wall 26 feet high, and 4 feet thick at base, of sufficient strength for present purposes.

The area enclosed contains two acres, and the various factories, shops, smoke-house, and lodging-prison, are of dimensions as follows:—The large building as you enter the yard on the right, is *forty* feet by *two hundred* and *twenty*; is two stories high, and built of brick, with a shingle roof. The ground floor is occupied with the engine and machinery, the carpenter, and the black-smith's shop. The second story is appropriated to tailors, harness-makers, carriage-trimmers, and finishers of the ornamental work upon carriages, chairs, &c., also to the coopers and bagging-weavers; these are directly above the smith's shops, and the atmosphere is loaded with smoke from below, and hemp dust from the looms, much, it seems to me, to the detriment of health and comfort.

A building on the side of the area opposite to this, *two hundred* and *four feet* by *forty*, two stories high, built of brick, and shingled, is occupied on the ground floor by the hacklers of hemp at one end, and the bagging-filling spinners on the other. The dust constantly filling the atmosphere like a dense cloud, is at times quite intolerable. The second story is occupied by the bagging chain spinners, through its entire length. A small building near this is used as the shoe-maker's shop; and in the centre of the yard is the stone-cutter's shed. The smoke-house is of brick, *thirty* feet by *forty*, two stories high, and is situated nearly opposite the entrance to the yard.

A new building of dressed stone and brick, *twenty feet* square, stands out in the yard, eight or ten feet from the men's lodging prison. Ostensibly, this is for the women's prison, though from its *plan* and *location*, it cannot be applied to that use, without outraging every decency of life. I feel fully justified in the assertion, that neither the respectable citizens of Kentucky, the Executive, nor the Legislature, will suffer its use, as a prison for women, after more than one experiment, if one ever should be made. It can by no possibility be converted into an Infirmary, which is greatly needed, for not one solitary arrangement rendering it suitable for such a use is planned, and the dimensions less even than the present Hospital, would negative such a proposition.

I do not speak unadvisedly, in saying that if this building is completed, it will be a standing monument of the misapplication of funds, to whatever purpose it may be applied, and if, (as is not probable) as a prison for women, it will without doubt be condemned as a nuisance by the first visiting Grand Jury.

The outer wall of the enclosing prison, is in length 210 feet, by 40 wide. The cell-prison is 190 by 20. The area is 10 feet wide on all sides.

The surrounding area being below the surface of the adjacent yard, and there being no floor over the ground on which the cell-prison is built, every storm of rain affords an influx of water, which produces a strata of mud, and much of the time, increases dampness over the area.* One iron stove serves to temper the atmosphere, but not to maintain at any time sufficient dryness and warmth. Several fires ought to be sustained here, at all seasons, at once to procure dryness and ventilation. One window on the outer wall admits through the gratings a glimmering light and some air. I have always found lampsor candles burning here at mid-day to yield so much light as the business of sweeping, &c., require. The interior of the cells, except immediately nigh the entrance, or opposite the window referred to, can be seen only by artificial light, at any season. And this is one reason possibly, why they are never properly white-washed and cleansed. The cell-prison within, contains 252 cells in three tiers, of 42 upon each side of the ground floor and galleries.

The dimensions of the cells are 3½ feet by 7, and 7 high from the centre of the arch. Of the ventilation I can only say that it is exceedingly defective. The ground floor cells have two ventilating passages, each about 4 inches diameter, but so constructed as to be of little, if indeed they are of any use; they terminate, I am told, in the attic. The cells of the second and third stories, while they required of course a larger supply of pure air, have but one ventilator, and that is of no avail. When the outer door of the prison is closed at night, whether in winter or in summer, the air must be very impure and deleterious, especially loaded as it is, with various offensive animal exhalations. †

The cells are furnished with a few cot-bedsteads, and other various substitutes for bedsteads, but the largest part are without either. The floor of the cells is of board or plank, and bed-clothing. such as it is, is thrown thereon. There are 176 prisoners, and more cells than convicts; yet for months, and I know not how much longer, two men have been lodged in most of the ground-floor cells on the front side. Two reasons have been assigned for this improper arrangement; one as given to the "House Committee," that "the last year and before, they were badly infested with fleas, and were thrown two in a cell, in order to scrub and cleanse the others thus left vacant!" Another reason, and one often assigned upon various and sufficient authority, is that the beds are poor, and the bed-clothing quite insufficient to maintain a tolerable warmth in the cells during the night; therefore, *this cheap method* of supplying substitutes for the sufficient furnishing of the cells has been adopted! I respectfully suggest that some appropriation from the "*Sinking Fund*," be made, in order to supply present wants, and enable the keeper to enforce the statute; which see. (An act to regulate the Penitentiary,) approved January 29, 1829., vol. 2, page 1315, No. 1829, Sec. 4.

---

* The roof is much out of repair, and admits so much water as greatly to increase this evil.

† This section of the prison was planned, and built before the present Lessee took possession.

"*Be it further enacted*, That when the said improvements shall have been completed, it shall be the duty of the Keeper of the Penitentiary, for all time thereafter, to cause the convicts to be locked up *separately* in the cells of the Penitentiary, during *each night*, and as far as practicable, prevent all conversation between them during the day." Also: "The said keeper shall prevent any two or more of the convicts from conversing, sleeping, or in any manner associating together, except when the nature of their employments require it." No. 1805, H. R. Stat., vol. 2, page 1811.

The cells necessarily, and with due consideration on the part of the keeper, are lighted for a time in the evening. This, especially, is a kind and judicious plan, when the very bad construction of the lodging-prison is considered. It is to be hoped that one of the first improvements here, will be breaking windows through the wall of the outer building, for the admission both of light and air, by day and by night.

Perhaps something might be saved in the construction of *the 20 foot prison* for this reasonable demand!

The dimensions of the lodging-cells in the Penitentiary at Frankfort, correspond with those of the prisons at Sing-Sing, Charlestown, and Wethersfield: in all of which the ventilation is considered very defective, although they have this obvious advantage over the Frankfort prison, viz: better constructed flues, and the recurrence of windows at small distances along the walls of the enclosing prisons. And again, at Wethersfield the most exact cleanliness is preserved, while both at Sing-Sing and Charlestown it is not overlooked. At Frankfort, the usage has been to white-wash, *once a year*. In most Penitentiaries where white-wash is not in daily use, it is employed once a fortnight, or once a month; but the prevailing usage is to charge several of the infirm convicts who are not possessed of bodily strength for hard labor, to keep the cells swept, scrubbed, and to apply white-wash, which is always kept prepared in buckets, to every part of each cell, when at all discolored. This is not expensive, and it conduces to health, to cleanliness, and to improved personal habits. I concede, that from all accounts from all quarters, friends and unfriends of this prison, that it is *better than ever before*. Let no pains be spared to render it greatly more comfortable than it now is in all the cell arrangements.

It must be obvious at a glance, that needed facilities for labor; for carrying forward work profitably, for convenience, for health, and finally, for greater security against conflagrations, urge an extension of the present prison bounds. To those acquainted with the situation of the prison and adjacent premises, it must be apparent that the lot of land extending from the prison wall on the   to   St., is a necessary addition to the property already possessed. Nor do the above named reasons afford the sole arguments for inducing the purchase of said property by the State. In process of time, the lot referred to will, if not already secured, be taken up and built upon by private individuals. Overlooking dwelling-houses or stores, would be a serious disadvantage to the prison, would inevitably interfere with discipline, and conduct to communication with the prisoners from abroad, which the officers would have it in their power neither wholly to control nor prevent.

An enclosure now used as a lumber yard and surrounded by an expensive wall might well be used for either constructing thereon a woman's prison, with suitable apartments for a *matron and assistants*, or an Infirmary might be constructed there, using the ground floor of the building as a store-room, and the second as a Hospital. The present Hospital and guard-room above might be converted, if needed here, into a women's prison, at small expense, throwing in light from elevated windows in the outer wall.

LABOR.—The men appear to be quiet and diligent in the several departments where their labor is assigned, and no extraordinary force seems to be exerted to maintain discipline and industry.

PUNISHMENTS, apparently in a measure discretionary; no record is kept or required; but the statute is intended to control abuses in this respect; the keeper being first authorized, with the approbation of the inspector (Governor,) to establish such rules and regulations for the government of the convicts as he shall judge necessary, is limited in the enforcement of said rules, by the following concluding clause of the section : " In case of disobedience by any convicts to perform his or her duty, or of a violation of any rule or order, the keeper may inflict punishment proportionate to the offence, by *confinement to the solitary cell,* or by *stripes, at his discretion :* Provided, *that in no case shall the number of stripes exceed ten for the same offence at any one time; nor the confinement exceed forty-eight hours at one time, for the same offence."* See H. R. No. 4088, vol. 2, page 1311, No. 1806, Sec. 4, Statute Law.

I have had no opportunities of absolute personal knowledge, but from very general observation should decide that this prison is under a free discipline. In relation to punishments, I find the following rule laid down by the present keeper for the direction of the officers: "The prisoner offending must be committed to the dark cell, till the co-operation of the keeper can be conveniently had, as the inflicting of corporeal punishment by an assistant, without the advice of the keeper, is positively forbidden.

DIET.—The food seems of good quality, and afforded in sufficient supplies. It is coarse, but substantial, and wholesome. " Allowance, 1¾ lbs. bread, made of corn meal. Meat, if bacon, ¾ lb., if beef, 1¼. Rye coffee without sugar, for breakfast. They are furnished with vegetables in their season, two or three times a week; Irish potatoes, turnips and cabbages, are supplied in abundance. Soup is served often, made of beef, potatoes, cabbages, and turnips, at which times the quantity of meat is lessened, but bread not. They are supplied with butter-milk during summer and autumn; and a special diet is allowed to the sick. See Physician's Report, 1846.

The prisoners eat in common, and in a temporary shed not impervious to the weather, since the destructive fire before referred to. An eating-room is to be built shortly, or in course of another year.

CLOTHING.—The clothing of the convicts seems sufficient for general comfort, and I have observed that the apparel wears a decent appearance as respects wholeness; most of the labor engaged in would be an impediment to cleanness, as a daily rule.

HEALTH.—The general health of the prison seems to be good. There have been few severe cases in the hospital of late, and one usually sees there only the feeble and infirm. The report of the attending Physicians, (who visit daily, and oftener if requisite,) shows during the year past 215 cases under treatment, and *one* death only, amongst all the prisoners. At the close of 1844, there were in confinement 151. Received into the prison during the past year, 75. Discharged by expiration of sentence, pardons, and one death, 50 : leaving, at the commencement of 1846, in confinement, 176.

INFIRMARY.—This very inconvenient and uncomfortable room should be replaced by a commodious, dry, and airy apartment, in the most quiet part of the yard, and so planned as to afford to the physicians and nurses facilities for the proper treatment and care of the sick, which the present apartment fails to give in any one particular. It is a low, dark, damp, triangular room, out of repair, and the sooner out of use altogether, the better for all parties. This room, squared, is about 18 feet by 32. In it at one time, were 39 men ill of measles!

INSANE—But two in this prison; one not a convict; comfortable.

THE GUARD-ROOM, is over the Infirmary, and is equally ill-placed, inconvenient, uncomfortable, and unsuitable for the purposes it is made to serve.

WATER.—There is an ample and unfailing supply of pure water immediately without the walls, which is available, if necessary, as well as within the prison-bounds. But one of these wells, at present, affords pure drinking water, through want of care in cleansing them. If this were done, and a few repairs directed, ample protection, so far as supplies of water are considered, would be afforded in the event of a conflagration, for the pumps would discharge as much water as the engines could throw per minute. But in addition, at a *very trifling cost*, several tanks could be constructed within each building on the second floor, and supplied, as is often done in public buildings, with rain-water from the roofs, this would be an additional means of security. As good carpenters, and coopers if needed, are on the ground, a *very small* outlay of expense would complete these precautionary measures. The Kentucky prison has decided advantage, in this respect, of full supplies of water, over almost every prison in the country, except those ordered on the separate system, where full supplies of water are invariably conveyed into, and through the water courses of every cell.

BATHS.—None, either warm or cold; only present means of bathing, probably, not adopted, viz.: immediately under the pump. Several basins and buckets on benches, afford the means of washing the face and hands. No cleansing room for prisoners when admitted, or afterward; of course, there is no bath for the sick, should such be recommended by the medical adviser. As this accommodation, this *necessity* rather than luxury, could be supplied here by an exceedingly trifling outlay of labor and money, it is hoped it may be speedily furnished for the advantage of every prisoner in the Penitentiary. I cannot but refer to the admirable arrangements by which these benefits are secured to the prisoners in the Eastern Penitentiary, at Philadelphia.

" The mode adopted," writes the late excellent Warden in last year's report, " is attended with very little expense, and is as follows:—The daily escape-steam from the engine, is passed into a tank containing about 80 hogsheads of water, which thereby is uniformly maintained at a temperature of 90°." This water, heated without expense, is conveyed through pipes into the bathing cells, " where each prisoner is furnished with fresh supplies of water, towels, and soap." Fifteen or twenty minutes suffices for bathing, and this might be done, I conceive, not only without disadvantage to the prison through loss of time, but would secure a positive gain; for who does not know that the physical energies are quickened, and the mind by sympathy, refreshed, through the invigorating appliance of water. In the prison above referred to, the prisoners use the warm bath once a week, and the cold daily, if inclined.

VISITORS.—It has seemed to me that the interests of this Institution imperatively require some check upon the indiscriminate admission of visitors, who, conducted solely by idle curiosity, resort to the prison, stroll through the yards, linger in the shops, gaze at, and make audible remarks upon the prisoners, and finally retire, having imparted no good, and it is to be feared have exercised while there, the reflective faculties, too little to have received any. There are prisoners who suffer seriously from this reckless scrutiny, and heartless observation; there are others who, indifferent and hardened, become yet more callous to their own degradation, and unfortunate condition; there are none, I boldly assert, who are made the better by it.

But aside from the moral influence, it is also adverse to the interests of the State, and of the Lessee. At times the concourse gives serious inconvenience to the officers, and interrupts and retards employment. All persons are admitted who make the request civilly, but it would appear that some check is desirable. I greatly disapprove of making an *exhibition* of *crime and misfortune*. If general visitors are received, I suggest that the sum of ten and twenty cents be required for the admission severally, of children and adults; that a record be kept of the number of those who enter, and that the proceeds thereof be appropriated, not to the treasury of the State, or profits of the keeper, but to the use of the prisoners, making a division quarterly, and allowing each who has not forfeited claim to indulgence by extreme ill-conduct, to have the same expended for books, which he may own himself, irrespective of the library; or allow to increase by quarterly additions, to be sent either to his needy family, or to furnish him with an additional sum at the time of his discharge, to the *five dollars* granted by law. I do not doubt that the Clerk of the prison would cheerfully add this to his other duties, although his office is no sinecure; and the Lessee of the Penitentiary has so often expressed wishes for advancing the good of the prisoners by all reasonable methods, that to doubt his hearty concurrence would be to impugn his sincerity; and beside, he is fully sensible of the need of a check upon the present influx of strangers within the walls.

I would suggest, that all officers of the State, the Executive and Cabinet, the members of both branches of the Legislature, State Commissioners, Judges of the Courts, and the Grand Jury be regarded as official visitors, for whom the prison is at all times to open for visitation and inspection. Also, that the Sheriffs of counties and keepers of Jails, as well as the relatives of the prisoners, under such restrictions as the keeper shall deem necessary, shall be admitted without fee. To these of course, would be added all strangers who should visit the prison from motives arising out of a desire for knowledge upon prison discipline, all ministers of religion, and persons competent to give instruction, at suitable times.

VISITATION OF CONVICTS.—Since referring to the impropriety of the free admission of visitors at the Penitentiary, I have found in the Statutes, vol. 2, H. R., page 1317, February 1833, the following act, to-wit: "No persons whatever, except the keeper, his deputies, servants or assistants, the inspectors, officers, and ministers of justice, members of the General Assembly, ministers of the gospel, *or persons producing a written license*, signed by one of the said inspectors, shall be permitted to enter within the walls where such offenders shall be confined," &c. This certainly is a wholesome enactment, and I cannot find that it has been repealed. The probability is, that it never has been enforced, not that it has fallen into disuse.

INSPECTORS.—The Governor, according to the Statute, is sole Inspector of the Penitentiary.

THE BOARD OF VISITORS, consists of the Auditor, Treasurer, Register, and Attorney General, whose duty it is, according to the Statute, " to visit the Penitentiary as often as they shall deem proper, and at least once in each month ; examine the state of the Institution, the health of the convicts, the manner of dieting them, the *cleanliness* of the *cells,* and the treatment of the convicts generally, and make such report to the Legislature as the conditions of the Institution shall require."

PERMISSIONS.—The prisoners " may converse on the business of the yard," (and the shops,) according to the by-laws. According to the Statute, the " keeper may furnish them with such quantities of tobacco as are necessary;" " may leave the bounds of the prison by direction, or permission of the keeper or guards, on specified labor connected with the prison business." I have repeatedly seen them thus employed removing materials consumed in the business of the yard.

A piece of ground is rented, outside the prison bounds, and cultivated by some of the more feeble convicts, as a vegetable garden. Indeed there are two lots so rented ; I am not sure that both are under cultivation. The vegetables so produced supply, in part, the consumption of the same by the convicts.

GENERAL, MORAL, AND RELIGIOUS INSTRUCTION.—Inquiries in the prison as to what has been attempted and is now doing under these three heads, have been very unsatisfactory. Referring to the Statutes, I find recorded from time to time, the passage of acts providing for the instruction of convicts in the Penitentiary, which afford evidence that the Legislature have for years been mindful of the improvement of the prisoners, and of their present and future well-being. No adequate appropriation has been made for securing the uniform services of a chaplain, who might unite here with special advantage, the offices of spiritual, moral, and mental instructor. In the Statutes, vol. 2, H. R., page 1315, No. 1829, A. D. 1829, the keeper is directed to procure, if possible, *one sermon to be preached by a regular minister of some religious denomination on each Sabbath,* and cause the convicts who are unlearned, in *reading, writing,* and *arithmetic,* to be taught in one or other of those branches, *at least four hours* on each Sabbath day ; and the keeper shall cause the convicts to be locked up in *separate* cells, during all the balance of the Sabbath day, not occupied in hearing, learning, or eating their regular meals : *Provided,* that the whole cost of such teaching and preaching, including guarding and all expenses, shall not exceed in the whole, two hundred and fifty dollars per annum." See also Statutes, Senate, Vol. 3, page 490. " The sum of two hundred and fifty dollars shall be *annually expended for* the *moral* and *religious* instruction of the convicts." Approved, February 24th, 1839. This is certainly explicit enough, and I should argue that being enacted without reservation as to objects, subsequent to the Statute before quoted, was to direct expressly and solely the sum of $250 to be paid for the moral and religious teaching at the prison.

The Keeper of the Penitentiary has made it his duty to secure as steadily as possible, the services of several of the resident clergymen of Frankfort on every Sunday, P. M., for a religious service. The duties of these gentlemen in connection with their respective congregations render it not practicable for them to adopt a regular course of daily visits at the prison, though

I have reason to know this is a work in which they would engage with much earnestness. There is no qualified minister or teacher, therefore, connected with the prison, rendering there those constant offices of moral and religious influences, as is now almost the universal usage in large prisons. It is true that the officers of the prison exert no counteracting influences, but it is believed quite the contrary: yet neither their duties, nor in general their habits of study and thought, qualify them for teachers and chaplains, especially where so much tact is requisite, to secure the regard and serious attention of the convicts. In 1836 the following act was passed, indicating the just views which were held by the Legislature upon affording the convicts the means of improvement through the use of books:—"That one hundred dollars be, and the same is hereby appropriated to purchase, under the direction of the Governor, from time to time, a small library of moral and religious books, for the use of the convicts now confined, and those who may hereafter be confined in the Penitentiary of the State; and the Keeper of the Penitentiary is hereby directed to have a case prepared, for the safe keeping and preservation of said books; and said Keeper shall have said books given out and returned every week, so that they shall be well taken care of." See Stat. vol. 3, Senate, page 484; also same vol., page 490, February, 1839:— " The sum of $100 is hereby appropriated to purchase, under the direction of the Governor, an additional number of moral and religious books, to be added to the present library in the Penitentiary," &c. The books heretofore purchased were all destroyed at the time of the fire, and none supplied as yet; the present year it is believed an appropriation may be made for furnishing such books as shall aid the convicts in acquiring a better common education, and advance their moral and religious knowledge. "To see your brother in ignorance," writes Jeremy Taylor, "is to see him unfurnished to all good works; and every master is to cause his family to be instructed, every governor to instruct his charge, every man his brother, by *all possible and just* provisions." Enlighten the mind, *but above all enlighten the conscience*, cultivate that knowledge, by study of the Gospel precepts, which restraineth from evil ways, and which sanctifies the heart and life; and so, assist the infirm purpose to a strong resolve, aid in reaching after virtue, and help to attain the narrow way which leads to eternal life.

The present state of Education in the Penitentiary, as reported by the Clerk, is shown by the following table:

Classical education, - - - - - - - -	1
Good English education, - - - - - - -	8
Common, viz.: read, write, and cypher, - - - -	60
Spell and read, only, - - - - - - - -	54
Entirely destitute of education, - - - - - -	53
	—-176
AGES.—From fifteen to twenty, - - - - - -	20
twenty to thirty, - - - - - -	93
thirty to forty, - - - - - -	39
forty to fifty, - - - - - -	11
fifty to sixty, - - - - - -	12
sixty to seventy, - - - - - -	1
	—-176

The above are all men; during the last ten years, eight women only, have been sentenced to the Penitentiary; most of these have received an early discharge by pardon. It is to be hoped that a House of Correction will be established in Jefferson Co. by that county, and to which the State may send such women convicts as are brought under the just penalties of the law, paying the expense to that Institution, rather than maintain them in the men's prison, at Frankfort.

SUPPORT OF THE POOR,

AND CONSTRUCTION AND CONDITION OF

COUNTY JAILS.

WOODFORD COUNTY Poor-House, removed from the immediate vicinity of Versailles, seems to receive an unusual amount of care and attention. Fortunately for the good government of this establishment, there are several citizens in the county heartily interested in the best well-being of the inmates; it is too often the case that these are forgotten, except when official business recals the fact of their existence. I think that the ordering of the general affairs of the House, as furnished in a document from the hands of the County Clerk, may be of both interest and use, and herewith copy it nearly entire.

"At November Court, 1844, the Superintendent of the Poor-House, was appointed by the following order:

" It is ordered that Silas Elliston be, and he is hereby appointed Overseer of the Poor-House, at a salary of $120, until November county Court, 1845, and he is to work the Poor-House farm for the support of the poor of said county, and of his own family, and to make any improvements which he can accomplish by his own labor that the committe of the Poor-House may direct, and any surplus of the produce of said farm shall be the property of the county, subject to be sold by the committee of the Poor-House, &c.

"The above contract was renewed in Nov. 1845. The committee is appointed from the Justices who compose the County Court. At November, $150 was appropriated to pay the Superintendent, and $200 was granted for the use of the poor.

" It is made the duty of two of the Justices to visit the Poor-House every sixty days.

"The Report of the committee of the Poor-House, made at November court, 1845, shows an expenditure for the poor, from the first of January, 1844, to first of November, 1845, (including $150 paid Overseer, at one time, and $120 subsequently:) of $520, the balance expended for clothing, food, sugar, coffee, &c., for the poor. Any of the poor who are aggrieved at the conduct of the Overseer, can appeal to the committee, or the visiting Justices, or to the Court.

"Other appropriations are made for the use of paupers who are partly supported by their friends. The number of poor at present in the Poor-House is about *seven*."

Six idiots are supported in this county by appropriations out of the State Treasury. As education advances, and *parental intemperance* diminishes, we shall have fewer of this hapless class of unfortunate dependents.

WOODFORD COUNTY JAIL, in *Versailles*, has been recently constructed; is built of dressed stone, cost $2,500, and is twenty-seven feet square. It is of one story, and consists of two arched rooms or cells, *nine feet* by *fourteen ;* these open upon a passage, through the outer wall of which is cut a window, rather too small, and secured by grates. There are no windows in either room, but a portion of light finds entrance, as also air, through the doors, which are grated. This jail is warmed, is secure, is tolerably convenient, furnished with some essential accommodations seldom found in jails, and may be rendered sufficiently comfortable. Prisoners here could not be separated, so as to prevent verbal communication, under whatever circumstances committed. This prison, with obvious deficiencies, and not perfectly ventilated, is yet a great improvement upon most which have met my observation.

A spirit of progress, of attention to education, and a desire for improvement, appears to exist in Woodford county, which is the promise of better things in coming days.

FRANKLIN COUNTY has no Poor-House, but has, as I am informed by the County Clerk, *eighteen paupers*, who receive for their support an allowance from the *County Court* the *sum of four hundred and forty-five dollars*, being about $24, 7¼ cents each! One idiot is supported here by the State.

FRANKLIN COUNTY JAIL, at *Frankfort*, is one of the best, if not the very best built jail I have seen in the State. It is fire-proof, and may last for a century. The plan, with a little modification, may be offered as a model for a county prison, where but few prisoners are likely to be in detention at one time. This should not be adopted for a city prison, nor for a populous county, even if the dimensions were doubled. The outside wall measures *twenty-five* by *thirty-five* feet. The Jail at Frankfort is situated in rear of the Court-house and county offices, and adjacent to the commodious building occupied by the keeper and his family. The passage conducting to both is paved, as is the yard. The jail originally was intended to consist of one story, but subsequently a second was added upon the flat *stone roof* of the ground prison. The first story is built of blocks of solid lime-stone rock, in width equivalent to the entire thickness of the wall, viz : *two feet three inches* ; deep, *fifteen* or *twenty inches ;* and long, from *five* to *eight* feet. The foundation is laid below the surface *four feet ;* the floor is formed of blocks of stone *eleven* feet long, and *two* feet deep ; the ceiling or roof, corresponds exactly with the floor, and is closely cemented through the joinings, forming thus a complete stone prison above, below, around. A floor of plank is laid over the stones, and plaster covers the walls, to guard against dampness. Ventilating flues pass up through the rear wall of each cell. The doors are of iron. There are three cells *thirteen feet* by *nine*, and *eleven* high—the separating walls being *eighteen* inches thick, as also the partition which sets off the front of the cells from the passage. Opposite to the strong grated door of each cell, is a window *sunk* in, or through the outer wall, and strongly grated. The passage or area, on which you enter from abroad, through heavy strong doors, is *thirty-one and a half feet* by *six* in breadth. This, and the cells are warmed by a stove. In the centre descends the waste drain. The brick story, added above this, is *ventilated, lighted, warmed, and is to be furnished.* This part of the prison contains one large well lighted, airy room, strong and commodious, to be used as a " watch-house" or " lock up." Cost of materials and labor from thirty-five to thirty-seven hundred dollars.

Scott County has a Poor-House some miles north of *Georgetown.* There are but few inmates, (eight or nine when I was there in December,) chiefly aged and infirm persons. These conduct the affairs of their two log houses, the men occupying one, the women the other; and receive supplies from the Overseer or Superintendent, who resides within a half or third of a mile of the place. The appearance of the different rooms indicated the means of living with tolerable comfort, and the disposition of the citizens is benevolent and liberal. I think the lodgings might be improved, and would be if visited by intelligent citizens from Georgetown. The establishment of Poor-Houses in a county where there are so few paupers, is not urgent, and as a general rule, except in the most populous counties, is not desirable. The State supports *fourteen idiots* in Scott Co.

Scott County Jail was destroyed by fire, not long since, and has not been replaced; it is hoped and believed when this shall be done, a model prison will be built, which will be creditable to the humanity and justice of the citizens. It should be constructed of brick or stone, and supplied by judicious architectural arrangements, with such recent improvements as these establishments claim, alike for the sake of the Jailer and those committed to his custody.

Grant County has a Poor-House, but no poor living there. Three individuals are aided who board in private families. Seven idiots in this county are supported by appropriations out of the State Treasury. I heard of several beside, as well as several insane, who are in charge of their relations.

Grant County Jail, at *Williamstown,* is built of logs: no prisoners in December. There is little use for this prison at any time. There are two rooms, reached by a flight of stairs to the second story, on the outside; the first entered is called the debtor's room; below this is the dungeon; dimensions of each, *fourteen* feet square, ventilated by an aperture *one foot* square, grated. Walls 2½ feet thick, filled in with rock between the timbers. Upper room warmed by a small stove; furnished with bed and bedstead: dungeon dark, damp, cold, and unfurnished. This jail is said to be secure, is unenclosed and isolated.

I conceive that all jails constructed as this, should be condemned as unfit for the imprisonment of any offenders, however guilty; since protracted confinement in dungeons so destitute of light, pure air, and warmth, must, as indeed we know is the case, often impair the health, both of mind and body. The criminal and the vicious must be restrained and punished, but not by such modes of correction.

Boone County has a Poor-House, but wholly unoccupied for a considerable time past. The citizens are very kindly disposed towards their indigent neighbors; indeed this characteristic of Kentucky social life, may be noticed through all quarters where I have journeyed.

Five idiots are supported by the State in various families in Boone county. Several cases beside, exist, both of idiocy and insanity, requiring hospital care. These I have found it difficult to class, from the fact of their scattered residences, and their being in private families, into which a stranger however excellent the motive, ought not to intrude, unless urged.

Boone County Jail, at *Burlington,* is built of two thicknesses of timber within, and of brick without; it is isolated and unenclosed. It consists of two rooms one above the other, eighteen feet by eighteen; one, *seven feet* high, the other *six and a half.* Ventilated by four small windows, *one* foot square,

3

double grated. The upper room is out of repair; the lower is warmed by a stove, and has some bed-clothing, and one bed on the floor. Prisoners, two, December 30th, one white, one black, well supplied with food. Jail said to be secure.

There appear to be many strong objections to unenclosed prisons, and also to those which are isolated, as this, from the residence of the Jailer.

KENTON COUNTY has few paupers, several insane wandering abroad, and three idiots chargeable upon the State.

KENTON COUNTY SEAT has been removed from Covington, formerly the shire town, to Independence, where a new and strong jail has been built of brick. The plan does not offer many advantages over other small prisons. The "lock-up," that is, the old jail at Covington, is still in use for temporary detention; it does not appear that the financial interests of the county at large, have been consulted by the transfer of the county-town from the river, though a few private individuals may derive advantage thereby.

CAMPBELL COUNTY has a Poor-House north of Alexandria; but one inmate in December, a lame sick man; the buildings are insufficient if numbers should gather, that is, more than three or six.

Campbell County has five idiots supported at the cost of the State.

THE COUNTY JAIL at *Alexandria* is constructed of brick without, and timber within, spiked; it is two stories high, in the second of which the Jailer and his family reside, while the ground floor is occupied as a prison. This consists of two rooms, entered from a narrow passage extending the entire length of the building. In one is placed a stove which communicates warmth to the adjoining room by means of a pipe and drum. Dimensions are *sixteen* by *sixteen*, and *eight* high. Two prisoners. Food, three sufficient meals daily.

PENDLETON COUNTY has a Poor-House, some miles distant from Falmouth. One inmate only. State supports two idiots in the county.

PENDLETON COUNTY JAIL, at *Falmouth*, is rather a roughly constructed building, not enclosed nor in repair. The Jailer resides in a part of the first and second stories. The building is of brick without, and heavy plank and timber within. Imperfectly lighted and ventilated; warmed by means of an oven in which fire may be lighted in the Jailer's apartment. Dimensions of the rooms about *fifteen* by *fifteen feet*, and *eight* high. No prisoners the first week of January.

The Jail in HARRISON COUNTY, at *Cynthiana*, has been condemned; it is old, inconvenient, and no longer answering the uses of a prison, is to be replaced by one for which the contracts are about to be made, if indeed they are not already concluded. It is to be hoped that the improvements which have been adopted in Franklin and Bourbon, will be imitated in Harrison.

BOURBON COUNTY POOR-HOUSE is some miles north of Paris, on the middle road from Cynthiana. It is said to be comfortably managed and has at times thirteen or fourteen inmates. The State supports two pauper idiots in this county.

BOURBON COUNTY JAIL, at *Paris*, is constructed of brick, timbers, and stone, and is one of the best planned jails in the State, though the masonwork is inferior to that of several in the northern part of Kentucky. The Jailor's house makes part of the building; the prison portion is enclosed by a high and well constructed stone wall, which affords a yard for exercise. The cells on the ground floor, as well as those in the second story, open upon an area of convenient size, in which is placed a stove which warms the prison comfortably. The prison is furnished with beds and bed-clothing upon bedsteads, but by what seemed to me a great error of judgment, the prisoners, instead of being required to occupy the separate cells, which are sufficiently lighted, ventilated, and supplied with fit accommodations, were living in association, and lodging altogether in the area on the ground floor. There are three or four cells below, and one less in the second story. The Jailer being absent, I did not enter the lower cells, but think they were pretty well kept, as I saw them through the gratings in the floor from above. Though the Jail at Paris is a very great improvement on most of the prisons in the State, it is not so perfect as to serve for a model. The best parts of this prison, and that at Frankfort together, would afford a better building, and with some better arrangements. It is highly creditable to the citizens of Bourbon that they have made so much exertion, and at so great cost, to produce a better style of prison architecture than has heretofore been adopted, and their public spirit and humane dispositions will stimulate other counties to follow in the work of amendment.

THE FAYETTE COUNTY JAIL, which I visited early in November, is connected with a large Hotel, of which, indeed, it seems to make a part. The prison consists of two cells on the ground floor, and one apartment above these, called the debtors' room. The cells are divided by a passage, running their entire length; at one end is the door by which entrance is gained from the public passage in a wing of the Hotel; the opposite extremity gives access to a small area or yard, which is enclosed by a high stone wall. The dimensions of the cells, estimated by those who attended me, without actual measurement, are about nine feet by eighteen or twenty, and ten high. Air and light are admitted through loop-holes, or very small windows, high in the wall, and these are secured by iron bars. A small stove is furnished in both cells. The substitutes for beds and bed clothing are indescribable. The cells had been swept, as also the passage and area. The cell on the right, contained *two women and one man;* that on the left, *eleven men,* and more recently, I am informed, has received *seventeen* at one time. Of all I saw, one only, I was told, by the person who conducted me through this department, was detained on a criminal charge—what was the nature of the offence, I did not enquire. I was informed that the supplies of food were sufficient.

Over the cells, and entirely disconnected therewith, is a large and comfortable apartment, called the debtors' room. This is entered from the passage common to the Hotel, and is little distinguishable from the apartments in that wing of the same, except by the guarded windows, and a strong lock to secure the door. The room was well furnished, decently arranged, and seemed to be in common use. A fire may be supplied, and such accommodations as are required.

This Jail is, in all respects, defective for serving the legitimate uses of a prison. The Jailor, as must be seen, has no means of separating or classifying his prisoners, providing he shall be charged to receive at one and the same time blacks and whites of both sexes, and all ages, and for all degrees of crime and misdemeanors.

This prison has been long built, and is, I am told, much objected to by many of the most enlightened citizens of Lexington. It is said that the County Court have had the subject of a new Jail under consideration, but as yet have arrived at no decision as to plan or location. In the event of a new prison, better adapted to the present wants of the county, I would respectfully suggest the expediency of connecting a Work-house, or house of Correction, with the Jail, rather than as now, associating the Work-house with the City Poor-house. It seems rather injudicious, if not unkind, in this way, to bring into immediate vicinity, though not into frequent personal communication, the innocent, who are subjects of the benevolent guardianship of the community, and the guilty, whose vices or crimes justly bring them under condemnation and restraint.

I believe it will be sufficient to direct the attention of the citizens to this mistaken arrangement, to secure the change which justice and humanity alike claim for the humble and dependent, but unoffending classes.

Referring again to the apparent inconveniences sustained in the Fayette County Jail, those affecting the necessary intercourse of prisoners with their counsel must be obvious; so, also, if governed by a sense of duty and influenced by sentiments of compassion, the ministers of the Gospel resort to the cell of the prison-bound, the devotional and preceptive ministrations must be exercised under the most disadvantageous circumstances. If contagious, or other sickness appear, the keeper has not the means of separating the healthy from the diseased—or of rendering those cares which common humanity demands. In fine, the Jailor cannot be accountable for the architectural defects of the Jail.

But I confess I am not sanguine in the expectation of seeing a well-constructed and well-ordered county Jail in Fayette, so long as the *county* appears to have so little use for a prison, *compared* with the accommodations it renders to any chance persons traversing the State, conducting their own affairs, or to the keeper of the prison himself. It would certainly be a remarkable exercise of liberality in the County Court, to order the construction of a commodious building, highly creditable indeed to the county as a prison, but which, under existing tacit permissions, should only more fully serve the purposes, to which the present edifice is chiefly applied;—purposes in which the citizens at large have no interest or concern—from which they neither directly nor indirectly derive advantage or benefit, and upon which, if they bestowed much thought, they would promptly, and almost unanimously, determine against. At least, if this assumption does not rest on correct premises, I have very greatly mistaken the sentiments of the tax-paying citizens generally.

FAYETTE COUNTY POOR-HOUSE, about twelve miles from Lexington, visited in November, exhibited a comfortable appearance externally. The lodging-rooms, were the numbers of occupants to increase, would require important additions of beds, bed-clothing, &c.: at present, there is no deficiency, and the establisament seemed to be supplied with all the necessaries, and many of the comforts of the table. The appearance and conversation of the persons who have charge of the house, were such as to convey the idea that they would perform their duty towards those committed to their care, so far as they should understand their obligations. There were here but two persons at public charge—one black, and one white.

The farm was said to be productive, contains about fifty acres, and belongs to the county. It is somewhat inaccessible for frequent visitation, but on the contrary, removed to such a distance from the temptations of a city as to obviate serious disadvantages.

LEXINGTON CITY POOR-HOUSE had twenty three residents on public charge at the time of my first visit in December; twenty whites, three blacks. The house is constructed of brick, and of convenient access, upon the confines of the city. It is designed that the Poor-House should be comfortably provided with food and clothing. Sufficient fires were maintained in the several lodging apartments. The eating-room is not conveniently situated, and is never warmed. The occupants of this establishment are chiefly aged and infirm persons, or those disabled by sickness, and young children, all proper subjects for the care here extended over them, and something in addition perhaps. Religious meetings are sometimes holden in the house, for the comfort of those who are too feeble to go abroad.

THE CITY WORK-HOUSE, injudiciously connected with this asylum for the poor and unfriended, contained but four prisoners, whose employment was hammering stone in an enclosed yard. The Keeper being absent on both my visits to the Poor-House, I did not see this department except from the overlooking windows of the main building. I heard this division of the establishment repeatedly censured by respectable citizens, and it seems to me with good reason. The ground-floor apartment is on one side very imperfectly protected by a canvass curtain, which is the sole substitute for a substantial partition. A fire is maintained here, but in severe weather is inadequate to the necessary comfort of the inmates. The lodging-room, which was above this partially enclosed day-room, was represented to me as neither weather-proof nor otherwise in good habitable order—while these prisoners justly suffer confinement at tasked labor, it seems to be no part of their sentence, under the municipal authority, to expose them to the rigors of the climate in severe weather without sufficient protection. I ask no indulgences for perverse transgressors—only justice.

Six indigent idiots of Fayette county, are sustained at the expense of the State. The number of the insane, out of Hospital care, I had no means of ascertaining correctly. The estimates were various and discrepant.

JESSAMINE COUNTY POOR-HOUSE, several miles from the shire town, had only two paupers at the time of my visit last autumn, both aged women, one white, one black. The place is owned by the county, and I was told that sixty dollars, beside the productions from this property, were allowed for each individual who should come, or be sent to this establishment. If possible, and I see not why it is not possible, the overseer of the poor, or some sensible and benevolent persons in town, would be accomplishing a good work and christian duty, to look more diligently into the condition of these poor persons, for whom certainly a liberal appropriation is made by the Court.

Ten idiots are supported by the *State* in Jessamine county.

JESSAMINE COUNTY JAIL, at *Nicholasville*, is constructed of brick, within an area of small dimensions, enclosed by a substantial, high brick wall. The prison consists of two stories; a dungeon on the ground floor, reached from a flight of stairs on the outside of the building; conducting you first immediately into the dismal prison room in the second story; next to a yet more dismal place below, entered through a strong massive trap-door. The dungeon is scarcely more damp, dark, and entirely unfit to receive human beings, for any considerable period than the room above. But it is not merely to these comfortless rooms I wish to direct the attention, the very serious attention of the citizens of Jessamine county. That they have permitted the construction of this substantial prison, on the plan referred to, was to say the least, a most unfortunate error of judgment; but when in addition to these wretchedly constructed dungeons, dark, though not totally dark, damp, and of course unhealthy, the visiter finds two expensive and *massive iron man-cages*, constructed of tire iron, the bars traversing perpedicularly and horizontally, affording a few inch spaces between each, strongly riveted and bound together, the door of course of sufficient size for a man to pass in, what conclusions must be drawn? I had supposed we had, at this period of civilization, outlived the *iron age* of dungeons, and that in these latter days at least, the humanizing influence of christianity was so blended with clear intellectual perceptions, that justice and mercy were seldom found asunder, so far as the commonest necessities of life are concerned. I would endeavor to speak gently on this subject. I know that the citizens did not purpose to revive illustrations of barbarous life. I have every reason to think them as kind and correct in their daily intercourse and social habits, as any persons in our country. But I think that a little reflection would render the fact apparent, that in the construction of this jail, no convenience or security has been effected for the benefit of the Jailer, and not the certain detention always of prisoners. To be sure, they could hardly escape but by attacking the Keeper, and this I conceive they would be very likely to do. It is hoped that both for the safe detention of prisoners, and the merciful detention of them, as well as for the personal safety of the officer, this prison will no more be used as it now stands.

MERCER COUNTY has a POOR-HOUSE, rather the poor are supported at the expense of the county, upon a farm some miles from Harrodsburg, which is owned by the person who is employed to take care of them, as I understood him to say; but on that point I am not positive. The farm contains one hundred and fifty acres, seventy-five of which are cultivated. I found here eighteen persons, sixteen whites, two blacks; men, women, and children. A forlorn and comfortless place. *Twenty-five dollars a year* is allowed for each pauper, and as the master truly said, "for that sum I can afford to give them no better lodgings, clothing, or food." It is not certainly creditable to this county, rich and prosperous as it is, to maintain its dependent poor under such circumstances. I should rejoice, if those of the respectable citizens I saw in Harrodsburg, would speedily unite their influence with others, to procure a more wholesome and just ordering of these affairs. The opinions expressed to me, certainly authorize a hope, that they will not suffer this discreditable state of things to be perpetuated.

This county has *twenty idiots* supported within its borders, by appropriations from the State Treasury.

THE COUNTY JAIL OF MERCER, at *Harrodsburg*, is maintained in good order, and is well built, though not convenient for prison purposes.

The Jail occupies the second story of a large building, on the first floor of which resides the Keeper and his family. The stairs which conduct to the prison, open upon an area, the dimensions of which are *twelve feet by forty-six*, lighted by seven large windows, and furnished with a stove. There are three strong rooms, closed by heavy doors, made of tire iron. Two small windows admit light and air; the rooms measure *fifteen feet by eighteen*, and *nine* high. Prison vacant. Usually but few prisoners, considering the population of the county, and the resort to this town, as a favorite watering place.

BOYLE COUNY has but few paupers. I was unable, at the season of both visits to this county, to see the Clerk, and procure statistics respecting the poor.

The State supports *five idiots* in this county.

BOYLE COUNTY JAIL, at *Danville*, has been built about two years. It is isolated, unenclosed, constructed of timber, clap-boarded, and painted. It consists of a small passage, in which is placed a bed for the guard, when any prisoner is in detention, and two rooms, one on the ground floor, another of like capacity above. Dimensions, *twelve feet by eighteen*, and *nine and a half high*. There are two windows opposite each other, *two feet by three*, glazed and guarded by a grating of bar iron. The room is warmed by a stove, and contains a bed. The windows opening upon an unenclosed space, offer means of indiscriminate communication from without, with all the idle or the curious who may choose to linger there. There were two prisoners in the ground-floor apartment ; a white man charged with murder, and a black man committed for larceny. Jail insecure.

LINCOLN COUNTY has few dependent poor. Here, as elsewhere, I find that those who suffer privation *through poverty*, are objects of a kindly charity from private sources.

Six idiots in this county are supported by the State.

LINCON COUNTY JAILS, at *Stanford*, are first the old prison, constructed of timber, &c. which is unenclosed, as is that more recently built, and connected with the residence of the Keeper and his family. The two rooms are reached by ascending from the dwelling within, to a small, low, unfinished room, imperfectly lighted by a small grated window. In the centre is a trap-door, locked and secured above; when rased, the dungeon is disclosed—no, not disclosed, unless total darkness is a revelation. I could not descend, as there were neither steps nor ladder, and I have not action enough as a Gymnast, to swing myself down into a depth of seven feet or more. I could not take the dimensions, but those with me said the place was "small, nine feet perhaps. perhaps something more." This dungeon is entirely unventilated, entirely dark, entirely without the means of being dried or warmed at any time; unfurnished, "except the Jailer give some bedding at his option;" "county does not pay for any thing, except food," and one in contemplating this dreadful place, almost questions if it had not been one mercy joined to many cruelties, to have withheld that. Desperate men, in desperate conditions, will effect seeming impossibilities, accordingly it has been found that this dungeon would at times "give up its dead." Prisoners have escaped. When I was at Stanford, a sick prisoner had been removed, by official order, under the representation of a physicion, to the tavern, and there guarded. He took advantage of the negligence of his Keeper, to escape. As I stooped over the dark dungeon referred to, I asked "is any one there?" A feeble voice answered, "yes." "How long have you been down there?" "I cannot count days." I could not see the person, but learned that he was young, and had been committed on a charge of larceny. Through the kind consideration of a professional gentleman, he had been discharged for a similar offence from the jail in the adjacent county of Garrard. Subsequently at two different periods, I have been informed on reliable authority, that he was a young man of infirm, imbecile mind, hardly a responsible being. Those who caused his arrest in Stanford, could not have considered his mental infirmity, or the doom to which they consigned

him in that dungeon, in which he was left through the cold weather, this unusually severe autumn. The same gentleman who plead for him at Lancaster, recollected him here one cold day, sought the Keeper, and desired
that he should be taken from the dungeon or he would inevitably freeze. After a little, the request was complied with, but he had, when they raised
the trap, "laid down to die." He was cold and chilled, and sleep had fallen
on him; it was some time before he was restored. That he should, in a few
days after, being recovered, escape, while still outside the dungeon, is not
remarkable. Imprisonment in this Jail has brought destructive effects on
both mind and body. Physicians have made oath that to incarcerate a
man therein, "was no other than judicial murder." Cases in point were adduced in evidence thereof. But a new prison the last year, was planned and
built. It was not wholly *finished* in November. Whether the entire original plan has been carried out I cannot tell. For the character of the members of the County Court we trust not. This is joined with or by the old
Jail; it has two rooms for prisoners: one in the second story, lighted by two
loop-holes; strongly built, but when I saw it, was not planned for being
warmed. The dungeon below, measured *twelve feet by eighteen,* and *eight*
high. This was constructed, with a due regard to strength and duration:
but here the merit of the work ended. The only light, warmth, and air
admitted, was to reach the prisoner through the massive grated iron door,
when the outer door, which opened immediately into the Jailer's family room
should be left open. It was proposed, I was told, ordered and in hand, to
have wrought two large iron cages, on the *Jessamine county* pattern, to
place on either side in this dungeon. Lately, I am infromed, that the altertion
in some sort, of this Jail has come under consideration, and that measures may be adopted for introducing a stove. Whether the project of com-
pleting the furnishing of the dungeon, by the introduction of the cages has
been abandoned, I cannot tell. An effort was made to direct serious attention to the barbarity of using them; and their real uselessness is apparent. Error of judgment and want of due reflection, have combined to
project these defective Jails; inhumanity, deliberate inhumanity, does not
characterize the citizens of Lincoln.

GARRARD COUNTY has a Poor-House some miles from Lancaster. I attempted to reach it, but the badness of the roads and inexperience of the
driver of my carriage, made it prudent to relinquish the attempt, after passing over several miles. The place is so remote from town as to render it
exceedingly difficult to maintain frequent supervision. The exact number
of inmates I did not learn, it was thought there were from nine to thirteen.
No idiots in this county supported at the cost of the State,

GARRARD COUNTY JAIL, at *Lancaster*, is unenclosed, but connected with
the residence of the Jailer. It is built of brick, consists of a lighted room
in the second story, and dungeon below, entrance through a trap-door; bed
and blankets, and sufficient food furnished. Few prisoners usually in detention. In November, one black man in on suspicion. The dungeon must be
as objectionable as in most prisons of the same sort: insufficiently lighted,
ventilated, &c., but here, as almost universally, the Jailer does all in his power
to guard against ill consequences.

WASHINGTON COUNTY has but few paupers; a kindly disposition prevails
for aiding the poor from private means. This county has thirteen idiots sup-

ported by an appropriation from the State, of six hundred and fifty dollars. I think one has recently died.

WASHINGTON COUNTY JAIL, in *Springfield*, is seldom used. There are two prison rooms on the ground floor, and opening from the apartments occupied by a family who have the building in charge. The rooms are lighted, ventilated, are of comfortable dimensions, and might be warmed. So seldom are they in request for county purposes, that I found them used as store rooms. They did not appear to be very strong, or capable of detaining a prisoner resolute to escape. I was told that if the county had more need of a prison, it would be considered worth while to erect a new one.

MARION COUNTY has few paupers; but four idiots, receive each an appropriation from the State of fifty dollars.

The COUNTY JAIL, at *Lebanon*, is said to be strong, it is built of brick, I could not see it within, in consequence of the absence of the family of the Jailer, who reside in the part of the building not appropriated to prisoners, and who had the keys with them. No prisonor in custody at that time, but few at any period. There are two prison rooms which two of the citizens described, "lighted, warmed, and aired;" no dungeon. Dimensions, *ten* by *eighteen* feet, and *nine and a half* high.

GREEN COUNTY has no Poor-House, but few poor, and these are boarded in the family of a farmer at a considerable distance from Greensburg. I did not visit them. Green receives from the State an appropriation for the support of *three* idiots.

The COUNTY JAIL, at *Greensburg*, is recently built, much more comfortable than most prisons in adjacent counties, though very inconvenient for the Jailer and his family, who reside on the first floor. The prison is considered secure, and is entered over a flight of stairs, which terminate in a lighted room or passage, upon which the strong rooms look, light being admitted chiefly through the grated doors. These prison rooms are *twelve* feet by *fifteen*, and *ten* high; unfurnished at present; the County Court make no appropriation for beds or blankets. The windows are high in the wall, *thirteen* inches by *fourteen*, and double grated. The walls are of stone, and heavy oak timber. Building unenclosed. I should not recommend this prison as a model in any respect, since with but little additional cost, one much better suited for prison purposes might be constructed. No prisoner in custody at the time of my visit, in November, nor any since May, 1845. The apartments were in general order. The keeper was represented as a person remarkably well qualified for the office he filled. The introduction of stoves is objected to from the frequent attempts at firing prisons. As yet none are so built, in this State, as to admit of being heated by means of hot air or steam from below, conducted through iron pipes.

A Poor-House has been established in BARREN COUNTY, not far from *Glasgow*; the situation was not fortunately chosen, and since I was there I am told it has been proposed to make some change. There was no pauper at the time of my visit—there are but few individuals entirely dependent in this county; a liberal spirit is exercised in neighborhoods, by rendering partial assistance to the poor, which spares much suffering. Three idiots in this county, are sustained by an appropriation from the State Treasury. The liberal county appropriation for support of the poor in the county Poor-House, has varied from $90, to $60, as now.

4

BARREN COUNTY JAIL is in *Glasgow*, and situated in a *sink* or hollow, a little on the outskirts of the public streets. The location does not seem to have been fortunately chosen for salubrious air. The building is of timber, weather boarded, and painted white. The dungeon on the ground floor, entered by a strong door, measures sixteen feet by eighteen, and ten high; the windows in the room above the dungeon, are guarded by three sets of iron gratings. Both apartments are warmed by means of stove heat. This jail is ventilated, secure, (though a guard is employed to lodge in the passage,) tolerably comfortable, not sufficiently furnished, prisoners well supplied with good food, Two occupants in November, a prisoner detained on a criminal charge, and an insane man held for safety, till the session of the Court, then to be transported to the Hospital, at his own charges.

ADAIR COUNTY has no Poor-House and farm, owned by the public. The poor are boarded in a respectable family, but the number who are at public charge is small, and often there are none at all. In November there were two boarded in a private family, both of them aged and infirm. Besides these, are nine persons crippled and infirm, who are supported by the county, but by special act, are not required to live at the "Poor-House," *so called*, as writes the county Clerk. Here, as throughout the State, private liberality saves, by partial support, many from the condition of pauperism. Four idiots in this county, are supported at the expense of the State.

ADAIR COUNTY JAIL, at *Columbia*, which I visited in November, is constructed of brick, and exteriorly presents a neat appearance. There is no enclosed exercise yard, and the keeper, with his family, resides in the left division of the building, on the left hand as you enter. The jail consists of a dungeon on the ground floor, totally dark, except the slab door is left open for a time, when a partial light is admitted, unventilated, not warmed, secure, but *very uncomfortable*. Dimensions correspond nearly with the room above, which is *twelve* by *fifteen*, and *eight* high; one large window securely grated, two by two and a half feet, opposite to one *nine* inches square; these admit sufficient light and air. The room is wholly unfurnished, and roughly finished, being like the dungeon beneath, constructed of solid heavy timbers, rough hewn, within the brick walls. But one prisoner in November; offence murder. This prison has received *forty three* inmates in a period of *two and a half years*: of course not all criminals.

RUSSELL COUNTY has no Poor-House; few paupers; when any, they are boarded in a private family. Two idiots in this county supported at the expense of the State. Few insane; these, as in adjacent counties, when not sent to the State Hospital, are under the direction and care of their kindred. Several epileptics.

The JAIL of RUSSELL COUNTY, at *Jamestown*, is fortunately not often occupied; in such an event, whether in cold or rainy weather, I should think it quite impossible for the prisoner not to suffer seriously in health. This prison was vacant at the time of my visit, November 17th. The jail is constructed of timbers, and not closed in all parts against the weather; of course the ventilation is always sufficient. The walls are three feet in thickness, double sets of timbers; floor three feet thick; one window *nine* by *twelve inches*. Dimensions of the dungeon, and room above, *thirteen feet* by *fourteen and a half*, and *six* high Straw or husk bed in the upper room; did not descend into the dungeon, which is reached through a trap door. No fire allowed at any time. The Jailer disposed to grant all he has authority to allow for protecting the prisoners when they come into his custo-dy. The jail has been built eighteen years, and is but little used.

WAYNE COUNTY has a Poor-House; in November four inmates. The county has few paupers at any time ; here as elsewhere, the rich impart of their abundance to the poorer classes, in times of especial necessity, and none go to the Poor-House, who by any efforts of their own, can live apart. Heard of several epileptics and partially insane persons, but none, at the present, requiring immediate removal to the Hospital. *Thirteen* idiots in Wayne supported by the State.

WAYNE COUNTY JAIL, at *Monticello*, has been built many years, and is somewhat dilapidated, and not secure. It is constructed of timber, that is, squared logs within, and weather boarded, and painted without. Access is had to the prison rooms by an irregular flight of steps. The dimensions of the upper rooms, are *sixteen* feet by *sixteen*, and *five* high: dungeon the same, and ventilated by a window twelve inches by eighteen. Not furnished, never warmed, detached from other buildings. Few prisoners are commit-ted here ; if any in severe weather, the Jailer usually, on his own responsi-bility, takes them to his own house to warm them. Food sufficient. A few years hence, and I think this jail will be replaced by a prison on a better plan. For example, one connected with the Jailer's residence, having an en-closed exercise yard, subdivided, warmed, lighted, ventilated, secure, and giv-ing employment to the prisoners, if it is no more than breaking stone to mend the public roads. These long months of idleness in prison, exert the worst influence over the habits both of body and mind.

CLINTON COUNTY has neither Poor-House nor paupers. Occasionally a few individuals are aided at the public cost. No idiots in this county sup-ported by the State, but several by their kindred. Several cases of insanity, one especially of great privation and suffering. The friends perhaps do not realize all the distress surrounding circumstances impose.

CLINTON COUNTY JAIL, at *Albany*, is a rude block-house, situated in a sta-ble or cow-yard, and consists of a single room, not readily accessible, and measuring *thirteen* feet by *thirteen*, and *ten* high. It is built of double tim-bers, walls two feet thick. Two windows on one side, *twelve inches* square, and double grated. Solid door, *two feet* by *four*. Floor two layers of tim-bers, ten inches thick, rock filled in between, in all two feet deep. This Jail is quite secure, not furnished, not ventilated, not warmed, in no wise com-fortable or safe for health. As in some other counties, the Jailer, on his own responsibility, takes such prisoners as he may have in custody, during the severe weather, to his own dwelling occasionally during the day, for warm-ing.

The general humanity and kindness of the citizens of Kentucky, is most singularly at variance with the ordering of the county jails. Surely these could be made to secure the safe keeping of the prisoners without such amazing disregard to the decencies, and ordinary and necessary comforts of life, as light, warmth, pure air, &c.

CUMBERLAND COUNTY has no Poor-House, the few paupers in this district, are supported in private families, at a given rate, under the direction of the County Court. There are in the county but few insane and epileptics; but *eight* idiots are supported at the expense of the State.

CUMBERLAND COUNTY JAIL, at *Burksville*, is isolated, unenclosed, neatly built of brick without, and heavy squared timber within. It was vacant in

November, and has usually but few occupants. It consists of two ground floor rooms, divided by a passage having at one end a window, which may admit light and air to the dungeon, two windows *eleven inches* square and grated, look upon the passage, otherwise it is not ventilated; the dimensions are *nine feet* by twelve, and *six* high. The walls are two feet thick, the doors strong, the prison secure. It is not warmed, not at present furnished, not considered sufficiently comfortable in damp or cold weather The debtor's room, so called, has two windows looking abroad, and is of the same dimensions as the dungeon.

Imprisonment for debt, except fraud is shown, is no longer permitted in this State.

MASON COUNTY has no Poor-House, few poor sustained at public cost, several insane out of Hospital care, one wandering from place to place, is said to suffer much from exposure, probably will be placed in the State Hospital at the spring session of court. No idiots supported at cost of the State: several by their friends.

I have often encountered in Kentucky, as elsewhere, the insane wandering abroad.

MONROE COUNTY JAIL, at *Tompkinsville*, was vacant. Constructed with double squared timber walls, *two and a half feet* thick. The debtor's room, lighted and ventilated by two windows in opposite walls—*twelve inches* by twelve. Dimensions, *fifteen feet* by *fifteen*, and *six and a half* high. Dungeon the same size. Secure, not warmed, not ventilateted below, not furnished, not comfortable. Entrance door very strong, *two feet* by *four*.

Though nearly every Jail in the State is very inconveniently constructed for enabling the Jailor to take charge of his prisoners, and though nearly all I have seen, and with very few exceptions, all which have been described to me by Judges of the courts and other citizens, are very defective in arrangements for securing the essential and ordinary comforts of the plainest life, bed-clothing, pure air, and fire, I have observed, with interest, that these defects are attracting notice and censure, and I percieve that in many places they will, at no distant time, give way to more *just* arrangements.

HART COUNTY has no Poor-House; the few individuals who are wholly dependent on the county Treasury, are distributed in private families, and from all I was able to learn, these receive a reasonable amount of care, and their daily wants are duly supplied. Supposed deaf and dumb, *ten;* blind, *four* or *five; ten* idiots, of whom one only is chargeable upon the State. Insane, believed, including epileptics, to be *ten;* nearly all these are supported by their own relatives.

HART COUNTY JAIL, at *Munfordsville*, has been built about four years, is founded on solid rock, constructed of squared timber, weather-boarded, and painted, and the walls are *three* and *four-twelfths feet* in thickness: floor laid on the rocks, three feet thick, transverse timbers. Inner door of heavy timber, ironed, and studded. This structure is isolated, unenclosed, and consists of two apartments, one called the dungeon, in which the two windows, each *twelve inches* square are double grated. The other apartment has two windows, *one* and *a half* by *two feet square*. The dimensions are of each room or cell, *twelve feet* by *twelve*, and *seven* high. That upon the second story, which is reached by a flight of stairs from without, is the closest.

This Jail seems to be entirely secure. It is ventilated; furnished with a straw bed ; but cannot be warmed, except as is sometimes attempted here, and elsewhere, by the dangerous expedient of introducing a pan of burning coals in the severest weather. Few prisoners are committed here, it was vacant at the time of my visit.

LARUE COUNTY, recently erected, sends the few paupers it is charged with, as I was informed, to Hardin county. Several idiots and insane supported by their families at home. None of the former by the State.

LARUE COUNTY JAIL, at *Hodgensville*, has been recently built, and consists of one small room, solidly constructed, of squared timbers, weatherboarded, and painted white. The Jail is isolated and unenclosed : it is entered through a massive door, through which, I was told, "it is designed some time to cut a window." The prison is not at all ventilated, not lighted, not warmed, not furnished—by that, I mean it is wholly empty.

I believe the strength and security of this Jail, so recently constructed, has never been called in question. I suppose one will not be considered too lenient in expressing the hope that no offender may ever be so severely punished as to be incarcerated for any considerable time in this dungeon: in such an event, I should apprehend that the County Court, which I think has absolute control in these affairs, might be in danger of incurring a similar charge to that urged against an official body, distant a few counties removed —that of judicial murder. In reality, I do suppose but little thought was given to the consequences which must follow such imprisonment.

HARDIN COUNTY has a Poor-House—but few inmates:the comforts of the establishment might be increased; and the general arrangements improved. There are five idiots in this county supported at the expense of the State.

HARDIN COUNTY JAIL, at *Elizabethtown*, has been built some years, is solidly constructed of brick without, and timbers within; the walls are three feet thick. The ground floor apartments are occupied by the Jailor and his family. The second story, which is the prison, is reached by a flight of stairs within, terminating upon a landing or wide and long passage, which is almost as large as the prison room opposite. There are two ground rooms, one has two windows *two* and *a half feet*, by *four and a half*, grated. At present, not furnished, not warmed, (except by handing to a prisoner heated stones or bricks;) quite secure, and weather-proof. One dark room or dungeon, not furnished, warmed, lighted, nor ventilated. A small aparture is cut in one of the two doors which close this cell. Dimensions of each room *twelve feet* by *twenty*, and *seven* high. No prison exercise-yard, but the building is said to be healthfully situated. Prison vacant when I saw it. I have no doubt that here all reasonable care and consideration are extended by the Jailor to any who, from time to time, he may hold in custody. The inconvenient construction of the Jail must make this a difficult task.

In GRAYSON COUNTY, is no Poor-House, but the poor are provided for by the County Court, according to their various claims and necessities. There are in the county several epileptics and insane, resident with their friends. Six idiots are supported at the expense of the State; several by their kindred.

GRAYSON COUNTY JAIL, at *Litchfield*, is constructed of stone without, strengthened by timber within. The first story is occupied by the Jailor and his family. The building is unenclosed; no prisoner at the time of my visit. The prison department occupies the second story, and is reached over a flight of stairs through a heavy trap-door. This mode of entrance, however secure as a barrier against escape when locked down, is exceedingly inconvenient and dangerous for the Keeper. The debtors' room is about *twelve feet* by *twenty*, and *ten* high, and is lighted and ventilated by two windows *two and a half feet* by *four*. Bed of straw or shucks on the floor allowed; no other furniture. All the doors strong and guarded. Dungeon lighted, not ventilated, not warmed. Prison considered secure.

The Jailor gives three meals per day, and I do not doubt renders all reasonable care to such prisoners as are committed.

BRECKINRIDGE COUNTY has no Poor-House. The County Court apportions such sums as the wants of those who claim assistance demand. It is intended that the poor should be made comfortable. But few cripples, blind, insane, or deaf and dumb in this county. Five idiots are State beneficiaries.

BRECKINRIDGE COUNTY JAIL, at *Hardinsburg*, is constructed of brick, lined with timber, is two stories high, the first floor occupied by the Keeper and his family, the second as a prison. There is the usual want of an enclosed exercise-yard for prisoners. Jail vacant at the time of my visit: this was every where the rule, occupancy the exception. As usual, two prison rooms, one called the debtors' room, from the chief use formerly made of it —the other the dungeon. These are reached by a stair-case passing up through a heavy trap-door, which is locked below, terminating upon a passage ranging the length of the two prison rooms. The dimensions of the rooms are *twelve feet* by *twenty*, and *nine and a half* high. The lighted room has two windows, single grated. Not warmed, furnished with straw bed and blankets, when necessary. Three meals per day. Allowance for board 37½ cents, as usual elsewhere. This prison is tolerably secure.

OHIO COUNTY has recently purchased a house for the poor, and small farm of about sixteen acres. Here are but few paupers; the Poor-House system throughout the State is exceedingly repugnant to the feelings of the poor, by whom it is considered often almost as disgraceful as to go to prison. Of course, the insane and epileptics who are not a State charge, remain chiefly with their kindred. Six idiots are paid for by the State in this county.

The OHIO COUNTY JAIL, at *Hartford*, is built of brick without, and timber within. It consists of two stories, the Keeper and his family residing on the first floor, while the prison occupies the second: the dimensions of each apartment are *twelve feet* by *twenty-one*, and *nine* high. One room is lighted by two windows *two and a half* by *three and a half*, grated within and glazed without. The only light and air admitted into the dungeon, is through a small aperture in the strong door about nine inches square. The prison is not warmed, not ventilated, not furnished; was vacant at the time I was there, and had been so since April. Doors heavy and the prison secure. The second story is entered through a trap-door which fastens below. Prisoners, when in custody, supplied with abundance of food.

MUHLENBURG COUNTY has no Poor-House. Eight poor persons receive support from appropriations by the County Court; the largest sum granted for one individual is seventy dollars, the lowest fifteen. Physicians charges' paid by the county. Three idiots supported by the State in this county. Heard of several insane in private families, and several epileptics.

MUHLENBURG COUNTY JAIL, at *Greenville*, is built of brick and lined with timber; is two stories elevation; family resides upon the first floor; no enclosed exercise yard; the prison is reached over a flight of stairs through a trap-door, opening on a passage of convenient size, which is lighted. The debtors' room has a fire-place, and two glazed windows, not grated, I think. Dimensions of each room, *twelve feet* by *twenty*, and *nine* high; dungeon, dark, cold, and airless. No prisoners early in December. Jail much out of repair, and very insecure. An appropriation has been made by the County Court to put it into better condition. May be furnished with straw bed and blankets. Food sufficiently supplied, and due attention from the Jailer, so far as the defective architecture of the prison permits.

Hopkins County has no Poor-House; but about *seven* paupers are supported at the cost of the county, at rates from forty to sixty dollars each. Six idiots supported in this county from the State appropriation; others, as well as epileptics and insane, supported by their friends.

The Jail of Hopkins County is at *Madisonville;* it is two stories, very well built of brick without, and timber within; is considered entirely secure. The ground floor is occupied as a saddler's shop. The jail is reached over a flight of stairs, terminating in a room, cheerful well lighted, warmed by means of a stove; window single grated, and glazed without. The dungeons are entirely dark, except the outer door is opened. Dimensions, *eleven feet* by *seventeen*, and *seven* high; the walls are *eighteen inches* thick, lined within the brick with four-inch oak scantling, and two-inch plank, closely rivetted with iron spikes wrought in. The floor is of solid joists, of scantling, and oak plank, bound together. Furnished with straw bed and blankets. Three meals each day. The doors are bar-iron, grated, and measure *three feet* by *five.*

One prisoner in December, charged with murder. I found him by a comfortable fire, occupying the strong room without the dungeon, by day; but the dungeon at night, as said the Jailer.

Caldwell Cunty Poor-House, has very few inmates. This establishment, though small, has fortunately some judicious overseers, who desire to promote its good management, and secure suitable care for all who are, or who may become its inmates. If Poor-Houses are established, they should be frequently visited by judicious persons, and good order, neatness and general comfort maintained. The cost of the poor is variously estimated, but as a charge upon the county it must be very moderate, for those who rely on public charity are few. The State maintains three idiots in this county.

Caldwell County Jail, at *Princeton,* is built of stone; plank within; one prisoner detained on suspicion, was in the dungeon, which is on the ground story. From the street, you enter through a strong door upon a wide passage, and ascend a staircase; the upper rooms are *ten* by *fifteen* feet, and *seven and a half* high. The dungeon, which is entered by a heavy trap-door, is fifteen by fifteen feet, and ten high. What light and air it receives is derived from a guarded aperture in the lower passage, which is partially lighted from above. The passage may be warmed by a stove, but is not; straw bed and blankets were supplied to the prisoner, but he was suffering; the weather was inclement, cold, and severe. It is said that at mid-day so much light penetrates this dismal place, as will enable a person whose vision is accustomed to it, to read. I think such must be endowed with *feline* sight. This jail seems to be secure; the doors and the windows in the second story are strongly guarded; the building isolated and unenclosed. I believe the citizens generally, will concur with me in condemning the prison.

The county prisons adjacent, west and south of Caldwell, which the exceeding inclemency of the season, and the state of the roads prevented my reaching, have been repeatedly described to me by gentlemen of the bar, whose professional objects take them often through these districts, and also by several Judges of the Courts, who unite to condemn them without exception, as unfit to be used as places of detention for any offenders, however guilty. Not having visited, I decline describing them. There are but few paupers in these districts, and for a long time, probably, there will be no need of Poor-Houses. The State supports in Union county one idiot; in Crittenden, none; in Livingston, three, of one family; in McCracken, two; in Ballard, one; in Hickman, four; in Graves, four; in Calloway, one; in Trigg, one; in Henderson, one.

CHRISTIAN COUNTY has had a Poor-House for about eighteen years; it was not occupied early in December, and has been, I am informed, but irregularly in use. I could hear of but two who were receiving support from the county, that is, a whole support. It was said to me that generally, about fifteen hundred dollars had been apportioned for the poor, but not so much latterly; at this time, from two hundred to two hundred and fifty dollars is paid out. Four idiots supported by the State.

THE JAIL OF CHRISTIAN COUNTY, at *Hopkinsville*, is decidedly a most *unchristian prison*. It is built of brick externally, timber within, is old, inconvenient, and condemned I am glad to say, by the citizens generally, which affords hope that it will be replaced by one more commodious, and fit for the detention of offenders. The question is before the County Court. A family resides on the first floor, and perhaps occupy the entire section of the building on the left as you enter. Dimensions of the room in the second story, *eighteen* by *nineteen* feet, and *seven* high; two small windows double grated, sashed outside the grates. Dungeon entered *when practicable*, through a trap-door, descending from this room—here is a double trap, as is frequent; the lock was out of order, and I did not of course descend the ladder beneath. No prisoners. Window six inches square in the wall of the dungeon. Jail not warmed; not secure; very comfortless.

TODD COUNTY has a Poor-House, and but few paupers. Heard through professional gentlemen of from seventeen to twenty insane in the county. County Clerk absent, could get no estimates of the cost of supporting the poor. No idiots at the State charge.

TODD COUNTY JAIL, at *Elkton*, is built of brick, timbered within. Keeper and family reside on the first floor. Prison tolerably secure, entered over a staircase usually covered with a trap-door, strong, and may be fastened beneath. Dimensions of the debtor's room, *fourteen feet* by *sixteen*, and *six* high. One window grated, two feet. Dungeon dark; when occupied, furnished with straw bed and blankets. If warmed at all, by a pan of coals, or heated bricks. Passage lighted and ventilated by guarded windows in opposite walls. The food is sufficient in quantity and quality, as I was told on reliable authority. The Jailer, a respectable and humane man, fulfils his duty, so far as the construction of the prison allows. So indeed do nearly all keepers of the county prisons which I have seen. There is at times, danger of oversight or neglect when the prisoner is quite isolated. Usually, if the buildings were fitly constructed, there would be little ground for censure. Jail vacant, at the time of my visit.

LOGAN COUNTY has a Poor-House, but few inmates. Seven idiots are supported by appropriations from the State Treasury.

LOGAN COUNTY JAIL, at *Russellville*, is constructed of stone; not enclosed, not altogether secure, walls lately repaired within; three stories high. A family, not that of the Keeper, reside on the first floor, and occupy a room on the second. The second and third stories are reached through trap doors above steep flights of stairs. The rooms which were accessible on the second floor, were about *fourteen* feet by *eighteen;* windows in the debtors' room only. No prisoners. The dungeons were in the third story. I did not see them, the Jailer being absent on a journey of business, and the trap locked down. Not warmed. I understand also, that they were not furnished or ventilated. It is *probable* that blankets are supplied when any offenders are in custody.

SIMPSON COUNTY owns a good farm and Poor-House thereon, and has on an average of late, about fifteen poor. Several insane reside with their relatives, and this is the case in every county. Some are quite comfortable; many suffer much for want of well directed management, and become hopelessly diseased from want of Hospital treatment.

The State supports in Simpson, three idiots.

THE JAIL IN SIMPSON CONNTY, at *Franklin*, was some months since destroyed by fire; it has since been substantially re-built, I am constrained to admit, but upon a plan so remarkably ill-devised, that for the sake both of Keeper and prisoners, one must hope there will be little occasion for its occupancy.

The building is two stories high, constructed of brick well laid, and of good quality. The largest part of this edifice is appropriated for the residence of the family of the Jailer. There is no enclosed yard. The prison, which was unfinished at the time I was there, consists of a single room, on the ground floor, about sixteen feet square, entered by a door from a passage imperfectly lighted, if at all when the doors are closed. The only light or ventilation received into this dismal place, is through two very small gratings cut in the wall, which opens on the passage. Whether now furnished, warmed, and occupied, I do not know. I saw no possibility of introducing warmth. The obliging gentleman who conducted me to see this prison, informed me that this dungeon was solidly founded upon rock, the floors of very heavy timber. The dungeon was a sort of *large cage, made of iron bars transversely and perpendicularly wrought together* and spiked to plank and timber, outside which was the substantial brick wall. Brick, timber, plank, iron, and stone, seem to have been brought together to construct this singular dungeon, which may be called a series of cages within cages; but the difficulty of classing and separating prisoners, never seems to have suggested itself. Should there be a dozen arrested, into this "Black Hole" must they all go. I suppose security from fire, and security from escape, are the only two objects which the architect proposed to insure.

ALLEN COUNTY has no Poor-House, but the paupers are supported in a private family, where the County Court pay their expenses.

THE JAIL IN ALLEN COUNTY, at *Scottville*, I did not examine, the Keeper being absent. It is constructed of logs, consists of a debtor's room, so call-

5

ed, and a dungeon, the latter lighted by two windows, about eighteen inches square, double grated, entered through a trap-door from the upper room; considered secure; the walls filled in with tan between the double blocks. No fire ever; bed allowed, and sufficient food. No prisoner in December.

WARREN COUNTY has a Poor-House, three miles from town, in which are not often more than two or three inmates. Before the establishment of the Poor-House, about one thousand dollars per annum was appropriated by the county officers to the support of the poor. This county has *three pauper idiots* supported by the State.

WARREN COUNTY JAIL, at *Bowlinggreen*, is constructed of brick and timber, filled in with rocks between the floor and between the walls, as I was informed when there. It is considered tolerably secure. The building is isolated, and stands on the Public Sqaure. I was told it had *no facilities* for warmth, light, ventilation, or other accommodations. I did not enter it, the Jailer being absent from town, and the keys not to be obtained. The prison was vacant. I was informed by a county officer, that the passage was lighted by two windows; the second story reached through a trap-door, and in the event of the detention of prisoners of a desperate character, a guard employed. Opinion seemed to differ especting this prison, several thinking it "quite comfortable enough;" while others denounced it as "unfit for the detention of man or brute." I cannot doubt that the sentiments of the citizens at large, will lead to the amendment of some of the most serious defects. Upon these defects opinion is correct, if action keeps measure therewith.

The extreme severity of the weather, but more the nearly impassible condition of the roads, deterred me from visiting the COUNTY JAIL OF EDMONSON, at *Brownsville*. It was repeatedly described to me as a "rough, poor prison, built of logs," (perhaps timbers?) "Seldom in use, and not fit for use." There are few paupers in the county, and no idiots chargeable upon the State.

Like reasons detained me from BUTLER as from *Edmonson county*. I was informed that the Jail at *Morgantown* was very defective; that there were few paupers dependent for support on county appropriations, and that there were three idiots supported from the State Treasury.

NELSON COUNTY has a Poor-House, tolerably well built. I am informed, that the number of inmates varies from ten to thirty. General sentiment is in favor of this establishment. I should suppose, that from all related, some modification would prove advantageous.

Three idiots in this county, are supported from the State Treasury.

NELSON COUNTY JAIL, at *Bardstown*, is a large stone building, two stories high; the ground floor occupied by the Jailer and his family, and the second story used as a prison. There are three prison rooms, one being a dungeon; these are *eighteen by twenty*, and *nine* feet high; lighted, ventilated, may be warmed, may be furnished; not so secure but that three prisoners escaped the day before I was there; two prisoners in detention, not criminals.

BULLITT COUNTY has few paupers, and *no idiots* chargeable upon the State.

SHELBY COUNTY has a Poor-House, but few paupers; *two idiots* only, are supported here at the charge of the State.

SHELBY COUNTY JAIL, at *Shelbyville*, was vacant in December. It is certainly not a prison to be offered as a model; whether humanity and justice are consulted in the use of it, I appeal to the citizens to decide.

JEFFERSON COUNTY has no regularly organized Poor-House, but one is to be established shortly, a few miles distant from Louisville, though I am not wholly assured whether this will embrace all the poor of the county, or those alone from the city. Citizens of benevolent feelings and of good judgment, are interested in the judicious planning and establishment of a Poor-House, and it is to be hoped it will be creditable to those who direct its affairs, and a comfortable asylum for the crippled, the infirm, the confirmed invalid, and the aged poor. The work-house, now standing on the confines of the city, is also to be removed to the country. A farm owned by the city will probably be devoted to the House of Correction and to the Poor-House, though they will not be thrown together. There were in the Work-House, when I saw it in December, from forty to fifty inmates, thirteen of whom were women, colored and white. The men, who numbered above thirty, were entirely idle, and were congregated in a dirty and uncomfortable room, "no work being on hand." One or two were reading, but most were rehearsing mischievous histories, while little boys from eight years of age to fourteen, were eager listeners; some had been committed for larceny, others were there because their parents had been committed, and "there was nothing else to do with their children." There are thirty-six lodging-cells, doors strong, window grated, *two feet* by *nine inches.* The cells measure *seven feet* by *ten*, and *nine* high. The women, who by day are employed in a separate building, are at night conducted to lodging-cells in the third story of the men's building, passing through the day room and passages referred to, in order to reach them. The men's building is enclosed by a wall twenty feet high: there is an unfailing supply of water in the yard. This establishment, take it all in all, could hardly procure worse influences, or effect less in the way of reformation. When the new institution, which is contemplated, shall be established, we may look for an amended order of things. The keepers are not, I think, blameworthy for the demoralizing influences of this wretched place; they have not the means, apparently, of carrying out a correct system even imperfectly.

There are two Asylums for orphan children in Louisville, into which many friendless and neglected children are gathered, and carefully trained.

There is also an excellently governed Hospital for the sick, where are found, besides patients under medical and surgical treatment, some infirm and other poverty stricken persons, who are very kindly, and I should say, judiciously cared for. The whole establishment was remarkably neat and well arranged, evidencing the good government which the Superintendent exercises.

No *idiots* in Jefferson county supported by the State.

JEFFERSON COUNTY JAIL, at *Louisville*, is constructed of stone, planned and built in view of carrying out the classification and separation of prisoners; unfortunately, the sensible purposes of those who proposed this system have not been sustained, partly in consequence of an error in not conveying heat, by means of iron cylinders, through the cells, and omitting several other requisites, when the building was going up. When I was there, in December, there were *thirty one* prisoners, of all ages, charged with various crimes and misdemeanors; these were divided, sixteen in one room, fifteen in another, on each side of the area which seperates the cells, as you enter the interior prison. These prisoners were thus associated for the advantage of a fire, it being impossible to heat the cells by placing a stove in the area. In the day rooms, therefore, they lodged and freely associated, *for* worse, not better ; "but," the Keeper remarked, "it is no great matter, for they are bad enough before they get here, and may as well learn of each other here what they have'nt got, as get it when they go out." The prison contains fifty four cells, in three tiers, and six day rooms, two upon each gallery. The dimensions of the cells are *seven* feet by *nine*, and *nine* high. They receive light and air through a perpendicular slit or fissure in the wall. The area in the centre is lighted and ventilated through large windows, opening at the end upon an enclosed yard. The apparatus for raising the water, is worked in the area, and throws the water into tanks in the upper story, whence it is conveyed through pipes below. I did not learn that any room was fitted up for the purpose of bathing and cleansing. With a little care and determination this prison might be made one of the best in the country. A Keeper, understanding the advantages of division, and employment for the prisoners, might make this a model prison ; rescue some of those who are committed here, from destruction, and afford to all the opportunity and means of improvement. While the citizens of Louisville are proposing amended plans for the Work-House, perhaps they will be induced to extend the reformation to this receiving and detaining prison, and offer a wholesome example to neighboring towns and cities

The citizens of Jefferson county decree their Jail to the *sole use* of the *county*, denying its use for the mere convenience of private individuals.

In concluding these notices of the State Penitentiary and County Jails, visited since October, I repeat the sentiment expressed in the beginning, I have faith in the improvement of all these prisons. I believe that those which are so unfit for custodial use, will not long be suffered to remain in the condition represented. They often open to receive persons of desperate character, and of a most unworthy class; but men are not made repentant through extreme privations and undue severity. Society certainly gains nothing by employing physical force, to the whole exclusion of moral influences. Too seldom is the heavy door of the dungeon unclosed to admit the Christian teacher, and too seldom is the attempt made by each and by all to seek and save those who are lost.

The Almighty, the all-benignant Father, sends his rain upon the just and upon the unjust, and makes his sun to shine upon the evil as upon the good; shall man be more just than God, be more pure than his Maker?

To visit the prisoner, to teach the ignorant, to enlighten transgressors, are included in the category of Christian duties. Raise up the fallen, console the afflicted, defend the helpless, minister to the poor, reclaim the transgressor, be benefactors of mankind!

Respectfully communicated.

D. L. DIX.

FRANKFORT, *February*, 1846.

APPENDIX.

—

(See dimensions of the Prison and State property, page 7.)

The official person who gave to me the dimensions of the prison, the area, yards, &c., through lapse of memory perhaps, omitted to state that, in addition to the larger and lesser walled grounds, the State owns, in connection with this property, about six acres, something more than one of which, lies immediately outside, and bounded by the prison walls on the north-east and east. A part of this tract, in summer, is used as a cow pasture; the other portions of the property were purchased a few years since by the immediate predecessor of the present Keeper, in two lots, of two individuals, at an entire cost of $550 dollars, and were subsequently transferred to the State, for the price originally paid.

The two tracts last referred to are separated from the lot which bounds the wall east, and from a lot owned as private property, by Shelby street. A contract has been concluded for the purchase of a lot situated on Clinton and High streets, for the purpose of extending the limits, buildings, &c.

EXTRACTS FROM "REMARKS ON PRISONS AND PRISON DISCIPLINE IN THE UNITED STATES, BY D. L. DIX."

"The six county prisons, of several hundred which I have visited and re-visited in the Northern and Middle States, and which most claim notice for their good discipline, are three on the silent system with labor, severally at South Boston, Mass.; at Hartford, and at New Haven, in Connecticut; and three established on the separate system, severally at Philadelphia, Harrisburg, and West-Chester. There are many other prisons, in the Northern and Middle States, which are well ordered as mere detaining prisons, but to which the very formidable exceptions must be made from indiscriminate association of all clases of offenders, and without employment either for the mind or the hands. These nurseries of vice claim early and efficient attention. Furnish them ever so well, keep them ever so clean, supply ever so sufficient, and well prepared food, as at fifty or a hundred prisons I could indicate, but what do these avail if the habits of daily life are becoming constantly more disastrous, and the soul is perishing for lack of the bread of life, and waters of salvation."

*   *   *   *   *   *   *   *

"Dauphin County Jail, at Harrisburg, is undoubtedly one of the best conducted county prisons in the United States. Like the jail in Chester county, it adopts the separate system with employment, and such instruction and advantages, as prisons constructed on this plan, secure to morals and habits. The provisions are excellent, and the food well prepared and supplied in sufficient quantities."

*   *   *   *   *   *   *   *

"Religious service is held in the Dauphin County Jail on every Sabbath afternoon, by the clergy of Harrisburg, who have volunteered their services, and so fulfil the law of Christ, preaching repentance and the forgiveness of sins 'unto the poor and prison-bound.' This instruction needs to be followed up by additional lessons. Many are profoundly ignorant upon the plainest principles of morals, so far as teaching and example have reached them. They need help in these things; more aid than the inspectors or warden can have leisure to give; and these official persons are both vigilant and interested to benefit and reclaim the prisoner. There is a well chosen library. Repeated visits to this jail have satisfied me of the kind and just discipline which prevails. Punishment is infrequent, and, when imposed, is of no greater severity or duration, than is absolutely necessary for securing compliance with the mild and needful regulations of the institution.

"The dimensions of the cells are 8 feet by 15, and 10 high, lighted at one end near the ceiling. Pure water is introduced through iron pipes, and the cells are maintained warm and dry by means of hot water thrown through small iron pipes in each cell. The bunks are furnished with a straw bed, replaced as often as necessary; and a sufficient quantity of clean bed clothing. The apparel of the prisoners is comfortable, and adapted to the season. I have found the prisoners in health and as good condition, physically, as the the same number of persons following like employments, and of steady habits abroad." * * * * * * * *

"The inspectors also remark, 'As to the efficacy of the system of separate confinement, *combined with labor*, being the most perfect yet devised for the punishment and reformation of offenders, our experience during the past year, fully confirms all that our remarks expressed in the last annual report —*giving precedence* to the 'Pennsylvania, or separate system.' The report concludes with a merited commendation of the warden, and other officers, for fidelity in the discharge of their duties. The fidelity extends to the inspectors, and it is as commendable as it is rare in county jails."

* * * * * * * * *

"Chester County Jail, at West-Chester, (Penn.) is built of stone, upon the plan of separate imprisonment. The cells are of good size, perfectly clean, and well aired. The provisions supplied are of excellent quality. The allowance is three meals daily, and as much as satisfies the appetite. There has been but one death, by disease, in four years, and this was by consumption, developed before admission; and one was pardoned in consumption, who was also sick when received. One man, who was received in a state of intoxication, committed suicide. I copy, from the warden's report to the board of inspectors, the following facts:

We had in prison on the 1st of May, 1843, - - - - -	32
We received, during the year, white males, - - - - -	41
Do do do females, - - - -	3
Colored males, - - - - - - - - -	25
Colored females, - - - - - - - - - -	4
Making in all, - - - - - - - - -	105
In prison on the 1st of May, 1844, - - - - - -	28

The total number sentenced to labor, during four years, since removed from the old prison, is 79. Of these, 47 could read and write; 24 could not read nor write; and 8 could read only. 33 of these prisoners were intemperate; 28 of them temperate, and 18 were moderate drinkers.

I visited this prison in July, and saw all the prisoners, of which there were 29. 20 of these were convicts, and 9 were waiting trial. They were in excellent health, often replying to my inquiry in the words, 'I am right hearty.' They conversed cheerfully, were clean in their person and apparel, and presented a remarkable contrast to the 68 prisons I have since visited, always excepting the Moyamensing prison, and that of Dauphin county. Some of the jails referred to were in Maryland, Virginia, Ohio, and Massachusetts." * * * * *

"The Suffolk County House of Correction, at South Boston, is well built, and is excellently planned for carrying out successfully the purposes of prison government, &c. In former years I often visited this prison; latterly more rarely, on account of distant journeyings. I never found it other than in good order; the law of the place, as of other city institutions within the stockade, being, apparently, that 'nothing is clean when it can be made cleaner.' The discipline is efficient, and as mild as the Auburn system of congregated labor will permit. The 3d of Sept., 1845, there were 225 prisoners, 74 of which were women, all sentenced by the municipal and police courts. Quite too many of the prisoners are discharged by pardons and remission of sentence; vastly too many escape imprisonment by the very injudicious imposition of fines, and the equally injudicious acceptance of bail. There are 360 cells which are perfectly clean and admirably ventilated. The stoves for heating the lodging cells and areas, in winter, are of better construction than any I have before seen in prisons.

The prisoners bathe in the salt-water, in a commodious bathing house, once a week during the mild seasons: and they bathe in warm water once a fortnight throughout the cold months. The health of the place is remarkable, and the deaths few, considering the previous habits of the convicts. The women's work-rooms are well governed and arranged. The cells are suitably furnished. The hospital is faithfully attended, and entirely comfortable. The laundry, bakery, and cook rooms, are in most admirable order. The food is of good quality, and well prepared.

The chaplain is diligent in the discharge of his duties, and holds two services on Sunday. There is, at an early hour, a Sunday School for the women. The teachers are from the city, and are much devoted to the improvement of the convicts, and extend a judicious care over all who, at the expiration of their sentences, give evidence of a disposition to lead an amended life. The library at this prison is not creditable to those whose duty it is to see the prisoners supplied with this means of improvement."

* * * * * * * * *

"I cannot conclude these remarks, without renewedly urging the reformation of the county jails. It is infinitely worse, to arrest offenders, and lodge them in jails where safe custody is the only consideration to which weight is attached, than to leave them at large. It is worse for offenders, and worse ultimately for society. In the first instance, they inevitably become more corrupt. They have no escape, if they wish it, from vicious companionship; and, when it is farther recollected, that these prisoners include the really guilty, the merely suspected, and those of both sexes and all ages, we cannot fail to see what is the imperative duty of the citizens of every county throughout the Union, in which this subject has not received so much deliberation and action as to have procured a remedy for neglects and abuses, worthy only of an age when vice was openly countenanced, and crime was at a premium. Hundreds certainly, more probably thousands, have for some first and trivial offence, been lodged in county prisons, exposed to the impure and contaminating influences of indiscriminate companionship. Here they have become hardened, here lost all self-respect, and have yielded, day by day, to the mind poisoning, moral miasm of these legalized receptacles.

From these great evils, society only can redeem the offender. If the offence is slight, or if suspicion alone attaches to the prisoner, there being no question of the justice of detention, the wrong is resolved into the injustice of compelling bad companionship, and making a jail a county free-school of vice. If the prisoner be already confirmed in vicious propensities and an evil life, it is manifestly very bad policy, all other considerations aside, to make him the teacher of what is mischievous and destructive of public safety, to those not confirmed in the practice of vicious excesses, and criminal mis-deeds. I have heard the observation that persons do not reach the jail till they are far on in paths of wickedness; this is a misapprehension, resulting from want of correct information. I could adduce a very large number of examples, especially of *young* persons and *children*. As such may be gathered in every county-town in the Union, not recently incorporated, it is quite unnecessary to enter upon details here."

MEMORIAL

TENNESSEE

1847

MEMORIAL

SOLICITING

ENLARGED AND IMPROVED ACCOMMODATIONS

FOR THE

INSANE OF THE STATE OF TENNESSEE,

BY THE ESTABLISHMENT OF

A NEW HOSPITAL.

BY MISS D. L. DIX.

PRINTED BY ORDER OF THE GENERAL ASSEMBLY,

NOVEMBER, 1847.

NASHVILLE:

B. R. M'KENNIE, PRINTER, WHIG AND POLITICIAN OFFICE.

1847.

MEMORIAL.

To the Honorable,
    the General Assembly of the State of Tennessee.

GENTLEMEN:

I ask to lay before you, briefly and distinctly, the necessities and claims of a numerous, and unfortunately, an increasing class of your fellow-citizens—I refer to the Insane of this State; the various distresses of whose various condition can be fully appreciated only by those who have witnessed their miseries. Pining in cells and dungeons, pent in log-cabins, bound with ropes, restrained by leathern throngs, burthened with chains—now wandering at large, alone and neglected, endangering the security of property, often inimical to human life; and now thrust into cells, into pens, or wretched cabins, excluded from the fair light of heaven, from social and healing influences—cast out, cast off, like the Pariah of the Hindoos, from comfort, hope, and happiness, such is the present actual condition of a large number of your fellow-citizens—useless and helpless, life is at once grievous to themselves, and a source of immeasurable sorrow to all beside.

In some cases, indeed, pitying friends strive to procure comforts, and exercise consoling cares: how little, under the cloud of this malady, these avail, many can bear sorrowful testimony. The only remedy or alleviation is to be found

in *rightly organized Hospitals*, adapted to the special care
the peculiar malady of the Insane so urgently demands.

Made conversant with the cruel sufferings and measure-
less distresses of which I speak, by patient investigations,
reaching through long and weary years, over the length
and breadth of our land, I represent the existence of troubles no imagination can exaggerate, and I have come now
to Tennessee, as the advocate and friend of those who cannot plead their own cause, and for those who have no friend
to protect and succor them, in this, the extremity of human
dependence.

I appeal confidently to the Legislature of Tennessee, in
which is vested the power, by the will of a whole people,
to interpose relief, and timely to apply a remedy to heal,
or at least to mitigate, the ravages of this cruel malady.

This subject, gentlemen, is not new to you. Good, humane, and liberal men in this State, more than eight years
since, discerned the necessities of the Insane, and applied
their energies to the establishment of a Hospital, in which
it was hoped and designed these should find relief through
the application of physical remedies and moral treatment.
Why the just and liberal spirit of the Legislature which
first acknowledged in Tennessee, the claims of the Insane
to become wards of the State, and through its generous
guardianship to find healing influences, has not been practi-
cally carried out, it is not my province to search into and
declare.

The intention on the part of the public was correct, and
the means ample; but that the experience of other States in
the construction of the Hospital, and in its internal organization, was not consulted, or, if consulted, not made instrnc-
tive, is evident, even to an uninformed and casual observer.

Most of the essential defects of the present edifice, which
is immediately on the confines of the city, do not admit of
repair or remedy; and even if this was not a demonstrable fact, the location, so singularly ill chosen, would present
a cogent objection to the permanent establishment by repairs and extended Hospital buildings, upon the present
site.

But again—though it might have been conceived by those entrusted with the responsibility of determining the extent of accommodations, that the present edifice was of sufficient capacity for the then understood wants of the patients, it is quite certain that now it cannot receive within its walls *one fourth* of all who are suffering immediately within your own borders, for such remedial treatment as a well-established Institution ought to afford.

I am not able to state the whole number of Insane, epileptics, and idiots in Tennessee, but it is certain that they are no longer to be numbered by *tens*, but by *hundreds*. Some calculators, predicating their estimates on the basis of ascertained facts in most other States, give an amount of from *ten to twelve hundred, in all.* I think this an excess, but allowing that there are but one-half or one-fourth of the above number, the need of much enlarged accommodations is not the less urgent.

There is less insanity in the southern, than in the northern States, proportioned to the inabitants of each; for this disparity several causes may be assigned: there is, in the former, comparatively but a small influx of foreigners, while they throng every district of the latter. In the Boston City Hospital for the Insane poor, were (in 1846) 169 patients; 99 of which were *foreigners*, 35 natives of other States, and 44 alone residents of the city. Of the 90 foreigners, 70 were Irish. In the New York City Hospital for the Insane poor, on Blackwell's Island, were (on the first of January, 1846,) 356 patients; of whom 226 were foreigners: at present the number exceeds 400. At the Philadelphia City Hospital for the Insane poor, and connected with the Alms House, there were received in one year 395 patients. The above Hospitals were established for the treatment of the Insane poor alone. But a more obvious cause is found in the fact of the much more numerous colored population here than there. The negro and the Indian rarely become subject to the malady of insanity, as neither do the uncivilized tribes and clans of European Russia and Asia. Insanity is the malady of civilized and cultivated life, and of sections and communities whose nervous energies are most roused and nourished.

Upon careful inquiry, it will be discovered that great suf-
ing is experienced in every county of this State, from the
want of a suitable Hospital for the Insane poor, as well as
for those who are in moderate or affluent circumstances.
This proposition admitted, it is clearly a duty to adopt such
measures as shall effectually remedy the evil.

Successive Legislatures have, biennially, for a considerable period, made such appropriations from the Treasury as
have been found to meet the most obvious wants which
have been revealed. The people at large, therefore, are
aware that Hospital care for the Insane is desirable, and
that it is sustained at least to a limited extent. I apprehend
that the insufficiency of this support for present necessities
is not widely known and appreciated. It will require no
subtle arguments to show that much more is to be done, and
it is not Tennessee which will offer the example of slight-
ing the claims of her afflicted children. *Here,* you will not
reveal yourselves less true, less honorable, less humane, less
just than are your sister States on every hand. Tennessee,
which in population and productions ranks fifth in the Union,
will not allow her younger or her senior sisters to excel her
in what is liberal and humane.* She is abundantly able to

---

*It may be interesting to some readers to possess the date and place of the
principal Hospitals in the United States now occupied, or in progress of construction.

The fiirst Hospital for the Insane was established in Philadelphia, being one
department of the Penn Hospital, in the year 1752. This was tansferred to
Blockley, 1832, a short distance from the city.

The second Institution receiving Insane patients, and the first exclusively for
their use, was at Williamsburg, Va., in 1773.

The third was the Friends' Hospital at Frankford, near Philadelphia, in 1817.

The next in succession were the McLean Hospital at Charlestown, now Somerville, near Boston, in 1818, and

Bloomingdale Hospital, near the city of New York, 1821.

South Carolina Hospital, 1822, at Columbia.

Connecticut Hospital at Hartford; and the

Kentucky Hospital at Lexington, 1824.

Virginia Western Hospital at Staunton, 1828.

Massachusetts State Hospital at Worcester, 1833.

Maryland Hospital at Baltimore, 1834.

Vermont State Hospital, ———, 1837.

New York City Hospital at Blackwell's Island, 1838.

do this good work—she *will* do it; and she will do it *now*, freely, unitedly, and well!

Allow me to state briefly the most prominent defects of the Hospital, at present devoted to the treatment of the Insane.

1st, The interior construction:—the wards in each wing are ill arranged for the proper classification of the patients: the excitable, the noisy, the sick, the languid, and the convalescent, are frequently associated in such sort as to prevent comfort, destroy quiet, and retard recovery. The highly excited patients shut into those wretched cells in the cellar, damp, cold, and unventilated as they are, are not fit for any human creature, much less for the treatment of the sick; and these patients are beneath apartments occupied by others requiring repose, and every comforting and cheering influence. Your superintendent in his last report anticipates my statements, declaring that "the cells belonging to this institution being under ground, and not susceptible of ventilation, are wholly unfit for the habitation of human

Tennessee Hospital at Nashville, 1839.
Boston City Hospital at South Boston, and
Ohio State Hospital at Columbus, 1839.
Maine State Hospital at Augusta, 1840.
New Hampshire State Hospital at Concord, 1842.
New York State Hospital at Utica, 1843.
Mt. Hope Hospital at Baltimore, 1844.
That of Georgia, at Milledgeville, some years since.

The Rhode Island State Hospital and Butler Asylum, at Providence, will probably be opened for patients, under the able conduct of Dr. Ray, early in 1848.

The New Jersey State Hospital. at Trenton, will be ready for occupation in the first or second month of 1848, under tho competent superintendence of Dr. Buttolph, so long the respected and indefatigable Assistant at the New York State Hospital.

The Indiana Institution, at Indianapolis, so ably advocated and established by Dr. John Evans, will probably be completed in less than a year.

The State Hospital of Illlnois, at Jacksonville, will be finished in about a year and a half.

The Louisiana State Hospital, at Jackson, will probably be occupied within two years.

The Missouri State Hospital will not be completed for two years.

We hope, confidently, in little more than that period, to see the new and much needed Hospital of Tennessee finished and open to receive two hundred and fifty patients to its fostering care and restoring benefits.

beings; and even supposing them to be of value as places of temporary confinement, they are nevertheless utterly useless for any remedial purpose." On a late visit at the Hospital, I found these cells occupied, and the most vehement excitement prevailing, unquestionably stimulated and protracted by the unfortunate circumstances surrounding the patients. The lodging-rooms above are of sufficient size, indeed might without disadvantage be made smaller, but they are either not warmed at all, or insufficiently heated, and not ventilated. In fact, the proper ventilation of the whole building appears to have been entirely overlooked in its construction, and it is not possible to preserve a pure and wholesome atmosphere throughout.

A new warming apparatus, lately introduced at a large cost, is apparently a complete failure: and by its defective construction, allowing the escape of deleterious gases, the patients are in worse condition than before the introduction of the furnaces. In no way, at present apparent, can the temperature either of the day-rooms or the lodging apartments be properly regulated for the feeble or more vigorous patients.

There are in the Hospital no bath rooms; and thus a most important remedial agent is not to be had, except under circumstances of great exposure, and unreasonable extra labor. Convenience is not consulted, nor personal cleanliness attainable in any special department. There are no clothes room, no store rooms, no labor saving arrangements of any description whatever—no convenient dining-rooms, with labor saving dumb-waiters, &c., &c.

The kitchens and laundry are so amazingly defective that the surprise is to witness the accomplishment of daily work in any manner so as to secure the order of domestic economy. There is no bakery, no meat house, no smoke-house, no ice-house, no corn-crib nor meal-bin, no spring-house, milk-house, nor sheds for storing coal, wood, &c., &c.

There are no cisterns, and no wells which afford a supply of water—there is never, I am told, at any season a sufficient supply for culinary and other domestic purposes, much less for the preservation of personal cleanliness. The superintendent informs me that they are often "mainly dependent on the quantity they can haul from the river with one horse, over a distance of a mile and a half!" Wood being used for fuel, a large, if not an ample supply might be saved from the roofs, but *there are no cisterns*, and the casks used are *so few* and so small, that water collected in this way of course fails to meet the demand. The superintendent states in his report, "that during a considerable portion of the year, they have not water even to drink," (*see report, page* 7.) It would require but a very moderate outlay to construct cisterns and tanks, and so furnish *without delay*, what appears indispensably requisite, a supply of wholesome, pure water.* To this plan it is indeed objected, that wood costs more than coal used as fuel—the next remedy then seems to be to economise in fuel, and conduct water through a sub-surface channel from the city waterworks, or from the river by horse power and a water-wheel. This should be a first care; for, finally, suppose the occurrence of a conflagration—no improbable event—there at your Institution, and no water at hand to check the progress of the destroying element—suppose it probable that the patients could be removed, (and this is doubtful when the number of care-takers is remembered,) why peril the loss of a valuable edifice, quite suitable to serve many uses, unfit though it is for the residence and proper treatment of the Insane.

There is another want too prominent not to attract notice. It is stated that for a number of patients, varying from *fifty*

---

*In the New York State Hospital, at Utica, while yet the number of patients was but 200, the daily consumption of water for all purposes was between *three and four thousand* gallons. The supplies were obtained as follows: In addition to rain water, flowing from the roof into six large tanks lined with lead, containing above four thousand gallons each, and placed in the attic stories of the wings, is furnished a well, distant five hundred feet in rear of the Asylum. This well is thirty-three feet deep, sixteen in diameter for twenty-three feet, and then eight feet for the remaining ten. The water is forced from this well by means of a pump, driven by horse-power to the attic story of the centre building, and thence distributed over the whole establishment. One horse will pump from forty to fifty hogsheads in an hour. This apparatus is simple, and applicable in all large Institutions. In nearly every Hospital, supplies are derived in similar or like manner.

to *sixty* and *seventy,* there are but *"three attendants or nurses."* Incredible as this seems, I am am assured it is the fact—indeed, a reference to the Report previously quoted, (*see page* 4,) exhibits at once the *fact and the assigned cause* in juxtaposition. "The *means at the disposal of the Institution*," writes the superintendent, "enable it to employ *only two male attendants and one female."* This admits an effectual and immediate remedy. Reference to the Treasurer's Report of the present year opens the following exhibit for the last two financial years: (see page 16.) "Attendants $2066 73;" and directly following, "Servants hire $1546 58." Perhaps the first charge embraces the salary of the Physician, matron, and steward. There is no table of officers, and it is not shown in either of the documents referred to, that there ever has been any organized body of this sort, as is usual in other Hospitals. I am sure that the Legislature do not purpose that the patients should suffer for lack of necessary care, nor that the Physician should be charged with a responsibility so great as that of guarding the patients from harm, and treating them remedially, without adequate means.

That present legislation is not requisite for authorizing remedy for many actual wants, is apparent in the Statutes for 1839–40: (see page 208, chap. cxx., sec. 4.)

"*Be it enacted,* That said Board of Trustees shall have power to make such orders and regulations as may be necessary for the government of their patients in the Hospital, its internal police, the supply of provisions, fuel, *water, clothing, books, and whatever else may be deemed necessary for the health, comfort, cleanliness,* and *security* of the inmates."

This act is certainly benevolent in its aim, and sufficiently full and explicit upon the subject treated.

In most of our State Hospitals, the *average* of nurses and attendants is one nurse to every ten patients. Sometimes the number of patients in charge of one nurse is larger, sometimes fewer, according to the state of the patients and other circumstances. (See numerous Hospital Reports.)—Paying patients may, according to the choice of friends, have special nurses wholly devoted to their service. The

night-watch nurses are always chosen with great care.
Too much caution cannot be taken in the choice and
selection of nurses for the Insane. Comparatively, the
number is not large who are suited to fulfil these duties.
Yet they can be found here as elsewhere. They must possess correct principles and self-control: they must be patient,
enduring, and forbearing; firm but kind; never requiting
injurious language and violent acts with passionate words
or vehement demonstrations. To return good for evil must
be the invariable rule. No excitement should be exhibited
under the wayward conduct and ungracious speech of an
intractable patient. Nor must the smallest deviation from
truth and sincerity be permitted. The conscietious nurse,
and no other, should approach the dependent Insane. None
should accept this responsible and careful office, alone for
the means of self-support, but because they may, while
laboring for their own subsistence, be at the same time rendering a priceless benefit to their fellow-beings. Money
alone can never compensate a faithful nurse: an approving
conscience must supply the deficiency. It is a rule closely
laid down, as far as I have witnessed, in all well-ordered
Hospitals, that no attendant shall, under any circumstances,
strike a patient. No blow shall ever be inflicted upon those
patients, who are so eminently *unaccountable* through the
malady under which they suffer—they must be guarded with
fidelity, guided with firmness and kindness, and respected in
their misfortunes. No attendant should be retained in office
one hour, after being known to offend by manifesting any
form of violent speech or act towards his patients. I would
never make one exception to a rule so necessary to be enforced, and of so searching obligation.*

---

*In procuring attendants, says Dr. Earle, "every endeavor is used to obtain
persons of kind dispositions, and of such character, that they may be looked
upon by the patients as companions and friends." Similar opinions are distinctly expressed by all our eminent Physicians. My visits at Hospitals have for
years been frequent, and under such circumstances as would show the true condition of the household organizations. I have rarely, very rarely found ill chosen
nurses, and I have never known such retained in a hospital claiming rank as a
curative Institution, save in two instances, and these, I trust, will not long be
quoted for deficiencies in the most important department of these Institutions.

I have represented chiefly the interior defects of the State Hospital, except one deficiency which exists to the same extent in no kindred establishment: I refer to the want of moral means to aid the skill of the Physician in procuring the mental health and boily vigor of his patients. They have neither suitable occupations nor recreations. There are no exercise grounds, no gardens, no fields, where productive and healthful labor in the open air may be carried on. There is no carriage for the use of the feeble patients, when daily exercise abroad would be highly beneficial.— There is no Library, no supply of periodicals fitly selected, for use and entertainment; no musical instruments; no sets of simple games, no work-shops—in short, life in the Hospital seems necessarily, under present circumstances, to be one dull unvarying round of like uninteresting events from day to day, and month to month. Under the head of Moral Treatment, the Physician of the Bloomingdale Hospital renders the following exposition, which in general corresponds with all the best organized and most successful Institutions of the country. I must somewhat abridge the statement:

"We have *religious worship* on the Sabbath; a *school* in the men's department during the cold season; *lectures* on scientific and miscellaneous subjects, by the superintendent, illustrated by experiments and painted diagrams. The *Library* which contains a thousand volumes; with current newspapers, magazines and reviews, furnishes reading for all who are disposed to use them, and the number is not small. Most of the patients walk out or ride daily in suitable weather.

"Some of the men work in the carpenters' shop, upon the farm, or about the grounds. Many of the women wash and sew, and assist in keeping their apartments in order. We use also ninepins, quoits, bagatelle, chess, chequers, dominoes, a swing in the grove, &c. We have social parties, from the different wards, but strictly within our own household of course, once a week. There is no undue exposure of the patients. or repetition of their insane conversations abroad. These are our chief moral means."

"Labor," remarks the superintendent of the Hospital at Utica, "especially gardening and farming, are to the men, in most instances, the favorite amusement. In addition, they resort to reading, writing, ninepins, battledore and ball. The women walk and ride abroad; quilt, complete all sorts of plain work, and almost every kind of fancy article that taste can desire.

"The school is beneficial to those who are convalescent, those who are melancholy, and to those whose mental powers seem sinking into dementia: their memories are thus improved, and they become more active and cheerful. Musical parties for those for whom a little excitement is good, are formed often at evening.

"The want of proper *mental* occupation has, till of late years especially, been much felt in Hospitals for the Insane; this end may now be supplied every where to a great extent."

The choir of singers at evening prayers, and at service on Sundays, is, in most Hospitals, composed of the patients aided by some of the attendants.

Very similar are the moral measures employed by Drs. Bell, Kirkbride, Awl, Allen, Brigham, Butler, Parker, Chandler, and others, as *remedial* means, too valuable to be dispensed with. Mere medical treatment, after the first few days, is usually altogether subordinate to diet, exercise, occupations, and amusements, employed of course always with discrimination.

In the Ohio Asylum, the ladies find great pleasure in cultivating their flower gardens in summer, and their houseplants in winter, and in the use of the needle in plain and fancy work. The most dull, inert, demented patient, may, with kind perseverance, be induced to take part in some work or sport. Dr. Allen, in Kentucky, has been eminently successful with this class.

Dr. Ray, who is high authority, and well known in Europe, as in our own country, for his excellent work, the "Jurisprudence of Insanity," remarks in one of his Reports, while yet he was superintendent of the Maine State Hospital, that "he would be a bold man, who should venture to say, that Pinel and Esquirol, whose medical treatment was confined chiefly to baths and bitter drinks, were less successful in their cure of mental diseases, than those numerous practitioners who have exhausted upon them all the resources of the healing art. Strictly medical means has less to do than some others, with the treatment of the Insane. In chronic disorders, especially those which are of a nervous character, the means on which the intelligent practitioner chiefly relies with most confidence, are *proper diet and exercise, change of air and scene, useful and agreeable* occupation of the mind, and various employments. Yet much must be done to prepare the system, by the *judicious* application of proper medical remedies, for the efficient action of moral means."

Dr. Trezevant, formerly of the South Carolina Hospital at Columbia, in a clearly written and valuable Report, remarks, that "there is not a year in which I do not see in patients brought to our Hospital, cases of constitutions shattered, and the recuperative energies of the brain entirely destroyed by the free use of the lancet and depleting remedies, before the patient is removed to our care."

In corroboration of these sensible views, I might proceed to adduce other opinions in accordance with them, from the highest authorities in our own country, in England, and in France; this is not here and now requisite: but allow me to direct your inquiries to your State Institution, so deplorably destitute of moral means for the benefit of the patients.

It appears to be universally conceded, that manual labor is eminently desirable for a large class of patients. To this end, it is important that at least one hundred acres of land be attached to the Hospital for cultivation, and other purposes.

The productions from the small farm attached to the Bloomingdale Hospital, at their fair market value, were estimated at $3,872 99—no inconsiderable sum in the item of table expenses; &c., in the Institution.

A careful, intelligent Physician will be cautious in giving active out-door work to recent patients, whose malady has been of short duration. All cannot be indiscriminately tasked, or rather employed: neither can the same patients, day by day, do an equal amount of labor. These things will always call for daily supervision, as do all things relating to the hygienic treatment of the patients.

Incurables who are able and willing to work, are more contented, and enjoy better health when employed. The following examples given in a Report of the Bloomingdale Institution, will pleasantly illustrate the benefits of employment for the curable patient. "Two farmers, each of whom possessed a good farm, were admitted into the Asylum, one about a week after the other. They were laboring under the most abject form of melancholy, and had both attempted suicide. In less than a month, their condition being already somewhat improved, they expressed a willingness, and one of them a strong desire, to work out of doors. Being furnished with implements, they daily went out together, and worked upon the farm with as much apparent interest as if it belonged to themselves. Under this course they both rapidly improved, and both were discharged recovered, one at the end of six weeks, and the other three months, from the time of their respective admissions.

"Another man was brought in the spring, in a state of active mania, his appetite was poor, and his frame emaciated. He was careless of his personal appearance, ruthless, turbulent, and almost incessantly talking in an incoherent manner upon the delusions attending his disease. When out of doors, he was wandering to and fro, talking to himself or digging the earth with his hands, without end or object, and generally having his mouth filled with grass. For some months there was but little change in his condition: at length, having become somewhat less bewildered, his attendant succeeded in inducing him to assist in making beds: shortly after, he was employod with the painters and glaziers upon the green-house, and then weut to the carpenters' shop, where he worked regularly for several weeks. Meanwhile his bodily health improved, his mind gradually returned to its former integrity, and he was discharged cured of his mental disorder, and weighing more than at any previous period of his life."

In the New York Hospital, a violent patient, after a few weeks special care and medical treatment, was invited to visit the carpenters' shop: he gazed round listlessly, but on a sudden seized a saw and declared he would make a sleigh and explore the frigid zone: he was allowed to carry out his fancy, worked laboriously with the carpenter for several hours daily, till his sleigh was finished—then declaring that there was not yet snow enough for good travelling, he resolved to commence another, and gave the first specimen of his skill to his fellow-workman, the carpenter. It was soon observed that his mind was resuming a healthful tone; his zeal in sleigh-making effectually diverted him from his delusions, and in a few months he returned to his family perfectly restored.

At another Institution, one lady quite recovered her health first diverted from her delusions by an interest in making work baskets of pasteboard and silk for her friends. Another was earnest to make a present to a friend, who was a student of natural history, and betook herself so zealously to copying birds from Audubon's Ornithology, that she forgot her troubles and recovered the use of her reason.

These cases are fair examples of the efficacy of a combination of medical and moral means.

Before the establishment of the City Hospital for the insane poor, in Boston, Mass., that department of the Alms-House assigned for their occupation, was a place of utter abomination. Scenes too horrible for description might be daily witnessed. These madmen and madwomen were of the most hopeless cases of long standing; their malady confirmed almost, by early adverse circumstances, and following gross mismanagement.

The citizens at length made sensible of great abuses, and conscious of the great injustice of herding these maniacs together, where day and night their shrieks and wild ravings destroyed the least appearance of repose, and where reigned all that was most loathsome and offensive,—resolved on establishing on correct principles, and at large cost, a special Hospital for their residence and treatment. The most sanguine friends of this measure hoped nothing more

for these most wretched beings than to procure for them
greater decency and comfort: recovery to the sound exercise of reason not being, under these circumstances, anticipated. The new Hospital was opened and its government
declared. The Insane were gradually removed from the
old department, disencumbered of their chains, and freed
from the remnants of foul garments; they were bathed and
clothed, and placed in cheerful, decent apartments, under
the superintendence of Dr. Butler—since made superintendent of the Retreat at Hartford, Conn. Thereafter, visit the
Hospital when one might, at neither set time nor season,
these hitherto most wretched beings would be found well
clad, usually tranquil, and capable of various employments in
the gardens and within doors, which were advantageous in
the economy of the Institution. Some might always be
found abroad, exercising under charge of an attendant, or
busy in the vegetable and flower gardens; others were in
the laundry, in the ironing-room, in the kitchen, &c. Care
was had not to allow fatigue by over labor, and the visitor
would see amongst those busy ones many of the incurables who had worn out years of misery in a dreary abode:
and though of this once miserable company, less than one-
sixth were restored to the right use of the reasoning faculties, with but few exceptions they were capable of receiving pleasure from employments and recreations, and of
being present in the chapel during religious service, where
they were serious and orderly. Than their's no condition
could be worse before their removal from the old Institution;
afterwards none could be better for creatures of impaired
faculties, incompetent as they were to guide and govern
themselves, yielding to beneficent influences, and gentle,
kindly cares.

In former times, it was judged that severity alone was the
power for governing the unfortunate beings who should
become subject, through bodily ailments, to loss of capacity
for self-care and self-government. It is true, indeed, that,
according to early writers, the priests of ancient Egypt received to their charge, persons drooping under deep melancholy, and languishing under nervous diseases, the symp-

B

toms of which were marked by deep depression or strange delusions. These were conducted to gay pavilions, charming gardens, surrounded by all that was cheerful and animating in nature, or captivating in art, and under a choice diet, often recovered, and went their way to their near or remote abodes! Not such was the discipline in the middle ages and later: no limit was placed before the terrors of the harshest treatment. The first radical reforms are traced to France, from thence have England and America brought the examples which now, in their practical results, bless humanity; restoring, through the exercise of benignant cares, and wise treatment, hundreds and even thousands to health, to usefulness, and all the blessings and benefits of domestic endearments, and social intercourse. With what blessings upon the name of the good Vincent de Paul do we learn of his self-sacrificing efforts to ameliorate the hard lot of the Insane, and then long years following we see Pinel, the benevolent, good man, the enlightened and skilful Physician, apply his noble mind to a thorough reform of those heretofore dreaded receptacles, the Hospitals of France. "It was, said the son of Pinel, in a memorial before the Academy of Arts and Sciences in Paris, "near the close of 1792, that Pinel, after reiterated importunities, induced government to issue a decree, permitting him to unchain the maniacs at Bicetre. After the most vexatious delays, he at last, by every skilful argument, induced M. Couthon, member of the Commune, to meet him at the Hospital, there to witness his first experiments. Couthon himself first proceeded to visit the patients, and to question them, but in return only received abuse and execrations, accompanied by terrible cries, and the clanking of chains. Retreating from the damp and filthy cells, he exclaimed to Pinel, 'Do as you will, but your life will be sacrificed to your false sentiment of mercy.'— Pinel delayed no longer; he selected fifty, who he believed might be released foom their chains without danger to others. The fetters were removed, first from twelve, using the precaution of having ready for use, jackets with long continuous sleeves, and closing behind.

"The experiments commenced with a French Captain,

whose history was unknown, save that *he had been in chains forty years!* He was thought to be dangerous; having with a single blow of his manacles at one time killed one of his keepers, so that ever after he was approached with caution. Pinel entered his cell unattended. 'Ah well, Captain, I will cause your chains to be taken off: you shall have liberty to walk in the court, if you will promise to behave like a gentleman, and offer no assaults!' 'I would promise,' responded the maniac, 'but you deride me, you are amusing yourself at my expense; you all fear me.' 'I have six men,' replied Pinel, 'ready to obey my orders; believe me, therefore, I will set you free from this duresse, if you will put on this jacket.' The Captain assented; the chains were removed, the jacket laced, the attendants withdrew, but left the door unclosed. He raised himself, but fell; this effort was repeated again and again: the use of his limbs so long constrained, nearly failed: at length trembling, and with tottering steps, he emerged from his dark dungeon. *His first look was at the sky!* 'Ah,' cried he, 'how beautiful!' The remainder of the day he was constantly moving to and fro, uttering continually exclamations of pleasure. He heeded no one: *the flowers, the trees, above all, the sky,* engrossed him. At night he volutarily returned to his cell, which had been cleansed, and furnished with a better bed; his sleep was tranquil and profound. For the two remaining years that he spent at the hospital, he had no recurrence of violent paroxysms, and often rendered good service to the attendants in conducting the affairs of the establishment.

"The next person released after the Captain, was Chevigne, a soldier of the French Guards, who had been in chains ten years, and was always difficult to control. Pinel, entering his cell, announced, that if he would obey his instructions he should be chained no longer. He promised, and executed the directions of his liberator with alacrity and address. Never in the history of the human mind was exexhibited a more complete revolution, and this patient, whose best years had been sacrificed in a gloomy cell, in chains and misery, soon showed himself capable of being one of the most useful in the establishment. During the horrors of the Revolution, this man repeatedly saved the life of his benefactor.

Next were released three Russian soldiers, who had been chained together for many years, but none knew when, why, or how they had been committed.

An aged priest next followed, who for twelve years had been a martyr to the most barbarous treatment. In less than a year, Pinel witnessed his entire recovery. He was discharged cured.

In the short period of a few days, this heroic and judicious Physician released more than fifty miserable maniacs: men of various rank and conditions, merchants, lawyers, priests, soldiers, laborers—thus rendering the furious tractable, and creating peace and contentment to a wonderful degree, where had for so many years reigned without interruption the most hideous tumults and outrages.

The efforts of Pinel were not limited to the Bicetre. At La Salpetriere, a ward bears his name, continually reminding the visitor of what France and the world owe to this great Philanthropist.

This rule of kindness, displacing violence and abuse, soon extended to England. The Retreat at York, founded by the society of Friends, was the first so distinguished, as in this country was their Hospital at Frankford the first to recognize and adopt humane laws. In England, the Middlesex Hospital, at Hanwell, under Sir William C. Ellis, first attained celebrity through humane methods of treatment.— His successor, Dr. Conolly, has advocated in his practice, and through his published works, an enlarged liberality and kind treatment.

In Germany, the principles of Pinel, and of his distinguished coadjutor, Esquirol, were established by the lamented Heinroth. The high rank of the Hospital at Leigburg, on the Rhine, under the direction of Jacobi, whose law and practice was "firmness and kindness," is every where known by all who are interested in the ameliorations I have described.

I might adduce innumerable examples witnessed in our Hospitals, and familiar to my own experience in poor-houses.

jails, and private dwellings, where the exchange of kindness for severity; care and nursing for abuse and neglect,
have been attended and followed with the happiest results.
I do not know of a Hospital bearing the least reputation or
trusted with confidence, where chains, severe restraints, or
any sort of abuse of *act* or *language* are permitted.

Dr. Conolly, connected with the celebrated Institution at
Hanwell in England, for so many years, in a recent letter,
published in the October number of the Westminster Review, expresses his idea of the obligations of the resident
Physician in a Hospital, while wisely objecting to the very
serious disadvantages of subjecting these Institutions to the
control of a "visiting, consulting Physician."

"The resident medical officer of an Asylum is, and must
always be, the most important person in it. No regulations, no caprice of committees, no appointments of other
officers, lay or medical, or however designated, can alter
his real position in this respect. He is constantly with the
patients; their characters are intimately known to him; he
watches the effects of all the means of cure to which he
resorts, and his own character gives the tone to the whole
house. The patients look to him as their friend, protector,
and guide. They know that he has authority to control
them, and power to confer many indulgences upon them;
he is always at hand to be appealed to, and his moral influence is complete. No arbitrary or prospective rule of treatment can be followed among the Insane, from day to day,
or even from hour to hour: their varying moods require constant consideration."

Skilful Physicians, of enlarged minds and liberal attainments in our country, spend the best strength of their best
years, in conscientious and diligent exertions for the relief
of patients entrusted to their care. Most of these men,
profoundly impressed with their great responsibilities, devote themselves without reservation to mitigate, by their
skill and their cares, the sufferings of the disabled mind.
Their interests, their labors, their lives are spent within the
Institutions over which they preside, with an earnestness of
self-devotion, which, so far as I can discern, bears fair

comparison with no other labors in any of the liberal professions.

It is knowledge of this fact which inspires me with confidence in the treatment of the Insane, in every correctly governed, rightly organized Hospital. Insanity requires a peculiar and appropriate treatment, which cannot be rendered while the patients remain at their own homes, or by even skilful Physicians in general practice. I confide in Hospital care for remedial treatment, and in no other care. One might quote volumes to show, that, however able the patient or his friends may be, to provide in private families every luxury and accommodation, it is hazarding final recovery to make even the experiment of domestic treatment.

Dr. Brighan, in one of his early reports of the New York State Hospital, remarks, that "when sufficient time has elapsed to show clearly that the case is Insanity, unaccompanied by acute disease, then *no time should be lost*, in adopting the most approved remedial measures, among which, as has often been stated, is *removal from home*, to a place where the exciting causes of disease are no longer operative." "Let the friends *fully satify themselves that the patient will receive kind treatment*, then, forbear all untimely interference with the remedial measures adopted in the Hospitals of their choice." An individual being Insane, *all ordinary considerations* should give place to the aim of recovery; and this should be steadily adhered to, however discouraging the circumstances, till it is entirely established that the case is beyond the reach of all available means of cure.

But, granting the patient *incurable*, hospital care and protection is hardly less necessary, whether we study the real comfort of the patient, the security and quiet of his family at home, or the safety of society. There are patients sunk into a state of low dementia, who may be considered under all ordinary circumstances harmless, but a numerous portion of those permitted at large, are liable to sudden access of vehement excitements, in which condition, depredations, assaults, suicides, murders, and arson, are committed, and not seldom under the most pitiable circumstances. Within the last *four* weeks I have seen the record of *thirteen* cases of self-destruction, homicide, and arson by the Insane, recorded under authority. I was induced to visit the ill-conducted jail at Pittsburg, three weeks since, and amidst a throng of disorderly prisoners of all ages, colors, and conditions, found an insane woman charged with the murder of her mother. The poor mother took care of her as best she could, for there was no Hospital within the reach of her means where to place the mad girl in safety, but ordinarily, I was told, she was "looked on as harmless," in a sudden and unexpected paroxysm she murdered her mother in a horrible manner; an attempt, strange to say, was made to bring the well known irresponsible creature to trial, but "she was too crazy for management in the court-room," and so was remanded to prison.

Your own Penitentiary, on the outskirts of this city, has one inmate, charged with the compound crime of murder and arson. The details are too sickening and horrible to relate. It is a most undoubted case of moral insanity, from which no recovery can possibly be expected.

More than two years since, a convict was sent to the Cherry Hill prison, under a long sentence, charged with assault and battery, with intent to rob on the highway; it was evident to every officer, that the man was insane; this was confirmed by the Physician on his first visit, but his sentence had been pronounced, he was legally committed, and could be discharged only by gubernatorial clemency. Some weeks went by, he grew worse, his friends traced him, his history was ascertained; he was a respectable operative in a neighboring manufacturing district: had sickened and became insane upon the sudden decease of a favorite son: his watcher slept, the excited patient escaped half clad, and after running some miles, suddenly leaped into a market wagon which was entering the city: the terrified owner gave the alarm—arrest followed, &c. Finally a pardon was obtained, he was restored to his family, and in a few months was perfectly recovered, and returned to his usual employments.

I might weary you with successive details; but I doubt not your own knowledge reaches in many instances to cases corroborative of my position. *It is not safe, nor is it humane,* to leave the Insane, *whether curable or incurable,* to roam at large, or abide in families, unguarded, unguided, and uncontrolled. For their own sake, for that of their friends, for that of the community, they should be rendered to the *kind, skilful, intelligent, judicious watch* of Hospital protection.

Beside the *propriety* and *general obligation* which I assert of placing patients in good Hospitals, there is the great probability of ultimate recovery of the healthy functional action of the brain.

Dr. Bell, of the McLean Hospital at Somerville—whose name commands a respectful confidence rarely exceeded, the skilful Physician, wise friend, judicious superintendent, the good man, he whose cares have restored so many sufferers to their homes, and the blessed affections centering there—has stated, in an early report, and repeated the proposition in succeeding documents, that, *"in* an Institution *fully provided with attendants,* there may be afforded to all except a few highly excited patients, any comfort to which they have been accustomed at home, *and all cases certainly recent,* whose origin does not date directly or obscurely back more than one year, *recover under a fair trial.* This being the general law, the cases to the contrary counting as the exceptions."

In the Hospital at Lexington, in 1845–46, of 19 *recent* cases, 16 were discharged cured.

That must indeed be an indiscreet State policy which forfeits the happiness of its citizens to fill its treasury, and even still more reprehensible, when a well defined economy suggests a contrary course. Legislators have not the leisure, as but seldom the opportunity to enter upon suitable investigations of this subject, and therefore facts are collected and placed at their disposal, giving them opportunity of pursuing an enlighted and *just* course.

Dr. Allen, the excellent and successful superintendent of the Kentucky State Hospital, at Lexington, after the experience of several years, concurs in the opinions quoted above, and urges in eloquent language, the *early* care of the Insane by qualified persons; recommending as the best economy as well as humanity, that a State can practice, prompt and entire provisional care of the Insane.

No fact indeed is better established in all Hospital annals than this; that it is *cheaper* (we now set aside the plea of humanity) to take charge of the Insane in a curative Institution, than to support them elsewhere for life.

In the Massachusetts State Hospital, at Worcester, then in charge of Dr. Woodward, in 1843, twenty-five *old* cases had cost ·······················$54,157 00
Average expense of *old* cases ··············· 2,166 20
Whole expense of twenty-five *recent* cases till recovered, ···························· 1,461 30
Average expense of *recent* cases············· 58 45
In the Maine State Hospital at Augusta, in 1842, twelve *old* cases had cost $25,300 00
Average expense of *old* cases················ 2,108 33
Whole expense of twelve *recent* cases········ 426 00
Average expense of *recent cases*············· 35 50
In the Ohio State Hospital at Columbus, in 1844, thirty-five *old* cases had cost the counties and State, ·······························$35,464 00
Average expense of *old* cases··············· 1,418 56
Whole expense of twenty-five *recent* cases,····· 1,608 00
Average expense of *recent* cases till recovered·· 64 32
In the Western State Hospital at Staunton, Va., twenty *old* cases had cost···············$41,633 00
Average expense of *old* cases··············· 2,081 65
Whole expense of twenty *recent* cases········ 1,265 00
Average expense of twenty *recent* cases till recovered ······························· 63 25

It appears unnecessary to multiply examples derived from other Hospitals, whether in locations near to or remote each from the other; but reference to other records may be made, if additional evidence is needed to prove *the economy* both to citizens individually, to counties, or to States, of establishing curative Institutions for the Insane.

I have endeavored to show that your State Hospital is defective for the objects which should be held in view, the *care* and the *comfort* of its inmates. I have tried to exhibit the unfitness of treatment in private families; a few lines will illustrate the only three remaining methods by which the Insane are brought under treatment or disposed of. I mean in the State prison, in the jails, and in the poorhouses.

First, the State prison is a totally unfit place of detention for the Insane, since there, they cannot be cured, if not incurable; they are not fit subjects of discipline; they are not amenable to the rules of a Penitentiary; they are not accountable for violent speech or criminal acts. Danger to officers, danger to convicts, and injury to themselves, accompanies their imprisonment. It is not many years since the Penitentiaries of Massachusetts, of Connecticut, of New York, of Pennsylvania, &c., &c., gave terrible examples to show how easily human life could be taken by the madman, and *of* the madman, in their workshops, in their corridors, and in their cells.

The criminal jurisprudence of Insanity has of late years engaged the careful consideration of some of our ablest jurists and most enlightened citizens. In Europe, France led the way to this wholesome reform, declaring with equal justice and perspicuity, *"that there is no crime nor fault when the party accused was in a state of insanity at the period of the act."* "Il n'y a ni crime, ni delit losque le presence etait en etat de demence au temps de l'action."

In the penal code of Louisiana, compiled by Honorable Edward Livingston, the same declaration appears, though less precisely worded. The penal code of New York lays down the same principle; and Massachusetts more recently and quite effectually protects this case, and declares in addition, (but it is since the murder of a warden in the prison,) that a convict becoming insane while serving out his term of sentence, shall, when the insanity is fully proven, be transferred to the State Hospital.

If a State Penitentiary is an unfit place of custody for a maniac, surely a county jail is not less so: here exist the

same objections as above advanced, only in much increased
force; but it is not always the supposed criminal insane man
or woman who is liable to be committed to the custodial
charge of the jailors: we find too often those unfortunates
incarcerated in dreary cells or loathsome dungeons, and this
for "safe keeping alone!"

Upon this monstrous abuse of human rights I need not
pause to comment.

Finally, in the poor-houses are frequently found the poor
who are insane, as well as other afflicted cases, there most
inappropriately bestowed. If violent, their phrenzied ravings disturb the members of the household, and disquiet
especially the sick, the infirm, and the aged, who should
find in these Institutions a comfortable asylum and tranquil
home. If blasphemous and unruly, their presence is demoralizing, as well as dangerous to the personal security of
other inmates. On the other hand, the Insane are continually exposed to injudicious treatment, to careless oversight,
to abuse and insult, nay more, as I have had too much opportunity to know, to gross outrages.

A very large proportion of the Insane of the United States,
are either in narrow circumstances or absolutely dependent.
In poor-houses they rarely recover the exercise of the reasoning faculties; especialty where rigorous discipline is
employed. Poor-houses should have every arrangement for
the comfort of the aged, the helpless, the cripple—those who
are altogether dependent on the public for support, who are
unable to care for themselves, or incapable of laboring for
their own subsistence, but not including in this class the
Insane, whether tranquil or violent.

I submit the question, Gentlemen, whether the poor-
houses of Tennessee are fit asylums for the curable or the
incurable Insane. If any doubt through want of knowledge from personal observation, I suggest that the poor-
house of Davidson county, which I visited last week, and
which I am assured is "one of the best in Tennessee"—be
visited for purposes of positive information. The Insane
will be found there, in ill-repaired out-houses and cold,
cheerless cells, though "some," lately inmates, I was told,

were "dead, and others had run away." In inclement weather the patients must suffer severely.

Gentlemen, the object of this memorial is accomplished if I have succeeded in showing you, that you are destitute in this State of that which it has also been my aim to convince you that you need, a *suitable curative Hospital* for all classes of the Insane, and attached thereto a department for such as are considered *incurable*.

"Incurable cases." writes an experienced superintendent, "instead of being immured in jails and county poor-houses, without employment or comfort, where they are continually losing mind and becoming worse, should be placed in good asylums, and have employment on the farm or in shops. In this way they would be rendered much happier, and their existence, if in one sense a blank to themselves, would not be useless to others."

Look over our country at the large class of incurables, oftenest made so by neglect and ill-treatment; see these wretched beings wearing out a mere animal existence through long and dismal years; place yourselves, if you have courage, only in imagination, and for but few hours in their condition, then ask what would you, that, in such circumstances, your fellow-men should do for you? In *act*, let your reply be—"do even so unto them."

Were I to recount but briefly, a hundredth part of the shocking scenes of sorrow, suffering, abuse, and degradation, to which I have been witness—searched out *in jails, in poor-houses, in pens, and block-houses, in dens and caves, in cages and cells, in dungeons and cellars;* men and women in chains, frantic, bruised, lascerated, and debased—your souls would grow sick at the horrid recital. Yet have all these been witnessed, and for successive years shocking facts have been patiently investigated; and why?—in order to solicit and *procure a remedy* for such heart-rending troubles: the only remedy—*the establishment of well-constructed curative Hospitals.* I desire not to nourish morbid sensibilities, nor to awaken transient emotions. The ills for which I ask relief, in the name of all who are suffering, are too real, too profound for transient emotions to work a remedy, or for

sudden sensibilities to heal. I ask you, gentlemen of the
Legislature, men of Tennessee, to think, to ponder well,
to discuss fairly this subject; then you will not need that I
urge other arguments to secure effective action. Fathers,
husbands, brothers, friends, citizens—you will require no
more earnest solicitations to incite to the accomplishment
of this noble work of *benevolence*, of *humanity*, and of
justice.

Go—look into the dreary cell—behold there the phrenzied, helpless maniac!—go thence, and look into the well-
disposed wards of a Hospital—or, rather, go to the home
made happy—and behold the Insane *"clothed and in his
right mind!"*

You will be prompt to admit that the sentiment of patriot-
ism, whether in its broadest or most limited interpretation,
is not to be associated with narrow views, selfish desires, or
aims after mere personal aggrandisement. You are here
to act from noble motives, pure and exalted principles of
integrity. Upon the fidelity with which the representatives
of a people discharge the duties of their grave and responsible office, depends the honor, and ultimately the prosperity of our States, and of the United Republic.

That all the affairs of Government ought to be administered with regard to a just and well-directed economy, none
can doubt. That a high moral courage should actuate those
who control public affairs, is undeniable, if those affairs are
to be administered so as to secure the *greatest good for the
largest numbers.*

In promoting the establishment of beneficent institutions,
the State discharges a just debt to society. The admitted
claims of the Insane, of the Blind, and of the Deaf and
Dumb, are almost universally acknowledged. And let it
be remembered, this is not the exercise of *charity*, but the
enactment of *justice*; and I repeat a previous affirmation,
that efficient provision for the Insane in State Institutions,
is the truest *economy*.

Shall I, in conclusion, gentlemen, anticipating the results
of your legislation upon this question, state briefly what is
needed to remedy existing necessities, and what will, at

the same time, be rendering justice to the humane sentiments, the obligations, the high-mindedness, and to the
Federal rank of the State of Tennessee?

The *first* step must be to secure a farm of from one to
two hundred acres, a considerable portion of which has
been reclaimed by cultivation. It is not desirable that
there should be any buildings upon that property, as they
would not be available, or in a very unimportant manner.
Office buildings must be adapted to a Hospital, not the Hospital conformed to the standing buildings. In the choice
of a farm, care must be had that it be reached over good
roads, that it be in such vicinity, say within a mile and a
half or two miles of the city, as to afford ready daily communication with the markets, shops and post-office, and
other accommodations affecting the comfort of the inmates
and convenience of the officers: also it should not be too
remote from the steam-boat landings, and stage-coach offices, as the transfer of patients would be more expensive and
inconvenient. A primary consideration in the choice of a
farm, having determined the distance from the town, is, that
it furnish an ample, never-failing supply of wholesome water for all domestic, agricultural, and general uses. There
must be no oversight here. If coal is to be used for fuel,
you must rely on springs and wells: in this country it seems
desirable to avoid the vicinity of creeks or any streams subject to overflow their banks. The Ohio Hospital is supplied
by cisterns and wells, as are most others; but at the Hospital
in charge of Dr. Kirkbride, near Philadelphia, they have on
the premises, in addition to those, a pure stream of soft
water, affording infailing supplies to the laundry and farm.

Your Commissioners will be instructed to build for *use*
and *comfort*, not for display and needless ornament. Every
thing which can minister to the recovery and accommodation of the patients should be supplied; all modern improvements in plan, in ventilation, in building, in labor-saving arrangements should be studied, compared, selected from, and
such adopted as are best suited to your *climate*, and to the
entire provision for not less than two hundred, nor more than
two hundred and fifty patients. Let every thing pertaining

to the construction of your Hospital be carefully estimated, only do not suffer wise economy to degenerate into meanness. All appropriations for State charities, or uses lavishly applied, is but robbery of the poor and needy, and brands the vice of extravagance as yet more vicious, through misapplication of the public monies. In building raise the walls of the edifice of brick rather than of stone; save some thousands of dollars by burning the brick upon your own grounds if you have at hand clay of good quality; and this, first, that the cost of transportation is saved, second it may be equally well made at much lower rates. It is the best economy to employ the best workmen in every branch of labor. It is well in all buildings, but especially is it important in the construction of Hospitals, to give the basement its chief elevation above the surface; otherwise dampness occasions many evils not needful to dwell upon here. The lodging-rooms for the patients should be well ventilated by flues and transon windows, and the outer sash so constructed as to be raised or closed without the patients interference. Hot air furnaces, full evaporation of water being secured in the air-chambers, are preferable for heating these buildings throughout, to steam apparatus, being less liable to get out of order if properly constructed than the other, and less liable to injurious accidents if the conducting pipes through any flaw in their make cause explosion.

Avoid in the construction of the Hospital windows, every thing giving the *appearance* of a prison. Build the wings of the Hospital three stories above the basement, thus giving advantages of light, and dry air, and another sound reason for adopting that elevation in preference to an extended area, is, getting the choicest aspects for the greatest number of rooms. I might add also that it is better economy, as there is much less roofing to keep in repair.

An English writer remarks that "there is no doubt that the average atmosphere is purer and better adapted for human breathing at a height of from fifty to one hundred feet above the surface of the earth, than it is at the surface, whether that surface be composed of clay or gravel;" if of vegetable mould it is yet more important to gain elevation for lodging rooms. The air is drier as you rise above the line of surface evaporation, and poisonous or unwholesome gases are less prevalent.

The Washing establishment, especially in a climate like this, should not be in the *main building*, but removed to a considerable distance, for reasons too obvious to require to be specified.

The Bath rooms as usual in all Hospitals, should be adapted to the accommodation of each class of patients upon each floor of the several wings.

There is another very important point to secure, that the building should be so placed as that the sun's direct rays, at all seasons, may, during some portion of the day reach all occupied apartments. It is not needful to discuss here the soundness of this position, sustained by philosohpy and plain reason as it is.

Perhaps I am tedious, but all these things are more important in securing health than is commonly estimated. And while we are seeking physical health for patients, through which perfect mental health alone can be ensured, we certainly do most wisely to adopt all those rules of hygeine which modern science and intelligence supply.

Tennessee has been called "the Mother of States!" Shall she not, by the *promulgation* of *wise laws*, the liberal encouragement of *schools* of *learning*, and the substantial *support* of *beneficent Institutions*, offer an example for the young States she has so largely and widely colonized? Embalming her memory in the hearts of her grateful children, they hereafter, reverting to their mother-land, with fond veneration and pride shall declare, how noble her example, and hasten to emulate her exalted aims!

Respectfully submitted,

D. L. DIX.

Nashville, November, 1847.

MEMORIAL

NORTH CAROLINA

1848

MEMORIAL

SOLICITING A

STATE HOSPITAL

FOR THE PROTECTION AND CURE OF THE INSANE,

SUBMITTED TO THE

GENERAL ASSEMBLY OF NORTH CAROLINA.

NOVEMBER, 1848

RALEIGH:

SEATON GALES, PRINTER FOR THE STATE.

MEMORIAL.

To the General Assembly of the
        State of North Carolina:

GENTLEMEN :—

I respectfully ask your attention to the subject
herein presented and discussed ; and solicit your prompt
and favorable action upon the same.

I come not to urge personal claims, nor to seek individual benefits ; I appear as the advocate of those who
cannot plead their own cause ; I come as the friend of
those who are deserted, oppressed, and desolate. In
the Providence of God, I am the voice of the maniac
whose piercing cries from the dreary dungeons of your
jails penetrate not your Halls of Legislation. I am the
Hope of the poor crazed beings who pine in the cells, and
stalls, and cages, and waste rooms of your poor-houses.
I am the Revelation of hundreds of wailing, suffering
creatures, hidden in your private dwellings, and in pens
and cabins—shut out, cut off from all healing influences,
from all mind-restoring cares.

Could the sighs, and moans, and shrieks of the insane
throughout your wide-extending land reach you here and
now, how would your sensibilities to the miseries of these
unfortunates be quickened ; how eager would you be to
devise schemes for their relief—plans for their restoration
to the blessing of a right exercise of the reasoning faculties. Could their melancholy histories be spread before
you as revealed to my grieved spirit during the last three
months, how promptly, how earnestly would you search

out the most approved means of relief; how trifling, how insignificant, by comparison, would appear the sacrifices you are asked to make; how would a few dimes and dollars, gathered from each citizen, diminish in value as a possession, compared with the certain benefits and vast good to be secured for the suffering insane, and for their afflicted kindred, by the consecration and application of a sufficient fund to the construction of a suitable hospital in which the restoring cares of skilfully applied physical and moral treatment should be received, and in which humane and healing influences should take the place of abuse and neglect; and of galling chains and loathsome dungeons.

North Carolina, hailed of her sons, " the glorious Old North,"—North Carolina, unburthe ned by State debts, untouched by serious misfortunes, is last and latest of the " old thirteen," save the small terrirory of Delaware, to make provision for the care and cure of her insane citizens, and almost the last embracing all the New States in our broad Union.

But it is not to the State pride of the intelligent citizens of North Carolina that my appeal comes ; it is to the liberal and humane hearts of this portion of my fellow citizens, its plea reaches ; it *cannot* be rejected, it dares not consent to be put off, it claims with earnest importunity that its merits may be discussed, it would merge in oblivion the multiplied miseries resulting from past neglects and procrastination, by wakening to action the efficient energies of humanity and justice.

At present there are practiced in the State of North Carolina, four methods of disposing of her *more than one thousand* insane, epileptic, and idiot citizens, viz : In the cells and dungeons of the County jails, in comfortless rooms and cages in the county poor-houses, in the dwellings of private families, and by sending the patients to distant hospitals, more seasonably established in sister States. I ask to represent some of the very serious evils and disadvantages of each and all these methods of disposing of the insane, whether belonging to the poor or to the opulent classes of citizens.

It may be here stated that by far the larger portion of the insane, epileptics, and idiots, are detained in or near private families, few by comparison, being sent to Northern or Southern State hospitals, and yet fewer detained in prisons and poor-houses, yet so many in these last, and so melancholy their condition, that were the survey taken of these cases alone, no stronger arguments would be needed to incite energetic measures for establishing an institution in North Carolina adapted to their necessities, and to the wants of the continually recurring cases which each year swell the record of unalleviated unmitigated miseries.

If the plea of suffering humanity is insufficient to quicken Legislative interposition, an argument based on indisputable evidence, may be advanced, whose force cannot be slighted; I mean the *economy*, directly to individuals, towns, and counties, and remotely, but not less actually to the State, of establishing without delay, a Hospital for the treatment and protection of the insane.

In order precisely and definitely to present this subject in an economical point of view, I quote from carefully prepared tables furnished by the experienced Superintendant of one of the most successfully conducted Hospitals in the Union. The cases affording the following results are taken in their order of successive admission. The first twenty were the first incurable cases which were received at the institution : the last, those latest received. The expense of the first, cost *before admission, one dollar and fifty cents* per week. They had in the aggregate cost to the State each, *one thousand five hundred and fifty dollars and fifty cents*. On the other hand, the actual expense of the last twenty cases which have been discharged from the Hospital *cured*, amounts only to *forty-seven dollars and a half each*. Hence, it appears that the expenses *already* incurred for taking care of twenty cases suffered by delay and neglect, to become incurable, has been more than *thirty-two* times greater than the same number of cases for which early and proper provision had been made. The recent cases are well; the old ones will doubtless continue a charge through life. Strange as it may appear, it is not the less true, that taking an average chance for cures, it would have been a pecuniary saving to the State to have had seasonable care of these old cases, though at an expense of *eighty dollars a week*, rather than by neglect to have incurred the necessity of supporting them to the present time, and till their decease.

The incarceration of insane men and women in County prisons, whether furiously mad or otherwise, is objected to, first as subverting the uses for which these prisons are constructed, second, as placing the innocent on a level with the guilty, making misfortune and crime, disease and health, go hand in hand. I said on a level, I mistake; the felon looks forward to a period of enlargement, and notes the time when his prison bonds shall be broken · the insane whose imprisonment is aggravated and prolonged by consequence of sickness, not for his crimes, anticipates no season of liberty, no period of release.

Again, many persons adopt the idea that the insane are not sensible to external circumstances, that to their perceptions the dungeon, chains, cold, nakedness, and harsh epithets are as acceptable as a comfortable apartment, freedom from shackles, a pleasantly tempered atmos· phere, decent clothing, kindly speech, and a courteous address. They assert that coarse, ill-prepared food is as palatable as that which is wholesome and well cooked, that cold and heat, sunshine and cloud, pure air and that loaded with noisome exhalations, liberty and confinement are all one and the same to the insane, producing like impressions and results on the deranged intellect. Greater error of belief was never adopted; more serious mistakes, and conducting to more fatal results could not be propagated. The insane in most cases feel as acutely, and distinguish as readily as the sane.

Nor are we to conclude that because a man is insane that he is not in a large majority of cases, able to appreciate the advantages of good associates, or that he is obtuse under the contact of ill-chosen companionship. I recollect a gentleman who had enjoyed a liberal education, and possessed a refined mind, who became insane and shortly furiously mad; for a little time he was conveyed to a jail, and exposed to the daily observation of a crowd of criminals, whose base language and coarse manners constantly exasperated his temper ; finally he was removed to a well ordered hospital, and after some months his recovery being complete, he was restored to his family and friends ; but he could not forgive them his detention in the prison; he spoke with bitterness and severity on his having been subject to such a degradation. On the contrary, he dwelt with tender gratitude upon his situation in the hospital, (that of Bloomingdale, near New York) and spoke with continual pleasure of the comforts which there surrounded him. But he never has relinquished the opinion that his malady would have yielded much more promptly to the mental and moral treatment in that Institution, had he been *at once* conveyed thither. "I object absolutely, says Ellis, to the inhuman custom of confining insane persons and idiots in the same buildings as prisoners and criminals ; the usage cannot be too strongly censured." Many examples might be adduced to illustrate the correctness of this position, and for other reasons than those already stated.

In 1844, I found a furious madman in one of the dungeons of the old jail in Fayette County, Penn. His disposition was homicidal ; he had been in prison nearly fifteen years. On one occasion a man was brought into the prison intoxicated, having committed some offence while under the influence of ardent spirits ; he was thrown into the cell of the maniac, who it is supposed was provoked by him, but no one knows : this only is certain, he fell upon the involuntary intruder and murdered him in the excitement of a most ferocious temper. When the jailer

entered, a horrible spectacle presented itself, the murdered drunkard, mangled and lifeless, the insane muderer
covered with gore, and exulting over the reeking remains
of his victim !

In Philadelphia, some months since, the officers of the
Moyamensing prison were roused from sleep by the cries of
murder proceeding from a cell occupied by an insane man
and a prisoner who had been committed for disorderly
conduct. This unfortunate man was found lying upon
the floor weltering in blood, while the murderer, in the
highest state of phrenzy stood over him, brandishing a
bloody knife. The head of the victim was nearly sever-
ed from the body, and the body covered with frightful
gashes. In reply to the enquiry what had led him to per-
petrate this horrid deed, he answered that it was that he
might not himself be killed.

An insane man has for many years been confined in
the jail at Germantown, Stokes County, in this State.
On one occasion some time past, a negro prisoner was put
into the same room as the crazy man; he did not like the
companionship, and murdered him in a shocking manner,
yet he seemed quite insensible to the turpitude of the
deed, and rather exulted in the entire success of the act,
as I was informed on a recent visit at the prison.

I admit that public peace and security are seriously endangered by the non-restraint of the maniacal insane. I
consider it in the highest degree improper that they
should be allowed to range the towns and country without care or guidance ; but this does not justify the public in any State or community, under any circumstances
or conditions, in committing the insane to prisons ; in a
majority of cases the rich may be, or are sent to Hospitals;
the poor under the pressure of this calamity, have the
same just claim upon the public treasury, as the rich have
upon the private purse of their family ; as they have the
need, so have they the right to share the benefits of Hospital treatment. Urgent cases at all times, demand, unusual and ready expenditures in every community.

If County Jails *must* be resorted to for security against
the dangerous propensities of madmen, let such use of
prison-rooms and dungeons be but temporary. It is not
long since I noticed in a Newspaper, published near the
borders of this State, the following paragraph: "It is our
fate," writes the Editor, "to be located opposite the County Jail, in which are now confined four miserable creatures, bereft of the God-like attribute of reason: two of
them females; and our feelings are daily excited by
sounds of woe, that would harrow up the hardest soul.
It is horrible that for the sake of a few thousand dollars
the wailings of the wretched should be suffered to issue
from the gloomy walls of our jails without pity and without relief. Were our law-makers doomed to listen for a
single hour each day to the clanking of chains, and the
piercing shrieks of these forlorn wretches, relief would
surely follow, and the character of our State would be
rescued from the foul blot that now dishonors it." In nearly every jail in North Carolina, have the insane at different times, and in periods varying in duration, been
grievous sufferers. In Halifax County, several years
since, a maniac was confined in the jail; shut in the dungeon, and chained there. The jail was set on fire by
other prisoners: the keeper, as he told me, heard frantic
shrieks and cries of the madman, and "might have saved
him as well as not, but his noise was a common thing;
he was used to it, and thought nothing out of the way
was the case." The alarm of fire was finally spread; the
jailer hastened to the prison: it was now too late;
every effort, (and no exertions were spared,) to save the
agonized creature, was unavailing. He perished in
agony, and amidst tortures no pen can describe.

In Wentworth, Rockingham County, is an aged crazy
man whose history even carefully abridged would fill too
many pages to be introduced here. The principal facts
of his troubled life are known to many in all the adjoining Counties. Can it be credited? crazed and wretched,
he has been the inmate of a prison for more than thirty
years! and that not for the commission of crimes.

In Stokes jail, at Germanton, was a very crazy man, confined in an unventilated, dreary dungeon. Being tolerably quiet about that time, his chains had been removed, and he was rejoieing in being able to reach the low grated door, because, said he "I can put my mouth close to the bars and draw in some air : dont you like fresh air," he enquired, " Oh it is so good"! " but oh is'nt it pleasant to look out and see the sky, and see the pretty fields; I cant see them here, now you are come to let me out; I know you have; I want to get out; I want to walk about; I don't want to stay here." Alas I could render no relief, the unfortunate man was incapable of self control, and endangered life and property when at large, and there was no hospital to receive him in Carolina—he was poor, and so could not be conveyed to that of another State.

I recollect, of many examples, one recorded in a Report to the Virginia Legislature, by Dr. Stribling, which serves to illustrate what might have been, in all probability, the benefits of timely Hospital care for theis suffering madman.

In 1841, a patient was conveyed from a jail in——— County, where he had been confined loaded with irons for six months. He had been temperate and industrious, but was unfortunate and insanity ensued. He was conveyed to the Hospital bound hand and foot, screaming vociferously, and seeming a very demon in look and act. For days he was furious, but his malady yielded, at first by medical means, and finally by moral influences. In one month he was freed from all restraints, passed in and out of the building at pleasure, and soon cheerfully occupied himself upon the grounds of the Institution, in useful labor, without even an attendant. In *four and a half months* his cure was perfect, and he was discharged. His gratitude and attachment to his physician and nurse seemed unbounded. He returned to his home and set. tled his affairs there, and after a few months returned to offer his services as attendant in the Hospital, and has continued in the daily and hourly exercise of those kind and humane cares which were so grateful and soothing in his own experience. He has the responsibility of guarding, protecting, employing, and amusing a class of fifteen patients, all of whom are devoted to him. Comment upon this case is needless.

In the miserably dilapidated jail in Surry, was also a crazy man, quiet at the time of my visit, but subject to access of violent and alarming paroxysms. Before committal he often declared to his wife that " he felt mighty strange, that he was bound to kill somebody, that he felt dreadfully, that he had a desire to kill her." He was not malicious, did not entertain emnity towards any one individual, but had a morbid and almost uncontrollable desire " to see blood run." Of course, being looked upon as dangerous to the lives of others, he was committed to the jail for an indefinite period, where the application of moral and medical means was unattainable. In a Hospital, he would have been an industrions and useful inmate, and probably in a short period might have been perfectly restored to mental and physical health.

Since I was in Rowan, an insane man, possessed of a moderate fortune has been committed to the jail ; I will not attempt to depict his sufferings in the dismal dungeon into which he has been cast.

From the comfortless, and old jail in Wilkes, an insane women had been discharged some time previously to my visit. At that period and since, I have received the following facts of her history. Mrs. B. is now above 35 years of age, and had for many years been eccentric, at last deranged, and finally has hecome a decided maniac. While her husband lived, he was ever kind and indulgent, and often said to his neighbors, in excuse for her wayward conduct and ill-speech, that they must not mind her, for she was deranged, as he believed. More than a year since, she had been ill for sometime, her husband was exhausted from loss of sleep, and, as he thought at a favorable moment threw himself down to rest. She perceived him sleeping, she went out and returned with a large stone, with which she beat him upon the head so as to cause almost immediate death. Her insanity was fully proved upon her trial, and she was remanded to jail; after considerable detention her brother decided to take charge of her, and removed her to his house. Recently in a state of high excitement she attempted the life of her sister-in-law, and but for the timely arrival of her brother would have accomplished the shocking purpose. Her physician has lately written to me, that he regards her as a confirmed maniac, and dangerous at all times to be at large, as well as dangerous to all who unguardedly approach her when she is excited.

An insane man has lately been discharged from the jail in Beaufort County, and sent to Hyde, where he belonged. One also from Carteret, as I am told. In Craven County, I found a crazy man incarcerated in a noisome, damp, cold dungeon; "placed there for safe keeping!" His condition was very wretched; and his prospects of relief and appropriate treatment no better: if left there he must become a confirmed madman.

In a dark, dreary and filthy dungeon, in Northampton County, I lately found an insane man who had been confined closely for several years. I did not persevere in entering this dungeon, though I examined others corresponding with it in dimensions, but cleanly kept. The keeper doubted the safety or decency of opening the doors, and no advantage could have been derived from doing so, merely to attempt the near survey of a place, that must assure permanence to disease; and agravation to bodily and mental disability. I am disposed to believe that the keeper conceived himself in the performance of his duty, to the extent such means as he possessed allowed. This case I recollect, was repeatedly described, before I reached Jackson, by humane and intelligent citizens in adjacent Counties, better possessed of facts than myself, and speaking from personal observation of his sufferings, noted in professional calls at the jail, during the session of the Courts.

If Jails are unfit institutions for the treatment and restraint of the Insane, County poor-houses are but a degree, if indeed at all more suitable.

At the present time, there are no insane persons either in the Jail or poor-house of Wake County, but a considerable number of individuals in private families, in more or less suffering and exposed states, according to the ability of their friends to provide for them, and several are wandering at large, gathering a precarious subsistence, and not safe to be trusted with their liberty. The case of several requires prompt care One woman, whose propensities are homicidal, resides with her family, to their manifest hourly peril.

The Jail of Orange is well built, and was in good order, comparing well with the best kept Jails in the State. The reverse exists, in regard to the poor-house, which was neither clean nor comfortably furnished. I believe, sufficient food is supplied, and in sufficient quantities. A little expenditure by the County, and a little care, would render the establishment more comfortable. There were six insane ; three in close confinement, and much excited. The most violent, a man long a maniac and caged, was clean, but so noisy as to disturb all on the premises ; a large part of the time, the room in which his cage was built, could be made light. but was commonly dark and close, " to keep him more quiet!" A negro girl, a most pitiable case, was in the opposite building ; and a white woman also, in a separate compartment, vociferous and offensive in the extreme. In the passage, between their cells or cages was a stove in which fire was maintained when necessary. The place was very offensive. The keeper could not altogether be blamed for this ; he was hired to direct a poor-house, and not qualified to rule a mad-house, and should not be expected to do it. Very many cases of insanity, in various conditions, exist in this County.

In Granville County poor house, is an unfortunate man, who for years has been chained to the floor of a wretched room ; miserable and neglected, his now deformed and palsied limbs attest the severity of his sufferings through these cruel restraints ; flesh and bone are crushed out of shape by the unyielding irons. He was a man of good character, industrious, frugal habits ; a good citizen, and respectable as respected ; he became insane, and soon the malady assumed a maniacal character : he was carried to the poor-house, loaded with chains, and left like a wild beast to live or perish ; no care was bestowed to advance his recovery or to secure his comfort !

Caswell Jail was in good order, safely constructed, and vacant of prisoners. The family of the keeper reside in the building. The county poor-house establishment, not distant from Yanceyville, consists of a series of decent one story buildings, kept remarkably clean and neat, and reflecting credit at once upon the county, and those who have the immediate charge. Of the four insane residents here, two were in close confinement; a woman in a room of sufficient size. Who was in a highly excited state. The insane man was in a sort of stall or cage, and at the season of my visit the place was clean. The noise, perversity, and bad habits of these unfortunate persons was a source of much disquiet in the establishment.

In illustration of the blessing and benefit of Hospital care in cases long and most cruelly neglected, I adduce the following examples recorded by Dr. Hill, and corresponding with many cases under my own immediate observation since 1840. "Two patients," writes the Dr. "were brought to me in 1836, who had been confined in a poor-house between eighteen and twenty years. During this period they had not known liberty. They had been chained day and night to their bedsteads, and kept in a state so filthy that it was sickening to go near them.— They were usually restrained by the strait-waistcoat, and with collars round their necks, the collars being fastened with chains or straps to the upper part of the bedstead, to prevent, it was said, their tearing their clothes. The feet were fastened with iron leg-locks and chains. One poor creature was so wholly disabled by this confinement, that it was necessary for the attendants to bear her in their arms from place to place after she was brought to the Hospital; she shortly acquired good habits, and was long usefully employed in the sewing-room. The other

was more difficult of management, but soon gained cleanly habits, and now occupies herself in knitting and sewing, and that, after having been treated for years like the
lowest brute. Another case was brought in chains, highly excited ; five persons attended her; in six days all restraints were removed ; and she walked with her nurse,
in the patients' gallery. In June, she was discharged
from the wards quite cured, and engaged as assistant in
the kitchen.

The Jail of Rockingham is in tolerably good order, the
poor-house, but a short distance from Wentworth, is singularly neat, and well-ordered ; the inmates sufficiently
well-clad and very neat and respectable. The buildings require repairs. The house is well kept, but more
comforts might well be supplied.

The Jail of Stokes is in tolerably good condition, but
badly constructed for the admission of light and air
in the dungeons ; there should be a stove in the passage,
to dry the walls in damp weather.

The poor-house about three miles from Germanton,
is extremely comfortless, the apartments are entirely too
much crowded, and the arrangements are not suited to
promote the comfort or good order of the inmates.—
Rooms of the poor all ill-furnished and out of repair.
Residence of the Superintendant very neat and comfortable. There was one insane woman then at liberty but
often confined in a cell, in all respects, unfit for one in
her condition. I cannot forbear the remark, that when
not in close confinement, she was very improperly situated in the room she occupied. There were several others in the house in a demented state.

The Jail of Surry, is an isolated old two-story wooden
building, and in some parts dilapidated ; the poor-house
is about three miles from Rockford, the Superintendent
resides in town, and keeps several negroes to look after
the poor, of whom there were in September, about 30.
There were no insane in close confinement, but two who
are allowed the freedom of the place.

The jail of Guilford, is isolated, but very well built and well kept : in addition to the dungeons ,and other strong rooms, was the unusual provision of a large chapel room for religious services, when circumstances should make it desirable to hold such therein. The old poorhouse several miles from Greensboro' is about to be abandoned, being utterly comfortless and out of repair. New buildings on the Hillsboro road are ,nearly completed, and there is no doubt that the establishment will be in all respects well-ordered, and fitly conducted.

The jail of Davidson, a new, secure, and substantial building was found in excellent order ; the common mistake of insufficient air and light in the dungeons exists here. The County poor house about six miles from Lexington, was pretty well ordered, but too little visited. The supplies of food and clothing seemed sufficient for both health and comfort : but there, as elsewhere, the insane were out of place, and in a bad state. For this no blame is to be attached to the superintendant, so far as I could judge. One very crazy man was chained to his bedstead ; he was noisy, filthy, and truly repulsive. A crazy woman, but quiet, was rolled in a quantity of soiled bed clothing. These like many others would be useful, and decent in their habits, if resident in the hospital expressly designed for the insane. Besides these are two demented patients.

Rowan jail, on the first floor of which resides the jailor, is a substanial building—not clean when I saw it : chiefly commended, I was told, as a secure prison. An insane man has recently been committed here. The poor house about two miles from Salisbury, requires so much to render it comfortable that it would be difficult to know how to enumerate its deficiencies : the house occupied by the keeper was quite the most comfortless abode, that I have seen in North Carolina, except repaired, certainly not habitable for the winter. No insane man in confinement in this institution.

Iredell jail, is isolated and had just passed into the charge of a newly appointed officer, it would hardly be just to remark severely upon its very dirty and neglected condition. The County poor-bouse. a few miles from Statesville, is situated in a singularly secluded spot, remote from supervision and often observation, and is a model of neatness, comfort, and good order; having a most efficient master and mistress, especially the latter, upon whose cares in these institutions by far the most is dependent. All in all, this was in much the best condition of any poor-house I have seen in North Carolina, neat, plain, and decent, it would do credit to any State; but it is no fit place for the insane. Since I was there, in September, a highly respected citizen writes me that a young woman has been sent to the poor-house so violently insane, that it is quite unfit she should remain there. Also a man has in that County, very recently become so violently mad as to be quite unmanageable, and having no Hospital in the State, they have confined him with, *chains and manacles, hand and feet,* and do as best they can. A subscription paper has been circulated for the purpose of raising funds to send him to Columbia, S. C. Other painful cases exist in this, as in the counties which I have visited, and from which I have heard; most of which I do not feel at liberty, through their domestic and social position, to designate; but they plead in heart-reaching language for the early establishment of a State Hospital.

Wilkes jail is an old building, and so far as the jailor is accountable, is well kept: it is isolated, and a wretched place whether for the prisoner, or the insane who are sometimes confined here. There is no poor-house in this County. Five or six cases of insanity have been reported to me. One, a man named Dowell, is said by a respectable physician of Wilkesboro' to have been crazy for more than 12 years: the malady is gaining force gradually, and now exhibiting itself in furious mania; he is a very dangerous person to be at large, has proved himself to be mischievous, and once attempted to commit homicide.

The Jail of Caldwell is well built, was in good order, and has sufficient light and air in every part. There are no violently excited insane in the poor house, which is some miles from Lenoir, and but few cases in the County.

In the Jail of Davie, is one insane man; in the poor-house beyond Mocksville, I was informed, was a case of insanity truly pitiable, beside many others in the County.

The Jail of Bertie is an exceedingly well built edifice, sufficiently lighted and aired, and well-kept; the Jailor and family reside on the first floor; the County poor-house, about three miles from Morganton, is not well situated; the buildings are out of repair, and ill-arranged within, for either comfort or convenience in times of sickness or of health. I should think that the Superintendent was kind and faithful in the discharge of all his duties towards the poor. Here as in most of the poor houses in North Carolina religious services are frequently holden.

The jail of McDowell, like most of the County prisons in this part of the State, I found well built and well kept; there is no county poor-house in or near Marion, and my inquiries reached but few insane in the County. One man often violently excited, but ordinarily for the last few years so tranquil as to be at large, I found beyond Pleasant Gardens. At one time he was closely shut up.

The jail of Buncombe is a large substantial building; formerly there was a county poor-house six or seven miles from Asheville, but its remote situation and serious discomforts through bad management led to the entire breaking up of the establishment some time since. A plan succeeded this, somewhat original, which when I was in Asheville, had not been fully carried into effect; having no perception of its merits and claims to commendation, I shall dwell but slightly upon the subject, merely stating on authority of several of the citizens, that it was considered in constructing the new jail, expedient to make it of sufficient capacity to accommodate at one and the same time and place, the vagrants and felons of the county, and the unfortunate poor. The enclosed yard, "at present unimproved," is of sufficient extent to permit the erection

of additional buildings "if needful." "It is belived," said
my informant, "that the wardens and overseers consult e-
conomy by this arrangement in various ways, especially as
one man can keep the prisoners and the poor, saving the
cost of hiring a second individual for the latter service."
"But one pauper has been sent to jail, and he ran away
dissatisfied with his quarters, in about three weeks."

Rutherford jail is an old and poor building, but now
serves sufficiently for the County. It is quite isolated;
but the jailer seemed fitted to fulfil his duties with humanity and fidelity. The County poor-house, a short
distance from Rutherfordton, is not so comfortable as
respects the buildings and furnishing as it should be
made. The Superintendant seemed a favorite of the
poor there.

Cleaveland Jail is excellently built, cleanly kept, and
the Jailer, as should always be arranged, resides in one
part of the building, having thereby the more immediate
and efficient care of the prison. The County poor-house
about three miles from Shelby, is a small but neatly kept,
and seemingly comfortable establishment. It seemed to
me that the Superintendent received an insufficient recompense for the difficult charge the situation of several
of the inmates involved.

Lincoln Jail is a well-built, well-planned prison, well
arranged, and apparently well kept. The poor-house,
several miles from Lincolnton, had but three inmates in
October; their condition was uniformly represented as
not good, and the establishment described as being objectionable. Perceiving influential citizens, prompt to
admit existing evils, I did not personally visit it. No insane at present are confined there. Several in distressed
conditions in the County, in private families.

Gaston Jail is as yet unfinished, but appears to be a
well-planned building. No poor-house in or near Dal-
las; but one such needed for the County poor. Several
insane in the County.

Mecklenburg Jail is remarkably well planned and well
built, but less well kept than are most County prisons in

North Carolina, as respects cleanliness. The County poor-house, several miles from Charlotte, was nearly deserted in October, having but two of the County poor ; a partially insane woman, and a paralytic man.

Cabarrus Jail is a large, well constructed building—in tolerable order ; the Jailor occupies commodious apartments upon the first story. The County poor-house about two and a half miles from Concord, is very deficient in means for promoting the comfort of the infirm inmates. In a miserably dilapidated out-building, perhaps ten feet square, open on all sides to the ingress of the winds, rain, and snow, I found a crazy man chained to the floor, filthy and disgusting. At times he is suffered to go at large, but is at once troublesome and dangerous to those he meets, or whose house he frequents. In a Hospital, this crazy man would, under judicious care, be able to perform more labor than would suffice for his own maintenance. I did not visit the insane scattered in private families.

Stanly Jail is a small new building, neat and secure, but the dungeons so planned and constructed as almost to assure the destruction of health to any who might be long in detention ; there is hardly a possibility for the admission of sufficient air to support the absolute demands of the animal structure. There are in the County several cases of insanity requiring Hospital treatment. At present, there is no poor-house in or near Albemarle.

Montgomery Jail, like that of Stanly, is a neat substantial building, and well-kept, but not well planned for health, as respects the admission of light and air, though it assures security.

The County poor-house, at Lawrenceville requires, it appeared to me, much more careful attention on the part of the Wardens, to supply comfortable and necessary attendance upon the aged and infirm, who alone occupy the buildings. Nothing could be more creditable to these feeble women than the neatness and care with which they kept their apparel and their apartments. An insane man had been removed to some other situation in the

County. Several cases of insanity were related to me on authority.

Moore jail seemed a secure prison; its want of cleanliness was excused on the ground of there being no prisoners, and being occupied as a lodging for servants. The dungeons, which did not serve this use, were by comparison with the majority of prisons in the State, in bad order. The County poor-house, not distant from Carthage was excellently kept by a conscientious and kind-hearted family, to whose cares the comforts of the inmates are ascribable, rather than to the provision made by county officials. The buildings are much out of repair and unfit for winter habitation, or for stormy days at any season. The custom so worthy of entire condemnation, that of setting off the poor in mass, by lots or singly, to the lowest bidder exists in Moore County. The poor are fed, clothed, supplied with bed, clothing and fuel and waited on at the rate of 8 *cents the day each*; a sum which cannot pay those who undertake this charge. That I found the poor well supplied with food and well clad, I repeat was certainly ascribable to the liberality and christianity of the present keepers, rather than to the just guardianship of the public.

Cumberland jail is an old building, well lighted and well ventilated: it is said that more attention will be paid to the preservation of cleanliness than heretofore, the keeper and famly now residing upon the premises. The county poor house within three miles of Fayetteville is well situated, and apparantly excellently kept: cleanliness, that crowning excellence in house-keeping, prevailed in every room save one, and I imagine might with the exercise of a sufficient determination, be secured even in that. In a log building well constructed, and admitting sufficient light and air, planned so as to be warmed in damp and cold weather, were two small apartments for the insane : at the time I was there one room was vacant, the other was occupied by a violently excited and noisy insane man, whose shouts and vociferations reached me at a distance from the poor-house. In a hospital this poor creature's energies would find exercise in useful employment ; in a poor-house it is not to be expected that the superintendants should have the qualifications which pertain to a judicious control of maniacs : moreover the noise and disturbance these create, banish comfort and repose from the infirm, the sick, the dying , and the demoralizing influence, through use of profane language and additional evils. In this poor-house religious services are regularly and frequently holden, and one has evidence that the ministers of the various religious denominations in the vicinity had not overlooked that scripture, " To the poor the Gospel is preached which foretold the advent of Jesus the Saviour, and comforter."

The jail of Sampson is said to be decently kept. The county poor are said to be well clothed and supplied with wholesome food. Several cases of insanity have been related in this county

The jail of Duplin is defective. The wardens of the county poor-house which is situated east of Warsaw, several miles from Kenansville, have the reputation of giving uncommon attention to the temporal and spiritual comforts and consolations of the poor. Religious services are holden at the poor house. At present there are no insane persons there.

The jail of New Hanover appeared to be tolerably well kept. It is a large commodious building. Too little light and air are admitted into the dungeons. The county poor-house on the confines of Wilmington is in a miserable and dilapidated condition ; fallen wholly from its former well deserved reputation of being one of the best Institutions for the poor in the country. Apparently the acting wardens are responsible for its decline. There are affecting and suffering cases of insanity in several private families in this County.

Wayne jail is an old dilapidated building, shortly to be replaced by a new prison. Found in miserable condition. The County poor house several miles from Goldsboro', seemed quite decently kept, and in many respects bore an air of comfort. There seemed to be neglect from abroad in the attendance upon the sick ; several individuals were evidently suffering from want of medical advice and prescription. This establishment is but seldom visited, and the comforts enjoyed seemed chiefly referable to the care of occupants. One of the poor, an insane man, had wandered away : an insane woman was so far controllable as to be steadily and usefully occupied.

Lenoir jail, a very old and isolated building, but strong, seemed pretty decently kept ; it has some very great defects of construction. The poor of the county are not numerous, by comparison with the adjacent Country.

Craven jail, a very large brick building, promising exteriorly a better condition than the interior revealed. The dungeons were very bad, offensive, dirty, ill-lighted, and not ventilated. A very insane man, considered dangerous to be at large, was in one of them ; he was cold, exposed, and suffering ; his condition was such as to assure agravation, if not permanent confirmation of his malady. There are no means of maintaining either dryness or warmth in the passages or in the dungeons. The county poor-house, a short distance from Newbern, is well situated, and has the reputation of being well kept in general. The keeper's house, and several rooms occupied by the poor, were neat and well-ordered; others were in a poor condition. A sunday school is taught here by persons from Newbern, whose Christianity is illustrated in their practice of its precepts. There are here in Craven County, many cases of insanity.

Beaufort jail is a neat brick structure ; the jailor occupies the lower floor in front. The plan of the prison is not good, though it assures security when properly attended to.

A letter received from a physician resident in Washington, informs me that since I left that town a week since, an insane man in a state of high excitement, has been committed to the jail there for public security, and occupies a dreary, wretched cell. I cannot question the willingness of the jailor to perform his duty as humanely as possible ; but there is no mercy nor humanity in committing the insane to prisons.

The unfortunate man above alluded to might, in a well ordered Hospital, undoubtedly in a short time be sufficiently recovered, if not cured, to pursue some useful and profitable employment.

Recently fifteen cases of insanity have been stated, existing in this section of the State—that is in Beaufort, and adjacent Counties.

An insane person with whom I was conversing two weeks since, dwelt with profound feeling upon the trials and sufferings she endured, conscious of her state, and sensible of all that occurred around her : that which most moved my feelings at the time was, the indescribable pathos with which she related the sufferings and hardships of a crazy man confined in the Jail in her native County. She concluded, " I, in my troubles, have friends—he has none."

The county poor-house not distant from Washington, and reached over a good road, is pleasantly situated, but in a spot well known for its unhealthiness, having been abandoned by the former owner of the property, for its liability to create fevers, and for the general insalubrity of the place. The establishment needs an efficient Superintendant, competant in mind and body to carry forward the interests of the place. Offering at first glance the appearance of a comfortable institution, it fails to show forth either private or public efficient and fit direction. The sick and the children certainly suffer ; and those able to work need a director to insist upon their action. I found one woman here insane, but quiet.

Pitt jail is a neat, two story building painted white, and sufficiently large for present county purposes. The poor of this county are said to be well cared for. Sad and distressing cases of insanity were brought to my notice existing in private families, in conditions of extreme suffering and exposure, of which I do not feel at liberty to give the history.

Edgecombe jail is a well constructed, isolated prison ; well and cleanly kept : its defects of plan and arrangement are fewer than ordinary in county prisons. I did not visit the poor-house of this county established some distance from Tarboro, but it bears a good reputation, and at present there are no violently excited insane there; cases are known abroad in the county.

Halifax Jail is a well built prison seemingly, though isolated, *securely* kept, but bears the reputation of being deficient in cleanliness. At present no insane detained there. The poor house nearly three miles from Halifax, has much need of competent care, and efficient superintendence. Most of the inmates are aged and infirm. The buildings are well situated and conveniently planned for the occupants, but deficiently furnished, except one room furnished by the individual who dwells in it. The sick need nursing, care, and comforts; and all require supervision.

Northampton Jail is well-built, but defectively planned—the dungeons, of which there are four, are insufficiently lighted and ventilated, and however cold or damp are never warmed and dried. Here is an insane man confined for years in this dreary abode; from his sight, the genial sun, the beautiful sky, and the green fields are forever shut out; darkness, and foul air, and solitude, heaviness and misery are his portion. Kindred and friends are put far from him, and his acquaintance into darkness. May the merciful God compassionate those who are so cruelly abandoned by their fellow-men, and may no heavy retributions crush those, who so unhesitatingly and unpityingly consign a helpless, crazed creature, to such a hapless doom.

The poor-house, a mile and a half from Jackson, consists of five dilapidated, unfurnished rooms, at present abandoned. The Superintendant who resides in a pleasantly situated comfortable house, distributes quarterly, to one hundred beneficiaries an allowance of meat, meal, and clothing, at a cost to the county of about $2,500 00. Several insane poor, and others in better circumstances are in this County.

The jail of Nash is a small two story decent building; no insane now confined therein. The poor-house I had not time to visit, but understand it is comfortable. Several cases of insanity were reported to me existing in the county.

Time would fail in the narration, even were it proper to unveil the miseries, protracted, and indiscribably varied, of the insane in private families, and the distress of families thrown into sorrow and trouble unequalled, through the affliction and sore perplexities arising out of care over the demented, the epileptic, and the maniac. A detailed description of their personal condition, horrible as it must be, could not present the half of the woes which exist in every county throughout North Carolina. Loathing and horror would overwhelm the reader, successively introduced to dreary apartments, loathsome cells, and foul cabins, whence issue the most horrible sounds and poisonous effluvia, and wherein are spectacles of protracted bodily and mental misery language is poor to represent.

Of the few examples *of many which exist*, to which I shall now refer in private families, the following have quite recently come under my observation : A poor but industrious farmer in the western part of this State, the father of a numerous family, became insane; it was in vain to control him in his own dwelling, he was furious and he was conveyed to the County jail; here his sufferings were aggravated and his malady exasperated: I cannot tell for how long a time the lone dark dungeon echoed to his moans and cries, nor at what cost the county maintained human life, unaiding its sufferings and necessities. In process of time the paroxysms of violence subsided, and finally he was transferred to the humble log cabin of his aged widowed mother, a lone woman dwelling upon the mountains. There I found the infirm, afflicted mother, and the insane son. Amidst tears and sighs she recounted to me her troubles, and as she wept she said, " the Lord above only knows my troubles, and what a heap of sorrow I have had in my day, and none to give me help. There *he* lay in the jail, cold and distressed, and mightily misused ; if I could have got money to send him off to where they cure such *spells*, for they do say crazy folks can be cured, I should have had him in my old age to take care of me, but I am poor and always was, and there is no help here. Ah well, many and many is the long night I am up with him and no sleep or rest, anyhow; this cant last always; I shall die, and I dont know what is to come of him then." It is for Legislators to determine whether such as these shall drag out troubled existences, and no succour until the Angel of death brings release, and seals the long record of "man's inhumanity to man." A respectable citizen in the same quarter of the county, by very slow degrees lost his reason. First was a nervous restlessness, next unwonted irritability, then a craving for stimulants, which were in time used to excess, and quickened the malady, yet none then traced the real cause of the growing evil; but the type of a deranged intellect was shortly developed beyond doubt, and in a few months the distress and trouble of the household knew no alleviation nor interval. Finally, removal from home, under most grievous circumstances, ensued, and I have not long since been witness to the afflictions of this worthy and respectable family whose efforts to sustain themselves are as affecting as praiseworthy. Had there been in North Carolina, a State Hospital, timely care might have secured a permanent cure. It is almost too late to assure this now, but instead of restoration is life-long expense, and life-long suffering.

In Lincoln County, near a public road, stands a decent dwelling; near by is a log cabin, strongly built, and about ten feet square, and about seven or eight feet high; no windows to admit light; the square logs are compactly laid; no chimney indicates that a fire can be kindled within, and the small low door is securely locked and barred. Two apertures at right angles, ten inches long by four wide, are the sole avenues by which light and air are admitted within this dreary cabin, so closely secured, and so cautiously guarded. You need not ask to what uses it is appropriated: the shrill cries, and tempestuous vociferations of an incarcerated maniac will arrest you on the way, and if you alight, and so far as the light received as before described will allow, examine the interior of this prison, you will discern a ferocious, filthy, unshorn, half-clad creature, wallowing in foul, noisome straw, and craving for liberty. The horrors of this place may not be more definitely descibed; they can hardly be imagined: the state of the maniac is revolting in the extreme. This creature, is a man—insane for more than thirteen years—for a long time suffered to range the country far and wide, addicted to mischief and disposed to violent acts. For assuring public and private safety, his family have adopted the only alternative of confining him upon their own farm, rather than seeing him thrown into the dungeon of the County jail. Of these two evil conditions, I confess, I see no choice. The family though enjoying the means of decent livelihood when unburthened by extra expenses, have not the means of sending him to a distant Hospital. The rich may partake the benefits such institutions afford: the poor must suffer, agonize, and bear heavily out, by slow-killing tortures, their unblessed life! Are there no pitying hearts, and open hands that can be moved by these miseries?

Well and truly may it be said of the insane: whose sorrows are like unto their sorrows, and whose griefs are like unto their griefs? Friend and companion are removed far from them, and their acquaintances are hid from their view!

Of thirteen cases of insanity in and near Raleigh, there is one to which my attention has within a few days been called, which especially illustrates the want of a Hospital for individuals in narrow circumstances. Mrs. ———— has for several years had rather feeble health. Sometime in February last, she manifested peculiar restlessness by day and night, became agitated and nervous, and her mind was subject to strange and harrassing delusions. From that time she became incapable of attending to the affairs of her household; neglected her child, and passed most of the time night and day in traversing the small apartments of her dwelling. Her husband, dependent upon daily industrious labor for a decent support, found himself embarrassed by the distresses of his home and the claims of business. He is unable to pay her expenses at any Hospital ; meanwhile, she is sinking into a condition of hopeless and permanent insanity. She who was neat, modest, industrious, and kind, is now through this most afflictive malady, utterly transformed ; her garments are rent in tatters, her person neglected, her hair dishevelled, falls in tangled locks about her head ; her speech is no longer gentle, true and kind; but violent, profane, and indecent ; in that humble, once pleasanthome, is now neither peace, nor rest, nor security : there is constant danger of destruction by fire, and acts of personal violence often recurring, indicate the increasing liability to deeds involving fatal consequences : in train with these alarming manifestations, are symtoms of a suicidal disposition. It has been found necessary at times to confine her movements by the application of painful modes of restraint upon the limbs ; which, though preventing present mischief, continually aggravate the malady. Hospital treatment might restore this patient to her family blessings, to society, and to usefulness.

Many cases of maniacal insanity have been removed to Southern and Northern Hospitals. Hitherto, North Carolina has been willing to be dependent upon other States for her afflicted children, while in possession of ample means to succor and heal their maladies within her own borders. But there are other objections to transporting patients to distant Hospitals for remedial care, beside the fact of encroachment upon the Institutions of other States. Expenses are vastly increased in making long and always difficult journeys under circumstances so harrassing and painful ; and an experienced physician of a celebrated Hospital has informed me that the fatigues, excitement, and exposures of several patients, conveyed long distances, have within the present year resulted in death. Want of sleep and exhaustion, have reduced them to the most dangerous condition before being received ; and not seldom depleting remedies injuriously adopted, have hastened dissolution. If there is cruelty and gross injustice in holding the insane in jails, poor-houses, and private families, there is serious risk of property and of life in leaving them to range at large. Plainly, there is but one remedy.

In Aberdeen, Ohio, an insane man, left in the room where a little girl three years old was sleeping, in the absence of the mother, threw down the Bible which he was reading, seized an axe. and deliberately chopped the little victim into five pieces.

In Rowan County, N. C., a maniac cut her husband's throat. In Wilkes County another beat her husband upon the head so as to cause his death. In Rockingham an insane man killed his neighbor. A man in Kentucky killed two of his children, and attempted the life of his wife. Another in Indiana cut his wife's throat and gashed her face so that she died. Besides these, I recollect more than thirty similar cases in which homicide was attempted and committed by individuals *known* to be insane.

I adduce a few, from many thousand examples on record, which illustrate the *benefits* of Hospital residence and of remedial treatment of the Insane, in both curable and incurable cases.

"There has been," writes Dr. Bates of the Maine State Hospital, "in this Institution for some years, an individual whose family is strongly disposed to maniacal insanity. By many years neglect this patient became incurable ; the powers of the brain seem to exist in fragments. He is, and probably always will be a public charge. Two of his sons have been attacked, *seasonably* brought under treatment, and cured. These young men during the absence of disease, were industrious and frugal citizens. They are both liable to a recurrence of the hereditary malady. If brought to the Hospital *soon* after each attack, there are nine chances in ten, that they will always soon recover and return to their occupations and former place in society ; if neglected until functional derangement changes to organic disease, they will become a public charge for life." These cases are selected plainly to illustrate the fact that economy not less than humanity calls for *early and efficient* action in assuring appropriate remedial treatment for the insane.

Dr. Stribling, the excellent physician and friend of the insane, and Superintendant of the Western State Hospital in Virginia, states several cases of much interest in his published reports to the Legislature From these documents I quote the following examples : In 1842, a young gentleman, twenty-one years of age, the son of a highly respectable individual who was formerly a prominent and efficient member of the Legislature of Virginia, was brought to our Hospital. Possessed of a good natural understanding, improved by education and such other advantages as wealth had supplied, and with a disposition uniformly cheerful, he was at all times a most interesting patient and companion. In the Autumn of 1842, he was attacked with bilious intermittent fever, which although speedily arrested, was followed by depression and neglect of all accustomed duties and care of property. In about two months the mind became harassed by the most distressing delusions, such as being surrounded by foes who were plotting his destruction; his friends were regarded as enemies, and he believed himself doomed to eternal punishment, &c. He remained in this state for some time, when suddenly he passed into the highest degree of cheerfulness and gaiety. Affection for his family revived ; he fancied himself by turns poet, philosopher, and statesman; at one time he was an angel in Eden, at another Noah defying the destroying flood, and finally he conceived himself the Creator of the Universe. He was removed to the Hospital where the application of moral and medical means in a short period assured his recovery : he left us rejoicing in the blessing of restored health.

A respectable gentleman who had been esteemed by all who knew him, as an affectionate husband and father, a generous friend and worthy citizen, was received as a patient in the Western Hospital, in 1843. He was a merchant, and through unavoidable misfortunes rather than ill management, sustained heavy losses : he became depressed, was attacked with bilious fever, which left his health materially impaired ; after some months his friends became satisfied that his mind was seriously diseased ; evidences of insanity were multiplied ; he became maniacal and his family under the advice of an intelligent physician, placed him in the Hospital. He was feeble, emaciated, sleepless, and suicidal. His delusions varied, and were of a most distressing character. Demons seemed to surround him and to multiply their torments. In a short time his malady seemed to yield to remedial measures. His physical health improved ; his mind gradually became tranquil ; one delusion after another disappeared ; his spirits revived, and soon he was pronounced cured, and returned to his family, and to his business, a cheerful and happy man." As he was from that class of society which possesses extensive influence, and who in this part of the country, unfortunately, are too apt to regard institutions for the insane with aversion, and who consent to place their afflicted friends therein only when all other means have failed, and all other sources of hope cut off, it may not be amiss to quote a passage from one of his letters received by a friend after his recovery and by him communicated to his physician.

"I am truly happy to inform you that my health is now perfectly restored. I cannot say too much in praise of this institution, nor too earnestly express my gratitude to my friends for having placed me here. Instead of a place approximating to a prison, as I once considered it, when influenced as many are by ignorance and prejudice, I now view the establishment in the light of a pleasant hotel. I gratefully acknowledge comforts supplied and kindness received."

"Last year the wife of a respectable and independant farmer was brought to the Hospital in a most painful condition. She was endued by nature with a clear and vigorous intellect, being emphatically, a strong-minded woman," remarkable for her industry, discretion, and good management. She had not encountered those difficulties and disturbing cares that often wear out the heart, but had led a life of peace and enjoyment. Some time in the year before insanity was manifested, her strength seemed to diminish without apparent cause. Finally her mind became a prey to the most harassing delusions ; she fancied herself given over to everlasting condemnation ; believed herself the destroyer of a friend ; attempted suicide, and after six months lost in unavailing attempts to restore her, she was placed in the Hospital at Staunton. There was a continual conflict between her feelings and her reason, her affective and her intellectual faculties, which rendered her case one of care and interest. In a few months she was perfectly restored.

In 1843, a young lady of cultivated mind and accomplished manners sunk into a state of agitated depression. Change of scene, cheerful society, exercise and medical skill were employed in vain. Her affections towards her friends passed into indifference, and so to settled aversion. To her distempered fancy her husband, parents, and sisters appeared transformed to demons. The distressed mother could not see her child transferred to a Hospital, and long resisted the entreaties of wise-judging friends. The disease became for seven months continually more aggravated, till finally amidst lamentations and anguish her family consented to her removal. Her improvement was rapid, and restoration finally complete, and instead of distress at the thought of finding herself the inmate of a Hospital for the insane, she often exclaimed, " Oh why did not my friends place me sooner here." To a relative she wrote, " this is no prison, but a refuge for the distressed, where every comfort is furnished, and only the most soothing attentions experienced. I will ever cherish the most grateful recollection of this Hospital and of the excellent physician through whose skill by Heaven's blessing I am recovered "

" A man born of respectable and pious parents instructed from his youth in lessons of morality and religion,
grew up a peaceable, industrious, and useful citizen.
His disposition was mild and gentle, his feelings affectionate, and his habits exemplary. The decease of his
mother overwhelmed him with affliction : he fell into a
state of what is termed religious melancholy, and gradually became agitated and furious ; suddenly attempted
the life of his wife and children, killed one of the latter,
and seriously wounded the others. He destroyed at a
blow a neighbor, who attempted with others to secure
him, and was at last with difficulty secured, and lodged
in the jail, and shortly brought to the Hospital. Months
passed and he continued excited and dangerous. Very
gradually a change took place ; his habits improved ; his
physical health improved, and from being one of the most
loathsome and offensive patients ever introduced into
the institution, he became decent, quiet, cleanly, and
finally rational, peaceable, and in all respects well
behaved. He remained in the Hospital five months after the recovery of his reason, to ensure the safety of his
return to society, and was finally, through the solicitation of his family and friends, upon their special application, discharged by the Court of Directors. Thus far
his recovery seems to be permanent." The danger of
delay in placing the insane under remedial Hospital
treatment cannot be too strongly insisted upon. Hundreds and thousands of cases attest the cruelty and the
folly of procrastination. However writers upon insanity, and medical men may differ upon some points, on
this question all agree, and deprecate with forcible arguments the dangers of procrastination. Esquitol, Pinel,
Falret, Jacobi, Conolly, Bell, Brigham, Awl, Kirkbride,
Stribling, and a host of others, have earnestly and repeatedly enforced, and continue to enforce this truth ;
and employ the most eloquent persuasions to induce
friends and guardians to take advantage of Hospital treatment in the early stages of the malady. Willis, the celebrated physician to George the III, dismissed the king's

family, courtiers, officers, and domestics; procured strangers as nurses and attendants, and thus first succeeded in controlling the delusions which distracted the insane monach. " To separate the insane from the objects surrounding them at the origin of the disease, writes M. Pinal, to entirely disconnect them from their habitual intercourse with their relatives, friends, and servants, is the imperative and indispensable plan for commencing a course of treatment which shall be attended with favorable results:" and Falret, says, " it is demonstrated by repeated experience, that the *kind of isolation preferable to all others*, is that of an establishment especially devoted to the insane." " Few," writes Hallaran, "very few patients are found to recover under domestic treatment." There can be but one opinion as to the solemn duty of the removal and non-intercourse of the insane, with their intimate friends and family, and their familiar homes. The superintendant of an English Hospital writes in 1842, as follows : "In a large proportion of cases admitted the present year, owing to long detention by friends. or by parish officers, the prospects of recovery have been entirely precluded, and in successful cases, *the period of treatment bears generally an accurate ratio* to the prior duration of the disorder." The visiting commissioners of the sane Hospital report, that "they cannot too strongly express their conviction, from experience, that the hope of cure is materially lessened, and *not unfrequently defeated*, by the delay which is suffered to take place in sending patients to the Hospital after first confirmation of their malady." The physician of the York Retreat, states in an annual report, that "*forty-nine* years of experience establishes the fact of recovery of four cases to one brought under cure within three months of the first attack, while it is less than one to four in cases of more than twelve months duration when admitted."

The superintendant of the Edinburgh Hospital shows that " to be treated successfully, insanity must be treated early; ill founded prejudices, and false sensibility often operate to prevent this being done." These remarks are

as general and as often reiterated as are the establishment of Hospitals and the issue of reports emanating
therefrom. Dr. Earle, shows from his experience in the
treatment of the insane, that, " after the three first
months of insanity are passed the probabilities of entire
restoration rapidly diminish." Not only do delays in
placing patients in suitable Hospitals involve the risk of
permanently establishing the malady, but the safety of
property and security of life is hazarded in a vast many
instances.

Dr. Galt records an example in point, as occurring in
Virginia. An insane woman, the mother of a family, became so much the victim of distressing delusions, that her
family perceiving danger from her being at large, took
her before the justices for examination in view of placing
her in the Hospital at Williamsburg. The following
letter was addressed by one of these to the President and
Directors of that institution. "Sirs—at the time an examination was had into the state of Mrs. ———— mind, she
seemed so lucid that one of the magistrates, who had not
seen her previously, dissented from the opinion of the
other two, imagining that the public were in no danger
from her going at large; and had the examination taken
place one hour later, no doubt would have been felt upon
the subject by that gentleman, as she became so furious
shortly after, as to render it necessary to confine her in the
public jail. After a few days she became importunate to
return to her husband and children : and a call of her husband at the jail increased her supplications to be set
free. He finally prevailed with the jailor to take her
home, promising to return the next day to give bond and
security for her restraint and safe-keeping. In the night
she rose unperceived, proceeded to the yard and procured an axe, and after calling the servant who slept in
the room, and finding him asleep, gave her husband many blows over the head, fractured his skull in several places, and left him senseless. She left the house
and ran unremittingly for several hours ; affirmed herself dead, and declares that she has been buried these

five years. I have made these remarks to illustrate her case and assist treatment of the same." Another case occurring in Eastern Virginia, seems worthy of notice; there are but too many parallel cases in North Carolina. The friends of the young woman referred to were in limited circumstances, and even by making considerable sacrifices could not succeed in rendering her comfortable at home: they entertained the strongest prejudices against Hospitals for the insane. She was violently maniacal, breaking in pieces and tearing every thing upon which she could lay her hands; and vociferated perpetually in the most harsh and discordant tones. She was almost constantly confined in a small closet or cell constructed in a small apartment in her mother's house: occasionally, for change, she was taken into the open air and confined to a tree by heavy chains. At the time she was removed to the Hospital, she had contracted the most loathsome habits, and had plucked the whole of the hair from her head. For more than two years she had exhibited a most pitiable spectacle, and every day her misery seemed to be increased. After several months residence in the Hospital, her improvement commenced: her recovery is slow, but it is hoped will ultimately be complete.

In a report from Dr. Stribling, the following statement is on record: "Of all the cases received, *ninety-seven* were recent cases, of whom *eighty-three* were restored to reason; *five* remain in an improved condition; *three* are unimproved; and *six* died before any opportunity was offered to test the use of remedies in their behalf. These results correspond with those of other institutions. Of *one hundred and fifty-eight cases* remaining in the Hospital at Staunton in 1845, and in all probability doomed for life to endure the weary burthen of remediless disease, how many might have been restored to reason, happiness and usefulness, had they been subject to *early* and *appropriate moral* and physical treatment. In many cases the morbid sentiment of friends led them to reject Hospital aid, and now the care and skill are all too late!

The following Table, writes Dr. Allen of the Kentucky Hospital, *shew the Cases of less than One Year's Duration admitted into the Asylum, from July 1st, 1836, to September 30th, 1847; the Number of those cured, Relieved, Unimproved and Died, and the Per Cent. of Cures to Admissions and Discharges.*

ADMITTED.		Recovered.	Relieved.	Unimproved.	Died.	Per ct. of Cures to Admissions.	Per ct. of Cures to Discharges.
Males,	127	94	16	8	9	74.15	91.23
Females,	73	51	13	2	7	69.86	87.93
	200	145	29	10	16	72 05	90.62

"I have intimated," says the same judicious physician, "that such public institutions for the insane, as afforded every facility for their successful treatment, and such as to invite the early committal of them to Asylum discipline, were demanded on the score of economy. I would not, in the mean time, have it forgotten, that the illustration of this position, applies to persons who maintain their insane friends at private charge, as well as to the State."

The following Table shows the truth of the intimation, and the reason why it is so :

*A Table showing the comparative cost to the State of twenty old and twen-
ty recent cases of insanity, illustrating the importance, in an economical
point of view, of placing such persons under treatment at an early period
of their disease, and of providing every means of treating them successfully in an Asylum.*

OLD CASES.				RECENT CASES.		
No.	Age.	Time spent in Asylum.	Cost of each case at 65 dollars per annum.	No.	Duration before admission.	Time spent in Asylum.	Cost of each case at 1 dollar and fifty cents per week
1	47	20 years,	$1,300	1	1 week,	36 weeks,	$54 00
2	48	20 years,	1,300	2	7 weeks,	16 weeks,	24 00
3	52	17 years,	1,105	3	3 months,	32 weeks,	48 00
4	54	16 years,	1,140	4	2 months,	40 weeks,	60 00
5	47	17 yenrs,	1,005	5	2 months,	20 weeks,	30 00
6	46	15 years,	975	6	2 months,	20 weeks,	30 00
7	51	14 years,	910	7	3 months,	12 weeks,	18 00
8	31	13 years,	845	8	1 month,	20 weeks,	30 00
9	33	11 years,	715	9	2 months,	28 weeks,	42 00
10	45	12 years,	780	10	3 months,	24 weeks,	36 00
11	37	10 years,	650	11	6 months,	24 weeks,	36 00
12	39	10 years,	650	12	6 months,	32 weeks,	48 00
13	33	12 years,	780	13	4 months,	28 weeks,	42 00
14	45	15 years,	975	14	4 months,	12 weeks,	18 00
15	48	16 years,	1,040	15	6 months,	8 weeks,	12 00
16	56	12 years,	780	16	1 month,	8 weeks,	12 00
17	44	13 years,	715	17	2 months,	24 weeks,	36 00
18	47	15 years,	975	18	1 month,	20 weeks,	30 00
19	36	13 years,	845	19	6 months,	12 weeks,	18 00
20	36	9 years,	580	20	1 month,	20 weeks,	30 00
			$18,030				$654 00

Aggregate cost of 20 old cases, $18,030 00.
Average time spent in Asylum by each, 14 years,
Average cost of each case,
$901 50.

Aggregate cost of 20 recent cases, $654 00.
Average time spent in Asylum, nearly five
months.
Average cost of each case, $32 14.

Moral treatment of the insane with a view to induce
habits of self-control, is of the first importance. Uniform firmness and kindness towards the patient are of
absolute obligation. The most exact observance of truth
should be preserved in all intercourse with the insane.
They rarely violate a promise, and are singularly sensitive
to truthfulness and fidelity in others. They rarely forgive an injury and as seldom betray insensibility to kindness and indulgence. Once deceived by a nurse or atten-

dant, they never a second time bestow their confidence upon the same individual.

Moderate employment, moderate exercise, as much freedom as is consistent with the safety of the patient, and as little apparent anxious watchfulness, with cheerful society should be sought. The condition of the patients must determine the number of nurses in a ward. The general opinion is holden that all patients do better without special nurses, wholly devoted to their care.

"The proper mental and physical employment of the insane," says Dr. Kirkbride, " is of so much importance that the full treatment of this subject would be to give at once a treatise on the insane and on insanity. Whatever it may be, it must embrace utility, and it is well to combine both physical and mental occupation. Active exercise in the open air, moderate labor in the gardens, pleasure grounds, or upon the farm, afford good results. Short excursions, resort to the work shops, carpentering, joining, turning, the use of a good library &c. &c., are aids in advancing the cure of the patient." Sedentary employments are not in general favorable to health. The operations of agriculture seem liable to the least objection. There is a limit to be observed in the use of labor as a moral means; for there are always some patients to whom it is decidedly injurious. This effect is manifested oftenest in recent cases.

Dr. Ray says that it is an error to suppose that the insane can labor as productively and as uniformly as the sane man. The working hours of a patient should seldom exceed six or seven per diem, and not seldom work is altogether intermitted.

The manner in which labor exerts a beneficial influence upon the insane mind differs no doubt in different forms of the disease. In highly excited patients the surplus nervous energy will be consumed, if no other way is provided, in mischief and noise ; but let it be expended in useful labor, and although the work may not always be perfectly well done, yet the patient thinks it is, and experiences the gratification of having done what he believes is a good thing, and consequently, so far as it goes it is beneficial.

This sentiment of satisfaction in being useful, the guardian of the insane cannot too carefully watch over and foster, since it conducts to self-control and self-respect. Incurables who are able and willing to work, are much more contented and enjoy better health when employed. Even some of the most demented and idiots are found capable of doing something. A young man became a raving maniac, and in three months was conveyed to the hospital, but was already declining into idiocy; soon complete imbecility supervened. He was classed with the idiots in the institution; and considered as past hope of benefit or cure. One day he was observed to amuse himself with some rude coloring and odd figures upon the walls of his room. He was supplied with colours, brushes, and canvass, and soon commenced a portrait: he was now roused, and eager to accomplish his new and attractive work. He was encouraged to renew and repeat his attempts, and finally his mind was restored to its early and rational condition. Thus, careful attention to the daily state of the patient, suggested a method of treatment which resulted in a decided cure. The diseased organs were suffered to rest and their recuperative energies recovered action.

The physician of the hospital at Staunton, in a report of his institution, says, that during the past year, the men patients were chiefly employed in cultivating the farm, working the garden, improving the gronuds, constructing fences, cutting wood, and attending to stock. The women were engaged in sewing, knitting, spinning, and assisting in various departments of house-work, and other occupations and recreations suited to their sex.

" A patient, insane for more than ten years, and beyond hope of recovery, considered dangerous to the public safety, and therefore detained at a hospttal, converses incoherently and raves wildly, yet finds constant and profitable employment upon the farm; has charge of a stock of cattle and hogs and is scrupulously faithful in the discharge of his duties. Instead of confinement in a county jail, from whence he was removed to the Hospital, in a most filthy, and abject condition, at a cost of little less than three hundred dollars per annum, he is here a genteel, orderly, and industrious individual, cheerful, happy, and useful : his labor more than pays all his expenses, and supplies him with sufficient indulgencies."

Prichard, in a work on insanity, says that "at the Richmond Asylum, out of 217 patients, 130 were actively and
usefully employed viz: 18 in gardening, 16 in spinning,
12 in knitting, 18 in needlework, 12 in washing, 16 in
carrying tools, white-washing the wards, tailoring and
wearing ; and 12 were learning to read."

The following table exhibits the results of productive
labor last year upon the Bloomingdale Hospital farm near
New York, 8 or 10 acres being only cultivated.

Potatoes, 1952 bushels	900 bushels, sound, at $0 75	675 00			
Sugar Beet,	180 "	" 0 37½	67 50		
Blood Beet,	100 "	" 0 50	50 00		
Turnips,	460 "	" 0 31¼	143 75		
Carrots,	28 "	" 0 50	14 00		
Parsnips,	120 "	"	60 00		
Onions,	45 "	" 0 75	67 50		
Corn,	150 "	" 0 37½	56 25		
Egg Plant,	20 "	" 0 50	10 00		
Radishes,	125 "	" 1 00	125 00		
Beans,	120 "	" 0 50	60 00		
Peas,	65 "	" 0 75	48 75		
Punkins,	75 "	" 0 37½	28 12		
Squashes,	130 "	" 0 "	48 75		
Spinach,	210 "	" 0 75	157 50		
Asparagus,	40 "	" 3 00	120 00		
Tomatoes,	140 "	" 0 50	70 00		
Cucumbers,	100 "	" 0 75	75 00		
Nasturtiums,	1 "	" 2 00	2 00		
Peppers,	4 "	" 0 75	3 00		
Rhubarb,	52 "	" 2 00	104 00		
Citron Melon,	75 "	" 0 10	7 50		
Celery,	2500 heads,	" 0 3	75 00		
Cabbages,	3000 "	" 0 4	120 00		
Leeks,	1000 "	" 0 0½	5 00		
Salsify,	2000 "	" 1 00	20 00		
Lettuce,	4000 "	" 2 00	80 00		
				1,293 62	
Hay,	40 tons,	" 10 00	400 00		
Pork,	1296 pounds,	" 0 6	77 76		
Butter,	663 "	" 0 25	165 75		
Milk,	4488 gallons,	" 0 16	718 08		
Eggs,	303 dozen,	" 0 12½	37 88		
Poultry,	150 lbs.	" 0 6	9 00		
				1,408 47	
FRUITS.					
Apples,	200 bushels,	" 0 50	100 00		
Pears,	20 "	" 1 00	20 00		
Cherries,	150 "	" 1 00	150 00		
Currants,	25 "	" 1 00	25 00		
Peaches,	15 "	" 1 00	15 00		
Grapes,	1200 pounds,	" 0 6¼	75 00		
Strawberries,	8 bushels,	" 2 00	16 00		
				401 00	
Total,				$4,103 09	

The able and distinguished Superintendant of the Rhode Island Hospital writes, that "no form of labor appears so well calculated to promote the comfort and restoration of such patients as have had habits of employment, as working on a farm, *and no institution can fully accomplish these purposes without plenty of land,* and attendants to assist in cultivation." All patients, whether men or women, whose minds have been cultivated, and who have had habits of active industry and employment, possess high advantages in chances of recovery from attacks of insanity, over the ignorant, the indolent, and the inert. So also those whose habits have been methodical, and temperate in eating and drinking, have better chances of permanent restoration than those who possess their opposites.

The standard of sound health is elevated by the disuse of stimulating food, and of all intoxicating drinks: and by avoiding the use of Tobacco in any forms.

Stimulants even not inordinately used, excite to undue mental and physical action. It might seem that the Apostle of old, apart from the *morale* of life, had comprehended animal physics when he exhorted brethren to adhere to *"moderation* in all things."

"We have a patient, writes the Superintendant of the Maryland Hospital, " who had for many months been in a state of profound depression from which no efforts on our part could rouse him. He had repeatedly attempted suicide. He was a farmer, and when well, was enterprising, industrious, and devoted to the pursuit. He walked out to the hay-field, and after much persuasion, he was induced to amuse himself by mowing a little. Finding his interest in the work increase, he continued to ply the scythe for two hours with short intervals. He now became cheerful and communicative; ate with appetite at dinner; after which he expressed a wish to return to the hay-field, where he continued mowing until evening. This labor was followed by a night of profound and refreshing sleep. The next morning he hastened to the field, and from that time was seldom unemployed; his convalescence was rapid, and in about four weeks he returned to his family entirely restored. Similar cases are of frequent occurrence. Of *ninety nine* men patients, *forty-five* are habitually employed in useful work: And of *fifty-seven* women patients, all save *eleven* are for a great part of the time employed in the halls, in the kitchen, the washing and the ironing rooms, or in mending and repairing garments and house-linen, and various sorts of needle-work. *Thirty-eight* of the women, and fifty-five of the men have been habitual readers, and find great benefit and satisfaction in the use of the library; indeed several patients seem to owe their restoration to adopting a regular course of reading and study.

In our times, when knowledge is so widely diffused, it seems almost superfluous to dwell upon the benefits of hospital treatment above all private and domestic management. It cannot be questioned, that suppose knowledge, experience, and all domestic arrangements favorable, one might decide in favor of treatment for the insane in their own families. This, however, cannot be assured even when all the appliances wealth may procure are at command, and therefore all persons who are familiar with these subjects, do not hesitate in advocating Hospital residence for the insane of all conditions in society, whether rich or poor, educated or ignorant. Some object that associations of a painful nature may dwell upon the recollection of the recovered patient. Whatever apparent force this idea may possess, it is a well established fact that patients rarely entertain other than pleasant and grateful memories of their residence in well-regulated Hospitals. When these are not well organized, and wisely and carefully conducted, no patient under any circumstances should be sent to them.

Jacobi affirms that "the magnitude of anticipated evils has been greatly exaggerated"; "as regards these," he says, "I can positively affirm that of six hundred cases which I have had the opportunity of accurately examining in this establishment, (that of Siegberg, in Germany) I have never witnessed a single one in which the patient sustained any material injury from his residence in the establishment as a lunatic asylum, or from any influence exercised upon him by other patients. Such ideas only are true of badly ordered Hospitals and these may always be known from those of good organization. The time has gone by, thanks to Heaven, when the unhappy insane could be cast into mismanaged Hospitals, and, as too often is the case, left, in jails, and poor-houses, festering in heaps of filthy straw, chained to the walls of dark and dreary cells, unworthy of solicitude, and victims of the idle and interested maxim that insanity is an incurable disease, and that insane people are unconscious of the treatment they receive, and the cruel miseries to which they are so needlessly subjected. Much has been done, but more, much more, remains to be accomplished for the relief of these sufferers, in our own United States, as in other countries. With a population rating at more than 22,000 000, our insane and idiots number at the lowest estimate 22,000 ; and not 4,000, at this time have the advantages of appropriate care in well organized hospitals, or comfortable situations adapted to their condition and circumstances elsewhere.

In 1844, the number of inmates in the hospitals of England and Wales was 11,272. Additional accommodations have been called for and provided to a large extent. The oldest hospital founded in England is that of Bethlem, which king Henry the VIII presented to the City of London, in 1547.

There are twenty State hospitals, besides several incorporated hospitals, for the treatment of the insane, in nineteen States of the Union, Virginia alone having two government State hospitals. The following is a correct list, omitting several small establishments conducted by private individuals, and several pretty extensive poorhouse and prison departments.

The first hospital for the insane in the United States was established in Philadelphia, as a department of the Penn Hospital, in the year 1752. This has been transferred to a fine district near the village of Mantua, in the vicinity of Philadelphia, since 1832 : number of patients 188.

The second institution recieving insane patients, and the first exclusively for their use, was at Williamsburg, Virginia, in 1773 : number of patients 165.

The third was the Friends' Hospital, at Frankfort, near Philadelphia, in 1817: number of patients 95.

The next was the McLean Hospital. at Charlestown, (now Summerville,) in Massachusetts, in 1818. This valuable institution is second to none in America. Number of patients 180.

Bloomingdale Hospital, near the city of New York, was established in 1821 ; number of patients 146 : South Carolina Hospital, at Columbia, in 1822 ; number of patients 74 : Conneticut Hospital at Hartford, patients 122 and Kentucky Hospital at Lexington, patents 247, in 1824.

In 1845–46, the legislature of Kentucky passed a bill to establish a second State institution in the Green River country.

Virginia Western Hospital was opened at Staunton in 1828 ; number of patients 217. Massachusetts State Hospital, at Worcester, was opened in 1833, and enlarged in 1843; it has 370 patients. Maryland Hospital, at Baltimore, was founded in 1834; it has the present year 109 patients. Vermont State Hospital, at Battleborough, was opened for patients in 1837, and enlarged in 1846-'47; it has at present 320 patients. New York City Hospital for the poor, on Blackwell's island, was occupied in 1838; it is now being considerably enlarged: above 400 patients.

Tennessee State Hospital, at Nashville, was opened in 1839. According to an act of the legislature the present year, this hospital is to be replaced by one of capacity to receive 250 patients. In the old hospital are 64 patients. Boston City Hospital for the indigent, which has 150 patients, and Ohio State Hospital at Columbus, were severally opened in 1839. The latter has been considerably enlarged, and has now 329 patients. Maine State Hospital, at Augusta, 1840; patients 130. New Hampshire State Hospital, at Concord, was opened in 1842, and has 100 patients. New York State Hospital, at Utica, was established in 1843, and has since been largely extended, and has 600 patients. Mount Hope Hospital, near Baltimore, 1844-'45; has 72 insane patients. Georgia has an institution for the insane at Milledgeville, and at present 128 patients. Rhode Island State Hospital opened, under the able direction of Dr. Ray, early in 1848. New Jersey State Hospital, at Trenton, 1848. Indiana State Hospital, at Indianapolis, will be opened in 1848. State Hospital of Illinois, at Jacksonville, will be occupied before 1849. The Lousiana State Hospital will be occupied perhaps within a year.

These institutions, liberally sustained as are most of them, cannot accommodate the insane population of the United States who require prompt remedial care.

Such being the facts, one can hardly employ language too importunate, arguments too persuasive, to secure such increased accommodations for the Insane throughout the United States, but especially *in those States in which no Hospitals have been established,* as shall assure their sufficient care and protection; their remedial treatment so as to procure recovery when recovery is possible; and their safety and guardianship in all cases where the terrible calamity of *incurability* crowds them forever from all the bland affections, and social enjoyments of domestic and friendly association.

As ye would that others should do for you in like circumstances, so do ye for these helpless ones, cast through the Providence of God, on your sympathy and care! Be the guardians and benefactors of those, who as a writer in the 17th century finely expresses himself, "*are a particular rent charge upon the great family of mankind; left by the maker of us all like younger children, 'who though the Estate be given from them, yet the Father expected the heir to take care of them!*"

To see the mind once brilliant, and in the exercise of fine energies, obscured and inert ; or if quickened to action, trans. formed from the consistent bearing of a being possessed of rational understanding to the fury of a demon, or to the raging of an untamed brute—this is fearful, this is truly to behold the drain ing to the dregs the cup of bitterness ! Oh with what ready zeal, with what wisdom and humanity should not every one direct himself to prevent miseries which no skill can wholly heal, & of which no foresight nor prudence can prevent the recurrence.

" Weep not pale moralist o'er desert plains,
Strewed with the wreck of grandeur's mouldering fanes,
Arches of triumph long with weeds o'ergrown,
And regal cities—now the serpent's own ;—
Earth has more dreadful ruins,—one lost mind,
Whose star is quenched, has lessons for mankind
Of deeper import than each prostrate dome
Mingling its marble with the dust of Rome" !

Bereft of reason, man loses every thing that renders life valuable. Naturally endowed with capacities for the highest enjoyment, he is suddenly through an attack of insanity, disabled from partaking the rational pleasures of life, and of exercising his noble faculties for his benefit or for the good of society.

Though plunged in the most profound grief,—assailed by every form of trial and misfortune, while reason is spared, hope may cheer his dreary hours,—and faith support him through every trouble ; but dethrone reason and he is utterly prostrate. The merest infant is not more dependant on parental care, than is the maniac upon the tender ministrations of kindred or of friends. In an hour he becomes the beneficiary of humanity : the helpless ward of his fellow-men : him must nursing, and watching, and skilful cares surround, else is he the most pitiable of human beings—out-cast and forlorn— smitten of a terrible malady, exposed to sufferings, and woes, and tortures of which no language however vigorously combined can be the representation. Have pity upon him, have pity upon him for the hand of God hath smitten him ! Talk not of expense—of the cost of supporting and ministering remedies for these afflicted ones. Who shall dare compute in dollars and cents the worth of one mind ! Who will weigh gold against the priceless possession of a sound understanding? You turn not away from the beggar at your door, ready to perish :

you open your hand, and he is warmed, and fed, and clothed : will you refuse to the maniac the solace of a decent shelter, the protection of a fit asylum, the cares that shall raise him from the condition of the brute, and the healing remedies that shall re-illume the temple of reason ? Who amongst you is so strong that he may not become weak ? Whose reason so sound that madness may not overwhelm in an hour the noblest intellect ?

You will not, Legislators of North Carolina—Senators and Representatives of a noble State, you will not forget amidst the heat of debate, the clash of opinion, and the strife for political snpremacy ; you will not forget the majesty of your station, the dignity of that trust confided to you by the suffrages of your fellow-citizens.

It is not often that you are solicited to exercise your functions in behalf of the unfortunate. That you possess the power, and now the opportunity of exercising a gracious, benignant, and God-like influence upon the present and future destiny of hundreds, nay of thousands, who pine in want and misery, under privations and sufferings, wearily borne through heavy months and years—the light of whose reason is quenched, and whose judgment is as the stubble upon a waste field ; this it is believed is a sufficient argument to determine your decisions in favor of justice, and of humanity, and of unquestionable civil obligation.

As benefactors of the distressed whose mental darkness may, through your agency, be dispersed, how many blessings and prayers from grateful hearts will enrich you ! As your last hours shall be slowly numbered, and the review of life becomes more and more searching, amidst the shades of uncompromising memories, how beautiful will be the remembrance that of the many of this life's transactions, oftenest controlling transient and outward affairs, frequently conducting to disquieting results, and sometimes to those of doubtful good, you have aided to accomplish a work whose results of wide-diffused benefits are as sanctifiying as they are permanent: blessing through all Time—consecrating through all Eternity !

Gentlemen, the sum of the plea of your Memoralist is embodied in the solicitation for an adequate appropriation for the construction of a Hospital for the remedial treatment of the Insane in the State of North Carolina.

Respectfully submitted,

D. L. DIX.

Raleigh, November, 1848.

MEMORIAL

UNITED STATES CONGRESS

1848

MEMORIAL

OF

D. L. DIX,

PRAYING

A grant of land for the relief and support of the indigent curable and incurable insane in the United States.

June 27, 1848.

Referred to a Select Committee, and ordered to be printed, and that 5,000 additional copies be printed for the use of the Senate.

To the Senate and House of Representatives of the United States in Congress assembled.

Your memorialist respectfully asks permission to lay before you what seem to be just and urgent claims in behalf of a numerous and increasing class of sufferers in the United States. I refer to the great and inadequately relieved distresses of the insane throughout the country.

Upon the subject to which this memorial refers, many to whose justice and humanity it appeals are well-informed; but the attention of many has not been called to the subject, and a few, but a very few, have looked upon some features of this sad picture as revealed in private dwellings, in poorhouses, and in prisons.

Your memorialist hopes to place before you substantial reasons which shall engage your earnest attention, and secure favorable action upon the important subject she advocates.

It is a fact, not less certainly substantiated than it is deplorable, that insanity has increased in an advanced ratio with the fast increasing population in all the United States. For example, according to the best received methods of estimate five years since, it was thought correct to count one insane in every thousand inhabitants throughout the Union. At the present, my own careful investigations are sustained by the judgment and the information of the most intelligent superintendents of hospitals for the insane, in rendering the estimates not less than one insane person in every eight hundred inhabitants at large, throughout the United States.

There are, in proportion to numbers, more insane in cities than in large towns, and more insane in villages than among the same number of inhabitants dwelling in scattered settlements.

Wherever the intellect is most excited, and health lowest, there is an increase of insanity. This malady prevails most widely, and illustrates its presence most commonly in mania, in those countries whose citizens possess the largest civil and religious liberty; where, in effect, every indi-

Tippin & Streeper, printers.

vidual, however obscure, is free to enter upon the race for the highest honors and most exalted stations; where the arena of competition is accessible to all who seek the distinctions which acquisition and possession of wealth assures, and the respect accorded to high literary and scholastic attainments. Statesmen, politicians, and merchants, are peculiarly liable to insanity. In the United States, therefore, we behold an illustration of my assertion. The kingdoms of Western Europe, excepting Portugal, Spain, and the lesser islands dependent on Great Britain, rank next to this country in the rapid development of insanity. Sir Andrew Halliday, in a letter to Lord Seymour, states that the number of the insane in England has become more than tripled in the last twenty years. Russia in Europe, Turkey, and Hungary, together with most of the Asiatic and African countries, exhibit but little insanity. The same is remarked by travellers, especially by Humboldt, of a large part of South America. Those tracts of North America inhabited by Indians, and the sections chiefly occupied by the negro race, produce comparatively very few examples. The colored population is more liable to attacks of insanity than the negro.

This terrible malady, the source of indescribable miseries, does increase, and must continue fearfully to increase, in this country, whose free, civil, and religious institutions create constantly various and multiplying sources of mental excitement. Comparatively but little care is given in cultivating the moral affections in proportion with the intellectual development of the people. Here, as in other countries, forcible examples may be cited to show the mischiefs which result alike from religious,* social, civil, and rev-

---

*Note.—I wish to mark carefully the distinction between true religion and extravagant religious excitements. The one is the basis of every virtue, the source of every consolation under the manifold trials and afflictions which beset the path of every one in the course of this mortal pilgrimage ; while that morbid state which is created by want of calm, earnest meditation, and self-discipline, by excessive demands upon the physical strength, by protracted attendance upon excited public assemblies, is ever to be deprecated. The following statistics show how large a part of the patients in some of our best hospitals labor under what is commonly termed religious insanity. I offer a pretty full list from the report, for 1843, of the Massachusetts State Hospital, for the sake of comparison : number of years not recorded :

Intemperance	239
Ill health	279
Domestic afflictions	179
Religious	148
Property	98
Disappointed affections	64
Disappointed ambition	33
Epilepsy	45
Puerperal	47
Wounds on the head	21
Abuse of snuff and tobacco	8

Many cases not recorded for two years previous to 1844.

Dr. Woodward remarks, that " the coincidence of this table with the

olutionary excitements. The Millerite delusions prepared large numbers
for our hospitals; so also the great conflagrations in New York, the Irish

---

records of other institutions shows, conclusively, that if we have failed
in ascertaining causes, we have fallen into a common error."

Seven consecutive and valuable reports by Dr. Kirkbride, exhibit the
following results in the Pennsylvania Hospital for the Insane. This is
not, like the first referred to, a State institution, but has a class of patients from adjacent States, as well as its own State's insane. It will be
kept in mind, also, that more than 350 insane patients are in the Blockley
almshouse in the vicinity, of which no note is here made.

In 1841-'42, admissions 299; of which 238 were residents of Pennsylvania, viz:

	Men.	Women.	Total.
Ill health of various kinds	22	24	46
Intemperance	20	0	20
Loss of property	17	6	23
Dread of poverty	2	0	2
Disappointed affections	2	4	6
Intense study	5	0	5
Domestic difficulties	1	5	6
Fright at fires, &c.	2	3	5
Grief—loss of friends	4	16	20
Intense application to business	2	0	2
Religious excitement	8	7	15
Want of employment	9	0	9
Use of opium	0	2	2
Use of tobacco	2	0	2
Mental anxiety	4	1	5
Unascertained, &c.	0	0	123
			299

In 1842-'43, of 439 cases, there were from religious excitement 12
men, 9 women—total 21. In 1843-'44, of 592 cases, religious excitement produced of men 17, of women 11—total 28. In 1844-'45, in 769
cases, religious excitement in men 19, in women 16—total 35. In 1846,
of 936 cases, of men were, through religious excitement, 22; of women,
20—total 42. In 1847, of 1,196 cases recorded, 26 men, 24 women—total 50, through religious excitement.

Dr. Brigham's first annual report upon the New York State Hospital
shows, of 276 cases within the first year, there were through religious
excitement, of men 29, of women 21—total 50; besides 5 men and 2
women (total 7) insane through " Millerism."

Of 408 patients in 1842, 57 became insane through *ill health*, 32 through
intemperance, 54 through *religious anxiety*, 50 through trouble and disappointment, and 55 through various minor causes.

Of 179 cases received at Bloomingdale in 1842, 19 were from intemperance, 15 various causes, 15 puerperal, 14 religious excitement, 14 love,
13 trouble.

Of 122 cases received in 1842 at Staunton, Va., 33 were ill health, 20 riots and firemen's mobs in Philadelphia; and the last presidential elections throughout the country levied heavily on the mental health of its citizens.

Abroad, discontents in Scotland, civil and religious; agitations in Wales, social and civil; wide-spread disturbances in the manufacturing and agricultural districts of England; tumultuous and riotous gatherings in Ireland—all have left abiding evidence of their mischievous influence upon the records of every hospital for the insane. France, too, unfolds a melancholy page of hospital history. Subsequent to the bloody revolution which marked the close of the eighteenth century, the hospitals for the insane were thronged, showing that where the effect of exalted mental excitement failed to produce insanity in the parents, it was developed in the children, and children's children—a fearful legacy, and sure !

The political disturbances which convulsed Canada, several years since, were followed by like results.

In law, idiots are ranked with the insane. I have remarked, throughout our country, several prevailing causes of organic idiocy; of these the most common, and the most surely traced, is intemperance of parents, and the marriage and intermarriage of near relatives and kindred. Abounding examples exist on every side throughout the land.

In calculating the statistics of mental aberration, from the best authorities, it is found impossible to arrive at exactly correct results; approximation to facts is all that can be attained.

There is less maniacal insanity in the southern than in the northern States, for which disparity various causes may be assigned. Two leading causes, obvious to every mind, is the much larger amount of negro population, and the much less influx of foreigners, in the former than in the atter. While the tide of immigration sets towards the north Atlantic States with almost overwhelming force, one cannot witness the fact and not note its sequence.

Our hospitals for the insane are already receiving a vast population of uneducated foreigners; and most of these, who become the subjects of insanity, present the most difficult and hopeless, because the least curable cases. Take for example the following records, which are gathered from the city hospitals for the insane poor, passing by for the present all the State and general hospitals:

In 1846, the Boston City Hospital for the insane poor received 169 patients; 90 of which were foreigners, 35 natives of other States, and 44 alone residents of the city. Of the 90 foreigners, 70 were Irish. The New York City Hospital for the insane poor, on Blackwell's island, which went into opera-

---

intemperance, 14 religious anxiety, 12 domestic afflictions, 10 pecuniary troubles.

Of 1,247 patients received at the Hartford Retreat, 103 became insane through intemperance, 178 through ill health, 110 through religious anxiety, 65 through trouble and disappointment, 46 puerperal.

Irreligion, and the abuse of religion, are frequently the cause of insanity and suicide. Pure religion, more than any other power, tends to arrest, and assists to cure insanity. Of this fact there is constant evidence and illustration abroad in society, and within the limits of every well organized asylum.

tion in 1839, had, in the autumn of 1843, about 300 patients. Of 284 admitted the following year, 176 were foreigners, viz: 112 Irish, 21 English, 27 Germans; and besides these were 38 natives of New York. On the first of January, 1846, there were in the institution 356 patients, of whom 226 were foreigners. In January, 1847, there were 410 insane patients, 328 of whom were foreigners. The cost to the city of supporting this institution, in 1846, was $24,179 67.

In the Philadelphia poorhouse hospital, at Blockley, there were received in one year 395 insane patients; at the present time there are actually resident there 350 idiots, epileptics, and insane. At the Baltimore city almshouse, there are at the present time more than 85 individuals in various stages of insanity, the whole number of inmates reported being 1,726; of whom 873 are Americans, and 853 Europeans. In the Charity Hospital at New Orleans, in 1845–'46, were above 73 insane; in 1847–'48 there were above 80, chiefly foreigners, and presenting mostly chronic cases. The whole number of patients received at this institution the past year was 8,044: of these, 1,773 were Americans by birth, 6,150 were foreigners, and 121 were not recorded.

The report of the Commercial Hospital at Cincinnati shows, for 1844–'45, that of 1,579 patients, 85 were insane and idiotic. The report of 1846 exhibits the following summary: " Of 2,028 patients, 102 were insane." The last returns show yet an increase of this afflicted class, notwithstanding the enlarged accommodations in the State Hospital at Columbus, and the new buildings for the insane at the excellent asylum for persons in necessitous circumstances in the same city. I might adduce additional records, but believe the above are sufficient to extablish the correctness of my position.

" Allowing," writes Dr. Luther V. Bell, " only 15,000,000 of white inhabitants in the United States, and suppose but one in every thousand to be insane, (an estimate below reality, I believe,) we shall have 150,000: one-third of these may represent those who may be properly calculated upon as subjects for hospital treatment, viz: 50,000." *About eleven twelfths of all the insane who absolutely require fostering and remedial care are wholly unprovided for in this country.* Dr. Bell also states, that from his own actual knowledge of facts in New Hampshire, where, some years since, he had part in collecting facts from each town, compared with the newest returns in the State, and in others where the closest approximations have been made, he is satisfied that fully one-third of the insane population should be resident in hospitals. Dr. Kirkbride, who has carefully reviewed this subject, writes as follows: " In regard to whole numbers, my own inquiries lead me to believe that one in every six or seven hundred inhabitants would be a nearer approximation to correct estimate than one in every thousand, which has heretofore been assumed as the common rule." According to the latest Parliamentary returns taken with the report of the Metropolitan Commissioners on Lunacy, which give the numbers of all classes of insane in the hospitals of England and Wales, it is ascertained that in these two countries " there is one insane *pauper* to every one thousand inhabitants alone."

The liability of communities to insanity should not, I suppose, be estimated by the number of *existing* cases at any one time; for insanity does not usually hasten the termination of life. Take for example Massachusetts, New York, and Virginia, where are found so large numbers of established, long-existing cases. These are counted again and again, every year, every five, or every ten years. A fairer test of the liability of communities to insanity is to be found in the *occurring* cases in *corresponding given periods*.

There are twenty State hospitals, besides several incorporated hospitals, for the treatment of the insane, in nineteen States of the Union, Virginia alone having two government institutions of State and incorporated hospitals. The following is a correct list, omitting several small establishments conducted by private individuals, and several pretty extensive poorhouse and prison departments, which cannot properly be classed with regularly organized hospitals, being usually deficient in remedial appliances.

The first hospital for the insane in the United States was established in Philadelphia, as a department of the Penn Hospital, in the year 1752. This has been transferred to a fine district near the village of Mantua, in the vicinity of Philadelphia, since 1832: number of patients 188.

The second institution receiving insane patients, and the first exclusively for their use, was at Williamsburg, Virginia, in 1773: number of patients 164.

The third was the Friends' Hospital, at Frankfort, near Philadelphia, in 1817: number of patients 95.

The next was the McLean Hospital, at Charlestown, (now Summerville,) in Massachusetts, in 1818. This valuable institution is second to none in America. Number of patients 180.

Bloomingdale Hospital, near the city of New York, was established in 1821; number of patients 145: South Carolina Hospital, at Columbia, in 1822; number of patients 74: Connecticut Hospital at Hartford, patients 122, and Kentucky Hospital at Lexington, patients 247, in 1824.

In 1845–'46, the legislature of Kentucky passed a bill to establish a second State institution in the Green River country.

Virginia Western Hospital was opened at Staunton in 1828; number of patients 217. Massachusetts State Hospital, at Worcester, was opened in 1833, and enlarged in 1843; it has 370 patients. Maryland Hospital, at Baltimore, was founded in 1834; it has the present year 109 patients. Vermont State Hospital, at Brattleborough, was opened for patients in 1837, and enlarged in 1846–'47; it has at present 320 patients. New York City Hospital for the poor, on Blackwell's island, was occupied in 1838; it is now being considerably enlarged: above 400 patients.

The grand jury this month (June, 1848,) have made the following presentment in relation to the Blackwell's island hospital for the insane poor: " We found no less than 425 afflicted children of humanity suffering under the most terrible of all privations, and, *we observed with regret, less adequately cared for than their situation and the dictates of humanity require.*"

The same document places before the public the concurrent testimony of Drs. Macdonald, Williams, and Ogden, who in a clear and true report show that " the accommodations for the insane poor of New York city are at present inadequate and miserable; and the imperfect manner of their treatment is such as to be a disgrace to the city, which otherwise is deservedly famed for its liberal benevolent institutions. In *the present state of affairs* it is useless to attempt the recovery of any patients here."

The same remark holds good of the department for the insane connected with the commercial hospital in Cincinnati.

Well organized hospitals are the only fit places of residence for the insane of all classes; ill-conducted institutions are worse than none at all.

The New York City Hospital for the Insane, and the State hospitals of Georgia and Tennessee, cannot take present respectable rank as curative or comfortable hospitals.

Tennessee State Hospital, at Nashville, was opened in 1839. According to an act of the legislature the present year, this hospital is to be replaced by one of capacity to receive 250 patients. In the old hospital are 64 patients. Boston City Hospital for the indigent, which has 150 patients, and Ohio State Hospital at Columbus, were severally opened in 1839. The latter has been considerably enlarged, and has now 329 patients. Maine State Hospital, at Augusta, 1840; patients 130. New Hampshire State Hospital, at Concord, was opened in 1842, and has 100 patients. New York State Hospital, at Utica, was established in 1843, and has since been largely extended, and has 600 patients. Mount Hope Hospital, near Baltimore, 1844–'45; has 72 insane patients. Georgia has an institution for the insane at Milledgeville, and at present 128 patients. Rhode Island State Hospital opened, under the able direction of Dr. Ray, early in 1848. New Jersey State Hospital, at Trenton, 1848. Indiana State Hospital, at Indianapolis, will be opened in 1848. State Hospital of Illinois, at Jacksonville, will be occupied before 1849. The Louisiana State Hospital will be occupied perhaps within a year.

I repeat that these institutions, liberally sustained as are most of them, cannot accommodate *one twelfth* of the insane population of the United States which require prompt remedial care.

It may be suggested that though hospital treatment is expedient, perhaps it may not be absolutely necessary, especially for vast numbers whose condition may be considered irrecoverable, and in whom the right exercise of the reasoning faculties may be looked upon as past hope. Rather than enter upon a philosophical and abstract argument to prove the contrary to be the fact, I will ask permission to spread before you a *few* statements gathered, without special selection, from a mass of records made from existing cases, sought out and noted during *eight years* of sad, patient, deliberate investigation. To assure accuracy, establish facts beyond controversy, and procure, so far as possible, temporary or permanent relief, more than sixty thousand miles have been traversed, and no time or labor spared which fidelity to this imperative and grievous vocation demanded. The only States as yet unvisited are North Carolina, Florida, and Texas. From each of these, however, I have had communications, which clearly prove that the conditions of the indigent insane differ in no essential degree from those of other States.

I have myself seen *more than nine thousand idiots, epileptics, and insane, in these United States, destitute of appropriate care and protection ;* and of this vast and most miserable company, sought out in *jails*, in *poorhouses*, and in *private dwellings*, there have been hundreds, nay, rather thousands, bound with galling chains, bowed beneath fetters and heavy iron balls, attached to drag-chains, lacerated with ropes, scourged with rods, and terrified beneath storms of profane execrations and cruel blows; now subject to gibes, and scorn, and torturing tricks—now abandoned to the most loathsome necessities, or subject to the vilest and most outrageous violations. These are strong terms, but language fails to convey the astounding truths. I proceed to verify this assertion, commencing with the State of Maine. I will be ready to specify the towns and districts where each example quoted did exist, or exists still.

In B., a furious maniac confined in the jail; case doubtful from long delay in removing to an hospital; a heap of filthy straw in one corner served for a bed; food was introduced through a small aperture, called a slit, in the wall, through which also was the sole source of ventilation and avenue for light.

Near C., a man for several years in a narrow filthy pen, chained; condition loathsome in the extreme.

In A., insane man in a small damp room in the jail; greatly excited; had been confined many years; during his paroxysms, which were aggravated by every manner of neglect, except want of food, he had *torn out his eyes*, lacerated his face, chest, and arms, seriously injured his limbs, and was in a state most shocking to behold. In P., nine very insane men and women in the poorhouse, all exposed to neglect and every species of injudicious treatment; several chained, some in pens or stalls in the barn, and treated less kindly than the brute beasts in their vicinity. At C., four furiously crazy; ill treated, through the ignorance of those who held them in charge. 47 cases in the middle district, either scattered in poorhouses, jails, or in private families, and all inappropriately treated in every respect; many chained, some bearing the marks of injuries self-inflicted, and many of injuries received from others. In New Hampshire, on the opening of the hospital for the reception of patients, in 1842, many were removed from cages, small unventilated cells in poorhouses, private houses, and from the dungeons of county jails. Many of these were bound with cords, or confined with chains; some bore the marks of severe usage by blows and stripes. They were neglected and filthy; and some, who yet remain in remote parts of the State, through exposure to cold in inclement seasons, have been badly frozen, so as to be maimed for life. Details in many cases will not bear recital.

In New Hampshire, a committee of the legislature was named in 1832, whose duty it was to collect and report statistics of the insane. Returns were received from only one hundred and forty-one towns: in these were returned the names of *one hundred and eighty-nine* persons bereft of their reason, and incapable of taking care of themselves; ninety men and ninety-nine women. The number confined was *seventy-six, twenty-five* of whom were in private houses, seven in cells and cages, six in chains and irons, and four in the jails. Of the number at liberty, many had at various times been confined. Many of the facts represented by this committee are too horrible to repeat, and would lead many to the belief that they could not be correct, were they not so undeniably authenticated. The committee remark that from many towns no returns had been made, and conclude their report with the declaration " that they could not doubt that the numbers of the insane greatly exceeded the estimates rendered."

Where were these insane? "Some were in cells or cages; some in out-buildings, garrets, or cellars; some in county jails, shut up with felons and criminals; some in almshouses, in brick cells, never warmed by fire, nor lighted by the rays of the sun." The facts presented to this committee not only exhibit severe unnecessary suffering, but utter neglect, and in many cases actual barbarity.

Most of the cases reported, I could authenticate from direct investigation. One very insane woman was confined all winter in a jail without fire; and from the severity of the cold, and her fixed posture, her feet were so much injured that it was deemed necessary to amputate them at the ankle, which was accordingly done.

" Another female was confined in a garret, where, from the lowness of the roof, and the restrained position, she grew double, and is now obliged to walk with her hands, as well as her feet, upon the floor." I recollect eight cases corresponding with this, produced from similar causes, in other States. A man was confined in a cellar for many years without clothing, and couching in a heap of wet straw, which was from time to time renewed; another in a similar condition is chained in an out-building; another is at this time (1846) chained to the floor in an out-building, glad to pick the bones thrown into his kennel, like a beast: one with sufficient property, and formerly correct in life, active and happy. This case was reported to the committee in 1832, who, summing up their report, state, that " in the extremity of disease, the maniac is withdrawn from observation, and is forgotten. His voice, in his raving, grates not upon the ear of the happy. They who have the custody of the wretched being are too prone to forget their duty, and his claims upon them for kindness and forbearance. Their sympathy is exhausted, and their kindness becomes blunted by familiarity with misery. They give up the feelings of the friend for the apathy of the jailer." They adopt a common error, that the maniac is insensible to suffering; that he is incurable; and therefore there is no use in rendering the cares his situation demands.

A committee reported (in 1836) to the legislature of New Hampshire, that their whole number of returns was 312: the number of towns returned having insane, was 141; the whole number of inhabitants in all the towns returned, was 193,569. The number returned as confined, including all in cages, jails, close rooms, by chains and hand-cuffs, &c., was 81. From these statistics, carefully collected, it appears that *one in every six hundred and twenty is insane.* The committee of 1836 conclude their report as follows: "Neither the time nor the occasion requires us to allude to instances of the aggravated and almost incredible suffering of the insane poor which have come to our knowledge. We are convinced that the legislature require no high-wrought pictures of the various gradations of intense misery to which the pauper lunatic is subjected; extending from his incarceration in the cold, narrow, sunless, and fireless cell of the almshouse, to the scarcely more humane mode of '*selling him at auction*,' as it is called, by which he falls into the hands, and is exposed to the tender mercies, of the most worthless of society, who alone could be excited by cupidity to such a revolting charge. Suffice it on this point, your committee are satisfied that the horrors of the *present* condition of the insane poor of New Hampshire are far from having been exaggerated; and of course they find great unwillingness on the part of those having charge of them to render correct accounts, or to have these repeated to the public."

The report of the nine trustees for the hospital, for 1847, states, that from authentic sources they are informed that "in eight of the twenty-four towns in Merrimack county, having an aggregate population of twelve thousand, there are eighteen insane paupers; part supported upon the town-farms, and part *set up and bid off at auction from year to year, to be kept and maintained by the lowest bidder.*" According to the data afforded above, there must be in the State several hundred insane supported on the poor-farms, or put up at auction, annually.

In Vermont, the same neglects, ignorance, and sometimes brutal severity, led to like results. Dr. Rockwell, his assistant physicians, and the whole corps of hospital nurses, bear accordant testimony to the sufferings of patients formerly brought to that institution from all parts of the State; and many even now arrive under circumstances the most revolting and shocking, subject to the roughest treatment or the most inexcusable and extreme neglects.

I have seen many of these afflicted persons, men of hardy frames and women of great capacity for endurance, bowed and wasted till almost all trace of humanity was lost in grovelling habits, and injuries through severities and privations, which those cannot comprehend who have never witnessed similar cases of misery.

Not many counties, if indeed any towns or parishes, but have their own tales of various wo, illustrated in the miseries of the insane.

In the eighth annual report of the Vermont hospital for 1844 is the following record, which being a repetition in fact, if not almost literal expression of my own notes, I adopt in preference: "One case was brought to the hospital four and a half years ago, of a man who had been insane more than twelve years. During the four years previous to his admission he had not worn any article of clothing, and had been caged in a cellar, without feeling the influence of a fire. A nest of straw was his only bed and covering. He was so violent that his keeper thought it necessary to cause *an iron ring to be riveted about his neck,* so that they could hold him when they changed his bed of straw. In this miserable condition he was taken from the cellar and conveyed to the hospital. The ring was at once removed from his neck. He has worn clothing, has been furnished with a comfortable bed, and has come to the table, using a knife and fork ever since he was admitted. He is most of the time pleasantly and usefully employed about the institution." "Another man, insane for twenty-four years, for the last six years had worn no clothing, and had been furnished with no bed except loose straw. He had become regardless of everything that was decent. In less than three months after his admission, he so improved that he wore clothing constantly, kept his bed and room neat, and worked on the farm daily.

" Another man, insane more than thirty years, *was sold to the lowest bidder. For many years* he was *caged,* and had his feet frozen so that he lost his toes, and endured cruel sufferings which no person in a natural state could have supported. He was five months in the hospital, wore his clothing, was furnished with a comfortable bed, and sat at table with other patients. He was a printer by trade, and for a long time employed himself in setting up type for the newspaper printed at this institution."

Another patient, a woman 61 years of age, was taken to the hospital. She had been confined for several years in a half subterranean cage, &c., which was nothing other than a cave excavated in the side of a hill near the house, and straw thrown in for a bed ; no warmth was admitted save what the changing seasons supplied. Her condition in all respects was neglected and horrible in the extreme."

Examples here, as in *every State of the Union,* might be multiplied of the insane caged and chained, confined in garrets, cellars, corn-houses, and other out-buildings, until their extremities were seized by the frost, and their sufferings augmented by extreme torturing pain.

In all the States where the cold of winter is sufficient to cause freezing of the human frame by exposure, I have found many mutilated insane, deprived either of the hands or the feet, and sometimes of both.

In Massachusetts we trace repetition of like circumstances. In the fifth annual report of the State hospital, it is stated that "many patients have been received into the institution who have been badly frozen; some in such manner as to have lost their limbs—others a part of them." " Within a week from the date of this report, a man was sent who had been confined three years in a cage, where he had been repeatedly badly frozen, and in the late severe weather so much so, that his extremities were actually in a state of mortification when he arrived. He survived but two days."

In 1841 and '42, I traced personally the condition of more than five hundred insane men and women in Massachusetts wholly destitute of appropriate care. In one county jail alone there were twenty-eight, more than half of whom were furious maniacs. In another jail, in an adjoining county, were twenty-two neglected creatures. It was to this jail— just presented by the grand jury as a nuisance, a place totally unfit for even temporary use—that a female patient was hastily removed from the poorhouse of D——, in order, as was said, that she might be more comfortable—in reality to evade and avoid searching investigations entered upon by strong authority.

Said the keeper of one county prison, in which were many insane, committed " not for crime or misdemeanor," but for safekeeping, or because dangerous to be at large, and in default of sufficient hospital provision for the same, " My prison resembles more the infernal regions than any place on the earth !" Almost without interval might be heard furious exclamations, blasphemous language, and the wildest ravings, howls, and shrieks. In three towns of one county alone (Essex) I found sixty neglected cases. The returns of 1842 exhibited an aggregate of one hundred and thirty-five in that county. On the 24th of December, the thermometer below zero, I visited a poorhouse; found one of the insane inmates, a woman, in a small apartment *entirely* unfurnished: no chair, table, nor bed—neither bundle of straw nor a lock of hay. The cold was intense. On the bare floor crouched the wretched occupant of this dreary place, her limbs contracted, the chin resting immovably upon her knees. She shuddered convulsively, and drew, as well as she was able, more closely about her the *fragments* of garments which constituted her sole protection against unfit exposure and the biting cold. But the attendant, as I passed out from this den, remarked that they used " to throw some blankets over her at night."

Inquiring my way to another almshouse which I had heard was greatly neglected, I was shown the road, and told that there were " plenty of insane and idiot people there." " Well taken care of?" I asked. " Well enough for such sort of creatures." " Any violently insane?" " Yes ; my sister's son is there—a real tiger : I kept him awhile, but it was too much trouble ; so I carried him there." " Is he comfortably provided for?" " Well enough." " Has he decent clothes ?" " Good enough." " And food?" " Good enough—good enough." " One word more: has he the comfort of a fire ?" " Fire, indeed, fire ! What does a crazy man want of fire? he 's hot enough—hot enough without fire !"

At another poorhouse I found three confined in stalls, in an out building. The vicissitudes which had marked the life of one of these desolate beings were singular, and may bring instruction to those whose reason now " is the strength of their life," but who are not exempt from this great calamity.

H—— belonged to a respectable family, possessed good abilities, and was well educated. He removed from I——, in Massachusetts, to Albany, N. Y., where for a considerable period he conducted with ability a popular newspaper. In time, he was elected senator in the State legislature, and was a judge in the court of errors. As a public man he was upright and respected. Insanity was developed while he filled public stations : he was conveyed to the hospital at Worcester ; his property was consumed ; and he was finally discharged as altogether incurable ; and being very violent most of the time, he was placed, " for safety," first in the jail at S——, finally removed to that in I——, and thence transferred to the almshouse where I found him. He had even then periods of partial restoration to reason, so as to comprehend where he was, and how cared for : inhabiting an unfurnished, dreary, narrow stall, in a dreary building of an almshouse !

In a prison which I visited often, was an idiot youth. He would follow me from cell to cell with eager curiosity, and for a long time manifested no appearance of thought. Cheerful expressions, a smile, frequent small gifts, and encouragement to acquire some improved personal habits, at length seemed to light up his mind to a limited power of perception. He would claim his share in the distribution of books, though he could not read, examine them with delight, and preserve them with singular care. If I read from the Scriptures, he was reverently attentive : if I conversed, he listened earnestly, with half conscious aspect. One morning I passed more hurriedly than usual, and did not speak to him. " Me book ! me book !" he exclaimed, eagerly thrusting his hand through the iron bars of the closed door of his cell. " Take this, and be careful," I said. Suddenly stooping, he seized the bread which had been brought for his breakfast, and pushing it eagerly through the bars, he exclaimed, in more connected speech than was known before, " Here 's bread; an't you hungry?" How much might be done to develop even the minds of idiots, if we but knew how to touch the instrument with a skilful hand !

Attempts to cultivate the higher faculties of these creatures, seemingly the merest animals, have been successfully adopted to a moderate extent in France, Germany, and Switzerland, and in the United States the subject has been discussed. Dr. Ray, of the Rhode Island hospital, not long since visited a school for idiots which has been established at the Bicetre, near Paris. He writes, that " as early as the year 1828, Femes* made the first attempt in France to develop the powers of idiots, which attempt has resulted in the present school of Voisin, and which exhibits to the astonished spectator a triumph of perseverance and skill in the cause of humanity, that does infinite credit to the heart and understanding of that gentleman." This testimony is supported by Dr. Conolly, who, visiting the hospitals near Paris, said, " I was conducted to a school exclusively es-

---

* A small volume entitled " Essays upon Several Projects, by Daniel de Foe," London, 1702, contains this remarkable passage : " *The wisdom of Providence has not left us without examples of some of the most stupid natural idiots in the world who have been restored to their reason, infused* after a life of idiotism ; perhaps, among other wise ends, to confute that sordid supposition *that idiots have no souls.*"

tablished for the improvement of these cases, and of the epileptic, and nothing more extraordinary can well be imagined." Dr. Hayward, of Boston, who visited, last year, the schools for idiots above referred to, expresses the opinion that the great benefits to the unfortunate classes whose good they are designed to promote can hardly be appreciated, and that no pains should be spared to establish similar institutions in the United States.

I visited the poorhouse in W——. In a cage, built under a wood-shed, fully exposed to all passers upon the public road, was a miserable insane man, partially enveloped in a torn coverlet. "My husband," remarked the mistress of the house, "clears out the cage and puts in fresh straw once a week ; but sometimes it's hard work to master him. You see him now in his best estate !"

In the adjacent town, at the poorhouse, was a similar case; only, if possible, more revolting, more excited, and more neglected. There were also other persons there in different stages of insanity.

In a county jail not distant was a man who had been confined in a close apartment for many years; a wreath of rags invested his body and his neck; he was filthy in the extreme; there was neither table, seat, nor bed; a heap of noxious straw defiled one corner of the room.

One case more must suffice for this section: I would that no others could be adduced even more revolting than are these so briefly referred to. In G——, distant from the poorhouse a few rods, was a small wooden building, constructed of plank, affording a single room; this was unfurnished, save with a bundle of straw. The occupant of this comfortless abode was a young man, declared to be incurably insane. He was chained, and could move but a little space to and fro; the chain was connected to the floor by a heavy staple at one end—the other was attached to an *iron collar which invested his neck*—the device, it seemed, of a former keeper. In summer the door was thrown open, but during winter it was closed, and the room was in darkness. Some months after I saw this poor patient, and after several individuals also had witnessed his sufferings, the authorities who directed the affairs of the poorhouse reluctantly consented that he should be placed under the care of Dr. Bell. The man who was charged to convey the patient the distance of rather more than forty miles, having bound and chained him, (I have the impression that, by the aid of a blacksmith, he was released at this time from the torturing iron ring,) conveyed him as far as East Cambridge, arriving at dusk. Instead of proceeding with the patient at once to the hospital, which was distant less than a mile, in Somerville, he chained him for the night to a post in the stable. After breakfast he was released and carried to the hospital in a state of much exhaustion. While the careful attendants and humane physician were busied in removing the strong bands which chafed his limbs, and lacerated the flesh in many places, he continually endeavored to express his gratitude—embracing them, weeping, and exclaiming, "Good men! kind men! Ah, good, kind men, keep me here."

After some months of careful nursing, he was so much improved that strong hopes were entertained of his complete restoration. These were crushed by an absolute decision of the overseers of the poor, remanding him to his old prison. Remonstrance was ineffectual. The last account stated an entire relapse, not only to the former state, but to a still more hopeless condition. He had become totally idiotic.

In November I visited the poorhouse in F——; weather severe for the season; no mode of warming the insane. I was conducted to an out-building, so enclosed as to secure the closest solitude to the patient. He had been returned from the hospital as incurable. He was said to be neither violent nor dangerous, but shut up lest he should run away. The door was opened, disclosing a narrow, squalid, dark, unfurnished cell. In one corner was a heap of straw, in which the insane man was nestled. He raised himself slowly and advanced with unsteady steps. His look was calm and gentle.

" Give me those books; Oh, give me those books!" he exclaimed, eagerly reaching his hands for some books I carried. " Do give them to me, do!" he exclaimed, with kindling earnestness. " You could not use them; it is dark with you here." " Oh, give them, do give them !" and he drew a little nearer, lowering his voice to a whisper: "Give them, and *I'll pick a hole in the plank, and let in some of God's light!*" Just then the master arrived; he said that he purposed getting an *iron collar and chain*—then he could fasten him in the air sometimes outside. " I had," he added, " a cousin up in Vermont, crazy as a tiger-cat; I got a collar made for him. After this, I kept the poorhouse at Groton, and I fastened up a crazy man there: he was fast then. I mean to have one for this fellow. I know how to manage your crazy men."

In Connecticut, the estimated number of insane, nearly eight years since, was 542; a number even then below the actual amount, and now very much below the true estimate. Of these, not one-sixth were under hospital treatment five months since : in fact, it is believed that not a ninth part will be found receiving suitable care. The sad case of Rubello is too well known to require repetition. The insane patients in M—— no longer drag their heavy chains abroad, when at labor laying stone walls, nor are they in other respects as much abused and abased as formerly. But no county is free from the reproach of having within its limits insane patients needing humane and judicious care.

Of the most miserable neglects in the case of large numbers carried for successive years to the Hartford Retreat, Drs. Brigham, Woodward, and Butler can, even now, bear sad testimony ; and to the observations of med-ical men may be added the evidence of that good man and true friend of sufferers, Rev. T. H. Gallaudet.

Rhode Island has nearly or quite four hundred insane, idiots, and epileptics. About 90 recently are receiving the benefit of hospital care, under the enlightened administration of Dr. Ray. In no State, however, have I found more terrible examples of neglect and suffering, from abuse or ignorance, than existed there in the year 1843, and some cases in 1845 –'47. In the jails were many pining in narrow, damp, unventilated dungeons. In the poorhouses were many examples of misery and pro-tracted distress. In private families these conditions were less frequent ; but the suffering, through ill-directed aims at securing the patients from escape, was in many instances equally revolting and shocking. Here, as in the five States first referred to, hundreds of special cases might be cited, did time permit. I offer but a single *well-known* example.

In the yard of a poorhouse, in the southern part of the State, I was conducted by the mistress of the establishment to a small building con-structed of plank ; the entrance into a small cell was through a narrow passage, bare and unlighted. The cell was destitute of every description of furniture, unless a block of wood could be called such ; and on this

was seated a woman—clothed, silent, and sad. A small aperture, opening upon a dreary view, and this but a few inches square, alone admitted light and air. The inmate was quiet, and evidently not dangerous
in her propensities. In reply to my remonstrances in her behalf, the
mistress said that she was directed to keep her always close; that
otherwise she would run away, or pull up the flowers! How is she
warmed in winter? I inquired. "Oh, we just heat a stone and give her,"
was the laconic reply. Your other patient—where is he? "You shall
see; but stay outside till I get a lantern." Accustomed to exploring cells
and dungeons in the basements and cellars of poorhouses and prisons, I
concluded that the insane man spoken of was confined in some such
dark, damp retreat. Weary and oppressed, I leaned against an iron door
which closed the sole entrance to a singular stone structure, much resem-
bling a tomb, yet its use in the court-yard of the poorhouse was not apparent. Soon, low smothered groans and moans reached me, as if from
the buried alive. At this moment the mistress advanced, with keys and a
lantern. "He's here," said she, unlocking the strong, solid iron door. A
step down, and short turn through a narrow passage to the right, brought
us, after a few steps, to a second iron door parallel to the first, and equally
solid. In like manner, this was unlocked and opened; but so terribly
noxious was the poisonous air that immediately pervaded the passage,
that a considerable time elapsed before I was able to return and remain
long enough to investigate this horrible den. Language is too weak to
convey an idea of the scene presented. The candle was removed from
the scene, and the flickering rays partly illuminated a spectacle never to
be forgotten. The place when closed had no source of light or of ventilation. It was about seven feet by seven, and six and a half high. All,
even the roof, was of stone. An iron frame, interlaced with rope, was
the sole furniture. The place was filthy, damp, and noisome; and the
inmate, the crazy man, the helpless and dependant creature, cast by the
will of Providence on the cares and sympathies of his fellow-man—there
he stood, near the door, motionless and silent; his tangled hair fell about
his shoulders; his bare feet pressed the filthy, wet stone floor; he was
emaciated to a shadow, etiolated, and more resembled a disinterred corpse
than any living creature. Never have I looked upon an object so pitiable,
so wo-struck, so imaging despair. I took his hands and endeavored to
warm them by gentle friction. I spoke to him of release, of liberty, of care
and kindness. Notwithstanding the assertions of the mistress that he would
kill me, I persevered. A tear stole over the hollow cheek, but no words
answered to my importunities; no other movement indicated consciousness of perception or of sensibility. In moving a little forward I struck
against something which returned a sharp metallic sound: it was a
length of ox-chain, connected to an iron ring which encircled a leg
of the insane man. At one extremity it was joined to what is termed
a solid chain—namely, bars of iron 18 inches or 2 feet long, linked
together, and at one end connected by a staple to the rock overhead.
"My husband," said the mistress, "in winter rakes out sometimes, of a
morning, half a bushel of frost, and yet *he never freezes;*" referring to the
oppressed and life-stricken maniac before us. "Sometimes he screams
dreadfully," she added, "and that is the reason we had the double wall,
and two doors in place of one: his cries disturbed us in the house!"
"How long has he been here?" "Oh, above three years; but then he

was kept a long while in a cage first : but once he broke his chains and the bars, and escaped; so we had this built, where he can't get off." Get off! No, indeed; as well might the buried dead break through the sealed gates of the tomb, or upheave the mass of binding earth from the trodden soil of the deep grave. I forbear comment. Many persons, after my investigations here, visited this monument of the utter insensibility and ignorance of the community at whose expense it was raised. Brutal, wilfully cruel, I will not call them, black as is the case, and fatal as were the results of *their care!* But God forbid that such another example of suffering should ever exist to be recorded.

New York, according to the census of 1840, had 2,340 idiots and insane. I am convinced that this estimate was below the certain number by many hundreds. In 1841, the Secretary of State reported 803 supported at public charge. In 1842, the trustees of poorhouses estimated the number of insane poor then confined in the *jails* and *poorhouses* at 1,430. In 1843 I traversed every county in the State, visiting every poorhouse and prison, and the insane in many private families. The hospital for the insane at Utica was opened in January, 1843, and during the year received 276 patients, all with the exception of six being residents of the State of New York. On Blackwell's island were above 300 ; at Bloomingdale more than 100 : 26 were at Bellevue. Besides these, I found, chiefly in the poorhouses, more than 1,500 insane and idiots, 500 of whom were west of Cayuga bridge. In the poorhouse at Flatbush were 26 insane, not counting idiots; in that at Whiteplains were 30 insane; at Albany between 30 and 40; at Ghent 18; in Greene county 46. In Washington county poorhouse, besides "simple, silly, and idiotic," 20 insane. Nearly every poorhouse in the State had, and still has, its " crazy house," " crazy cells," " crazy dungeons," or " crazy hall;" and in these, with rare exceptions, the inevitable troubles and miseries of the insane are sorely aggravated.

At A——, in the cell first opened, was a madman. The fierce command of his keeper brought him to the door, a hideous object; matted locks, an unshorn beard, a wild, wan countenance, disfigured by vilest uncleanness; in a state of nudity, save the irritating incrustations derived from that dungeon, reeking with loathsome filth. There, *without light,* without pure air, without warmth, without cleansing, absolutely destitute of everything securing comfort or decency, was a human being—forlorn, abject, and disgusting, it is true, but not the less a human being—nay more, an immortal being, though the mind was fallen in ruins, and the soul was clothed in darkness. And who was he—this neglected, brutalized wretch? A burglar, a murderer, a miscreant, who for base foul crimes had been condemned, by the justice of outraged laws and the righteous indignation of his fellow-men, to expiate offences by exclusion from his race, by privations and sufferings extreme, yet not exceeding the measure and enormity of his misdeeds? No; this was no doomed criminal, festering in filth, wearing wearily out the warp of life in dreariest solitude and darkness. No, this was no criminal— " *only a crazy man.*" How, in the touching language of Scripture, could he have said: " My brethren are far from me, and mine acquaintance are verily estranged from me: my kinsfolk have failed, and my familiar friends have forgotten me: my bone cleaveth unto my skin and my flesh. Have pity upon me, have pity upon me, for the hand of God hath touched me!"

I turned from this sickening scene only to witness another yet more pitiable. In the far corner of a damp, dark dungeon on the right was a human creature—" a woman dreadful bad," said the attendant, who summoned her in harsh tones to " come out:" but she only moved feebly amidst the decaying mass of straw, uttering low moans and cries, expressive both of physical pain and mental anguish. There she lay, seemingly powerless to rise. She, too, was unclothed; and in this dungeon, alone, in want, and pain, and misery; no pure air, no pleasant light, no friendly hand to chafe the aching limbs, no kind voice to raise and cheer, she dragged out a troubled existence. I know nothing of her history; whether forsaken by able kindred, or reluctantly given over to *public charity* by indigent parents, or taken in, a wandering, demented creature. I only know that I found and left her reduced to a condition upon which not one who reads this page could look but with unmitigated horror. Do you turn with inexpressible disgust from these details? It is worse to witness the reality. Is your refinement shocked by these statements? There is but one remedy: the multiplication of well organized hospitals; and to this end, creating increased means for their support. In the same poorhouse, in the " crazy cellar," were men *chained to their beds,* or prostrate on the ground, fettered, and painfully confined in every movement. There were women, too, in wretched, unventilated, crowded rooms, exhibiting every horrible scene their various degrees of insanity could create.

In B——, the cells in the crazy cellar admitted neither light nor pure air.

In T——, the cells for the insane men were in a shocking condition.

In A——, were above twenty insane men and women in the poorhouse, mostly confined *with chains and balls attached to fetters.* " By adopting this plan," said the master of the poorhouse, " I give them light and air, preventing their escape; otherwise I should have too keep them always in the cells." A considerable number of women,. mostly incurables, were " behind the pickets," in an out-building: there was a passage sufficiently lighted and warmed, and of width for exercise. There was no classification; the noisy and the quiet mutually vexed each other. One woman was restrained by a barbarous apparatus to prevent rending her clothes: it consisted of *an iron collar investing the throat,* through which, at the point of closing in front, passed a small bolt or bar,. from which depended *an iron triangle,* the sides of which might measure sixteen or eighteen inches. To the corners of the horizontal side were attached *iron wristlets;* thus holding the hands confined, and as far apart as the length of the base line of the triangle. When the hands and arms were suddenly elevated, pressure upon the apex of the triangle, near the point of connexion at the throat, produced a sense of suffocation; and why not certain strangulation, it was not easy to show.

Not distant from the poorhouse I found a woman in a private dwelling, supported by two invalid sisters; she was in the highest state of phrensy, and nearly exhausted the patience of love in those who toiled laboriously for her and their own scanty maintenance. She had once been transferred to the poorhouse; but patience was never there exercised in behalf of the unruly; and bearing the marks of harsh blows, she was taken again by her sisters, to share " the little they could earn so long as they or she should live."

In E——, the insane, as usual, were unfitly disposed of. To adopt

2

the language of a neighboring farmer, "those damp dreary cells were not fit for a dog to house in, much less for crazy folks."

At R——, and M——, and L——, and B——, were repetitions of the like dismal cells—heavy chains and balls, and hopeless sufferings. After my visit at L——, I found one of the former inmates at the hospital in charge of Dr. Brigham. *He bore upon his ankles the deep scars of fetters and chains, and upon his feet evidence of exposure to frost and cold.*

In B——, several idiots occupied together a portion of a most comfortless establishment. *One gibbering, senseless creature* was the mother of an infant child.

At A——, the most furious were in narrow cells, which were neither cleaned, warmed, nor ventilated. In O—— was an insane man, so shockingly neglected and abused that his limbs were crippled, so that he could neither stand nor walk; he was extended on a miserable dirty pallet, untended and little cared for.

At E——, the insane were confined in cells crammed with coarse, dirty straw, in the basement, dark and damp. "They are," said the keeper, "taken out and *washed*, (buckets of water thrown over them,) *and have clean straw, once every week.*"

In H——, were many furiously crazy. Several of the women were said to be the mothers of infants, which were in an adjoining room pining with neglect, and unacknowledged by their frantic mothers.

I pass over hundreds of desperate cases, and quote a few examples from my notes in New Jersey; altogether omitting Canada East and West, as being without the limits of the United States; though corresponding examples with those in New York were found in almost every direction. In 1841, there were found in New Jersey, upon a rather cursory survey, *two hundred and fifty-two insane men, one hundred and sixty-three insane women, and one hundred and ninety-six idiots,* of both sexes. I traversed the State in 1844; the numbers in every county were increased, and their miseries were also increased. Sixty patients had been placed in the hospitals in New York and Pennsylvania, but hundreds still occupied the wretched cells and dungeons of almshouses, and of prisons. In the winter of 1845 several froze to death, and several perished through severe exposure and alarm at a fire which consumed a populous poorhouse. At S——, of eight insane patients, several were heavily chained, and two were furiously mad.

In one poorhouse was a man who had been chained by the leg for more than twenty years, and the only warmth introduced into his cell was derived from a small stove-pipe carried through one corner.

On a level with the cellar, in a basement room, tolerably decent but bare of comforts, lay upon a narrow bed a feeble, aged man, whose few gray locks fell tangled over the pillow. As I entered he addressed one present, saying, "I am all broken up—broken up!" "Do you feel much weaker, *Judge?*" "The mind, the mind is going—almost gone," responded he, in tones of touching sadness. This feeble, depressed old man, in a lone room in the poorhouse—who was he? I answer as I was answered. In his young and vigorous years he filled various offices of honor and trust in his county. His ability as a lawyer raised him from the bar to the bench. As a jurist he was distinguished for uprightness, clearness, and impartiality. He was also judge of the orphans' court, and was for many years a member of the legislature. He was somewhat eccentric, but his habits were always correct. I could learn nothing remembered to his discredit, but much which commends men to honor and respect. He had passed the meridian of a useful and active life. The property, honestly acquired, on which he had relied for comfortable support in his declining years, was lost by some of those fluctuations in monetary affairs which so often procure unanticipated reverses. He became insane : soon, insanity took the form of furious mania : *he was chained*, "for safety;" and finally, for greater security, committed to the county jail—a most wretched place—dreary, damp, and unfurnished. Time passed : a more quiet state supervened. He was placed at board in a private family, till the remnant of his once sufficient property was consumed, and then he was removed to the poorhouse. Without vices and without crimes, he was at once the victim of misfortunes and the prey of disease. A few months subsequent to my visit the almshouse was consumed by fire. The inmates, barely rescued, were hastily removed, and such cares rendered as the emergency demanded. Fires were kindled in the court-house, and a portion of the poor removed thither. Of this number was Judge S. His pallet was laid within the bar, below the bench where he had once presided. The place perhaps revived painful memories : he was conscious of his condition; spoke of his trials; languished a few days; and, in the good providence of God, was then released from the pains and afflictions of this mortal life, and, it is believed, passed to that state of existence where all tears are wiped from all eyes, and where troubles are unknown.

In P——, the *cells in the cellar for the insane* were in a most wretched condition. In M——, the insane, and many imbeciles, were miserably housed, fed, and clothed. In the vicinity of the main building was one of brick, containing the poor cells, *from eight to nine feet square*. A straw bed and blanket on the floor constituted the furniture, if I except the *ring-bolts and iron chains for securing the patients*. In P——, I found the insane, as usual, ill provided for. One madman was chained, clothed only with a straight jacket, laced so as to impede the motion of the arms and hands: cold, exposed, and offensive to the last degree, his aspect, wild and furious, was as shocking as his language was coarse and blasphemous. Such care was bestowed as the keepers of the poorhouse best could render; but an hospital alone could afford fit treatment for one so dangerous and so unmanageable.

At M—— were five idiots and insane, ill kept, and very turbulent most of the time. Said one poor maniac, whose fetters and manacles I had ordered to be removed, and whose aching, bruised limbs I was bathing, "Ah, now I am a human creature again : God is good—he sends you to free me : I will pray for you forever, and bright days shall shine for you." One woman, whose limbs bore marks of the cankering iron, worn for many years, said, "I could curse those who chain me, but the *soft voice* says, 'Pray for your enemies;' but, alas! my soul is dark, and the thoughts are black."

In the western part of the State I found a young man chained near his father's house, his bleeding limbs cut by the iron rings which confined the ankles; he moaned, and howled, and cursed, and raved, so that horror filled the neighborhood.

A middle-aged woman, who was often greatly excited, was for months at a time *confined in a smoke-house*. Her condition was filthy to the last degree; she had neither change of raiment, nor water for bathing, for months. " She'll be found frozen to death some of these nights, I reckon," said the " care-taker." Ten miles distant I found another case similar, but if possible more miserable.

In Pennsylvania, in 1839, careful inquiry, followed by authentic reports, placed the number of insane and idiots at over *twenty three hundred:* of these it was computed that more than *twelve hundred* were in the county poorhouses and prisons. I visited every county and considerable town in the State in the summer and autumn of 1844, and am satisfied that the number was much above the estimate of 1839.

In L—— I found above fifty insane, not counting idiots. The cells in the poorhouse, forty-four in number, measured *four feet by seven, and twelve feet high;* " *chains and hobbles*" were in constant use.

In Y—— were above thirty insane: those in the basement of the poorhouse occupied cells of sufficient dimensions, being *fourteen by ten,* and ten feet high; *hobbles* and *chains* in use. The physician estimated the number of insane in the county at more than one hundred, and added that cases of exceeding neglect and suffering often came to his knowledge. Sufficient provision in hospitals might save thousands of honest citizens from becoming a life-long burden to themselves and others, through permanent insanity. In this county above one hundred insane were found; there probably were other cases. In the poorhouse at G—— the insane were exposed and suffering; the basement cells measured *eight by eight feet, and eight feet high.* Chains, hobbles, and the miscalled " *tranquilizing chain*," were in use. There were more than forty insane in the county.

In C——, above twenty insane and idiots in the poorhouse; one was chained near the fireplace of a small room; a box filled with straw was near, in which she slept. Above 60 insane and idiots in this county. In B—— I found nearly 40; some chained, others confined in narrow cells. In S——, several insane in the jail; one, *heavily ironed,* had been in close confinement there six years—another for eleven months. In this county the insane and idiots were estimated to be 76 in 1840. I heard of more than 100. One woman has for months wandered in the woods and fields in a state of raving madness.

At G——, several cases in the jail; one chained: above forty in the county.

In N——, in the jail, two madmen in chains; no furniture or decent care. One was rolling in the dust, in the highest excitement: he had been in close confinement for fifteen years. On one occasion he became exasperated at the introduction of a drunken prisoner into his cell, who perhaps provoked him. No one knows; but the keeper, on entering, found the insane man furious, covered with the blood of the other, who was murdered and mutilated in the most shocking manner. Another insane man had been in confinement seven years, and both are to this day in the same prison. In the poorhouse were above twenty insane and idiots; four chained to the floor. In the adjacent county were above fifty insane and epileptics; several cases of misery through brutal usage, by " kicks and beating," in private families.

In W—— were seven very crazy, and above twenty simple, insane, and idiotic. One, who was noisy, was in a small building in a field. The condition of all was degraded and exposed. In P——, the insane in the jail were subject to great miseries. Many in the county were harshly confined; some wandering at liberty, often dangerous to the safety of all they met. The twelve counties next visited afforded corresponding examples. The nine next traversed had fewer insane, and fewer, in proportion to whole numbers, in chains. In H——, one case claimed special sympathy. Adjacent to a farm house was a small shanty, slightly constructed of thin boards, in which lies an old feeble man, with blanched hair, not clad either for protection or decency; " fed," as said a poor neighbor very truly, " fed like the hogs, and treated worse." He is exposed to the scorching heats of summer, and pinching cold of the inclement winter; no kind voice cheers him, no sympathizing friend seeks to mitigate his sufferings. He is an outcast, a crazy man, almost at the door of his once cheerful, comfortable home. I pass by without detail nearly *one hundred* examples of insane men and women *in filthy cells, chained and hobbled*, together with many idiots and epileptics wandering abroad. Some were confined in low, damp, dark cellars; some wasted their wretched existence in dreary dungeons, deserted and neglected. It would be fruitless to attempt describing the sufferings of these unhappy beings for a day even. What must be the accumulation of the pains and woes of years, consigned to prisons and poorhouses, to cells and dungeons, enduring every variety of privation—helpless, deserted of kindred, tortured by fearful delusions, and suffering indescribable pains and abuses. These are no tales of fiction. I believe that there is no imaginable form of severity, of cruelty, of neglect, of every sort of ill-management for mind and body, to which I have not seen the insane subject in all our country, excepting the three sections already defined. As a general rule, *ignorance* procures the largest measure of these shocking results; but while of late years much is accomplished, and more is proposed, by far the largest part of those who suffer remain unrelieved, and must do so, except the general government unites to assist the several States in this work.

In Maryland, large numbers are at this hour in the lowest state of misery to which the insane can be reduced. At four different periods I have looked into the condition of many cases, counting hundreds there. Chains, and want, and sorrows, abound for the insane poor in both the western and eastern districts, but especially in the western.

In Delaware, the same history is only to be repeated, with this variation : as the numbers are fewer, so is the aggregate of misery less.

In the District of Columbia, the old and the new jails, and the almshouses, had, till very recently, their black, horrible histories. I witnessed abuses in some of these in 1838, in 1845, and since, from which every sense recoils. At present, most of these evils are mitigated in this immediate vicinity, but by no means relieved to the extent that justice and humanity demand.

In Virginia, very many cases of extreme suffering now exist. The most observing and humane of the medical profession have repeatedly expressed the desire for additional hospital provision for the insane. Like cases of great distress to those in Maryland and Pennsylvania were found in the years 1844 and '45. In every county through which I passed were the insane to be found—sometimes chained, sometimes wandering free. In the large, populous poorhouse near R—— were spectacles the most offensively loathsome. Utter neglect and squalid wretchedness surrounded the insane. The estimate of *two thousand* insane idiots and epileptic patients in this State is thought to be below the actual number. The returns in 1840 were manifestly incorrect.

In the report upon the Western State Hospital of Virginia, at Staunton, for the year 1847, Dr. Stribling feelingly remarks upon the very insufficient means at command for the relief of the insane poor throughout the State. "We predicted," he says, "that during the present year, those seeking the benefits of this institution would far exceed our ability to receive. This anticipation, we regret to say, has been painfully realized, and we are now called upon to report the fact that within the last nine months *one hundred and twenty three* applications have been received, whilst only *thirty nine* could be admitted. What has become of the remaining eighty-four, it is impossible for us to report." I regret to say there is but one conclusion deducible from this statement: the rejected patients are suffering privations and miseries in different degrees in the narrow rooms or cells of poorhouses, or in the equally wretched sheds, stalls, or pens, attached to private dwellings, while some have been temporarily detained, for security, in the jails. The laws of Virginia forbid a protracted detention of the insane in the county prisons, at this period. Formerly, I have traced the most cruel sufferings in the confined apartments, uncleansed and unventilated, and in the still more neglected dungeons, into which the insane have been cast. The hospital physicians report patients often sent to their care painfully encumbered with cords and chains.

North Carolina has more than twelve hundred insane and idiots. I do not know by personal observation what is their condition; but within a few months, sad details have been communicated from respectable and reliable sources.

South Carolina records the same deplorable abuses and necessities as New York. I have found there the insane in pens, and bound with cords and chains, and suffering no less than the same class in States already referred to at the north, except through exposure to the cold in winter, the climate in the southern States sparing that aggravated misery. One patient was removed to the hospital after being confined in a jail more than twenty years. Another had for years been chained to a log : another had been confined in a hut ten feet square, and was destitute of clothing and of every comfort of life. A young girl was confined in a dismal cabin, filthy, and totally neglected. Her hair was matted into a solid foul mass; her person emaciated, and uncleansed ; nothing human could be imagined more entirely miserable, and more cruelly abandoned to want.

Georgia has, so far as I have been able to ascertain, fewer insane, in proportion to population, than either North or South Carolina, but there is not less injudicious or cruel management of the violent cases throughout the State; chains and ropes are employed to increase security from escapes, in addition to closed doors, and the bolts and bars which shut the dreary cells and dungeons of jails and other receptacles. I have seen the deep scars of former wounds produced by chains and blows ; and those who have received patients transported to the State hospitals, are as much at a loss for any decent language for describing the condition of these unfortunate beings as myself. Their condition is indeed indescribable. Patients have not seldom been transported to the hospital in open carts, chained and bound with heavy cords.

Alabama reveals in her jails, and in many poor dwellings, corresponding scenes. In 1846 and 1848, I traced there poor creatures in situations truly revolting and horrible. To record cases is but to repeat sad histories differing only in time and place, not in degrees of misery. So also in Louisiana and Mississippi, in the same years. There are not, at the lowest estimate, less than fourteen hundred in these three last named States.

In Texas it is said insanity is increasing. I have seen several patients brought hence for hospital treatment, bound with cords and sorely bruised.

In Arkansas the insane and idiots are scattered in remote districts. I found it often exceedingly difficult to ascertain precisely their circumstances : these were no better—and worse they could not be—than were the indigent, and not seldom the affluent, in other States.

In Tennessee the insane and idiotic population, as in Kentucky, is numerous and increasing. *The same methods of confinement to cabins, pens, cells, dungeons, and the same abandonment to filth, to cold, and exposure, as in other States.*

In Kentucky I found one epileptic girl subject to the most brutal treatment, and many insane in perpetual confinement. Of the *idiots* alone, supported by the State at a cost of $17,500 62, in indigent private families, and of which class there were in 1845 *four hundred and fifty*, many were exposed to severest treatment and heavy blows from day to day, and from year to year. In a dreary block-house was confined for many years a man whose insanity took the form of mania. Often the most furious paroxysms prevented rest for several days and nights in succession. No alleviation reached this unhappy being; without clothes, without fire, without care or kindness, his existence was protracted amidst every horror incident to such circumstances. *Chains in common use.*

In Ohio, the insane population, including idiots, has been greatly underrated, as I am fully satisfied by repeated but interrupted inquiries in different sections of the State. The sufferings of a great number here are very distressing, corresponding with those referred to in New York and in Kentucky. *Cells and dungeons, unventilated and uncleansed apartments, severe restraints, and multiplied neglects, abound.*

Michigan, it was stated, had sixty three insane in 1840. I think it a moderate estimate, judging from my investigations, reaching no further north than Jackson and Detroit, that the number in 1847 exceeded two hundred and fifty. I saw some truly afflicted and lamentable cases.

Indiana, traversed through its whole length and breadth in 1846, exhibits the usual forms of misery wherever the insane are found; and of this class there cannot be, including idiots and epileptics, less than nine hundred. *I found one poor woman in a smoke-house, in which she had been confined more than twenty years.* In several poorhouses the insane, both men and women, were chained to the floors, sometimes all in the same apartment. Several were confined in mere pens, without clothing or shelter ; some furious—others for a time comparatively tranquil. The hospital now about to be opened, when finished, will not receive to its care one patient in ten of existing cases.

Illinois, visited also in its whole extent in 1846, has more than four hundred insane, at the most moderate estimate. Passing into a confined room in the poorhouse at G——, I saw a cage constructed upon one side of the room, measuring six feet by three. "There," exclaimed the keeper, with emotion, "there is the best place I have to keep a madman; a place not fit for a dog—a place where they grow worse and worse, and, in defiance of such care as I can give, become a nuisance to themselves and every one in the neighborhood. We want hospitals, Miss; we want hospitals, and more means for the crazy everywhere." I found crazy men and women in all sorts of miserable conditions; sometimes, as in Georgia, &c., &c., strapped upon beds with coarse hard strips of leather; sometimes chained to logs, or to the floor of wretched hovels; often exposed to every vicissitude of the climate: but I limit myself to one more example. It was an intensely hot day when I visited F. He was confined in a roofed *pen,* which enclosed an area of about eight feet by eight. The interstices between the unhewn logs admitted the scorching rays of the sun then, as they would open way for the fierce winds and drenching rains and frosts of the later seasons. The place was wholly bare of furniture—*no bench, no bed, no clothing.* His food, which was of the coarsest kind, was pushed through spaces between the logs; "fed like the hogs, and no better," said a stander-by. His feet had been frozen by exposure to cold in the winter past. Upon the shapeless stumps, aided by his arms, he could raise himself against the logs of the pen. In warm weather this wretched place was cleansed once a week or fortnight; not so in the colder seasons. "We have men called," said his sister, "and they go in and tie him with ropes, and throw him out on the ground, and throw water on him, and my husband cleans out the place." But the expedient to prevent his freezing in winter was the most strangely horrible. In the centre of the pen was excavated a pit, six feet square and deep; the top was closed over securely; and into this ghastly place, entered through a trap-door, was cast the maniac, there to exist till the returning warm weather induced his care-taker to withdraw him: there, without heat, without light, without pure air, was left the pining, miserable maniac, whose piteous groans and frantic cries might move to pity the hardest heart.

In Missouri, visited in 1846 and 1847, multiplied cases were found in pens, in stalls, in cages, in dungeons, and in cells; men and women alike exhibited the most deplorable aspects. Some are now dead, others still live only to experience renewed troubles of mind, and tortures of the flesh.

Let these examples suffice; others daily occur. Humanity requires that every insane person should receive the care appropriate to his condition, in which the integrity of the judgment is destroyed, and the reasoning faculties confused or prostrated.

Hardly second to this consideration is the civil and social obligation to consult and secure the public welfare: first in affording protection against the frequently manifested dangerous propensities of the insane; and second, by assuring seasonable and skilful remedial cares, procuring their restoration to usefulness as citizens of the republic, and as members of communities.

Under ordinary circumstances, and where there is no organic lesion of the brain, no disease is more manageable or more easily cured than insanity; but to this end, special appliances are necessary, which cannot be had in private families, nor in every town and city; hence the necessity for hospitals, and the multiplication, *not enlargement,* of such institutions. The citizens of many States have readily submitted to increased taxation, and individuals have contributed liberal gifts, in order to meet these imperative wants. Hospitals have been constructed, and well organized. The important charge of these has been in most instances confided to highly responsible and skilful physicians—men whose rank in morals and in intellect, while commanding the public confidence, has wrought immeasurable benefits for hundreds and thousands of those in whom, for a time, the light of reason had been hidden.

But while the annual reports emanating from these beneficent institutions record eminent successes in the cure of *recently* developed cases, the provision for the treatment of this malady in the United States is found wholly insufficient for existing necessities, as has been already demonstrated in preceding pages.

To confide the insane to persons whose education and habits do not qualify them for this charge, is to condemn them to a mental death. The keepers of prisons, the masters of poorhouses, and most persons in private families, are wholly unacquainted with bodily and mental diseases, and are therefore incapable of the judicious application of such remedial measures, moral, mental, and medical, as are requisite for the restoration of physical and mental health. Recovery, even of recent cases, not submitted to hospital charge, is known to be very rare ; a fact readily demonstrable by examples, and by figures, if necessary. It may be more satisfactory to show the benefits of hospital treatment, rather than dilate upon the certain evils of prison and almshouse neglects or abuses, and domestic mismanagement.

Under well-directed hospital care, *recovery is the rule—incurable* permanent insanity the exception.

Dr. Luther V. Bell, in one) of his reports, shows that *" all cases certainly recent, whose origin does not date back, directly or obscurely, more than one year, recover under a fair trial."* And, again, in his report of 1843-'44, he remarks, that *" in regard to the curability of insanity,* in its different manifestations, there can be no general rule better established *than that this is in direct ratio* of the duration of the symptoms."

Dr. Ray repeats and confirms these opinions.

Dr. Chandler stated, in 1843, that his experience proved that the earlier the patient was placed under hospital treatment, *the more sure and speedy* was the *recovery.*

Dr. Brigham repeatedly states, in his reports, that more than *eight out of ten recent cases recover,* while not more than one in six of the old cases are cured.

Dr. Rockwell's reports corroborate these views.

Dr. Butler states that *delay* of appropriate treatment rapidly diminishes the chances of recovery.

Dr. Kirkbride declares that the general proposition that " truly recent cases of insanity are speedily curable, and chronic only occasionally, ought to be everywhere understood."

Dr. Awl, writing on this subject, says : " *Public safety, equity, and economy,* alike require that this should be so."

Dr. Earle shows that " *there are few acute diseases from which so large a per centage of the persons attacked are restored.*"

Drs. Woodward, Stribling, Parker, Allen, Buttolph, Stedman, and others, also support, in this country, the same opinions ; while the long list of able and well-known distinguished writers on insanity, and the physicians of the hospitals, on the other side of the Atlantic, place the question beyond doubt.

The following tables, prepared from the records of one hospital, afford a single illustration of the views above advanced, and show the duration of insanity before the admission of the 280 patients received in five consecutive years.

Table showing the duration of insanity before admission to the hospital.

	Total.	1833.	1834.	1835.	1836.	1837.
Less than one year -	280	48	56	49	54	73
From 1 to 5 - -	181	20	29	37	37	58
5 to 10 - -	86	27	14	17	13	15
10 to 20 - -	71	31	8	6	11	15
20 to 30 - -	23	12	4	1	2	4
30 to 40 - -	8	3	1	1	2	1
Unknown - -	36	12	6	7	6	5

Table showing the comparative curability of a given number of cases healed at different periods of insanity, as introduced to hospital care.

	Total cases.	Total of each sex.	Cured or curable.	Not cured, or incurable.
Less than one year's duration -	232			
Men - - -	–	123	110	13
Women - - -	–	109	100	9
From one to two years' duration -	94			
Men - - -	–	49	31	18
Women - - -	–	45	32	13
From two to five years - -	109			
Men - - -	–	65	18	47
Women - - -	–	44	18	26
From five to ten years - -	76			
Men - - -	–	40	5	35
Women - - -	–	36	4	32
From ten to fifteen years -	56			
Men - - -	–	35	2	33
Women - - -	–	21	1	20

An author of profound research and high intellectual endowments, in a work which was first published some years since in several foreign languages, and has since been reproduced in this country, states that " *the general certainty of curing insanity in its early stage* is a fact which ought to be universally known, and then it would be properly appreciated and acted upon by the public."

Dr. Ellis, director of the West Riding Lunatic Hospital, England, stated in 1827, that of 312 patients admitted within three months after their first attack, 216 recovered; while, in contrast with this, he adds that of 318 patients admitted, who had been insane for upwards of one year to thirty, only 26 recovered. In La Salpètriere, near Paris, the proportion of cures of recent cases was, in 1806–'7, according to Dr. Veitch's official statement, as nearly *two* to *three* cured, while only five out of 152 old cases recovered. Dr. Burrows stated, in 1820, that of recent cases under his care, 91 in 100 recovered; and in 1828, that the annual reports of other hospitals, added to his own larger experience, confirmed these observations. Dr. Willis made to Parliament corresponding statements. At the Senavra hospital, near Milan, the same results appeared upon the annual records.

But *cure* alone, manifestly, is not the sole object of hospital care: secondary indeed, but of vast importance, is the secure and comfortable provision for that now large class throughout the country, the incurable insane. Their condition, we know, is susceptible of amelioration, and of elevation to a state of comparative comfort and usefulness.

Insanity prevails, in proportion to numbers, most among the educated, and, according to mere conventional distinctions, in the highest classes of society. But those who possess riches and a liberal competency are few, compared with the toiling millions; therefore the insane who are in necessitous circumstances greatly outnumber those whose individual wealth protects them usually from the grossest exposures and most cruel sufferings.

I have seen very many patients who had been confined for years in stalls, cages, and pens, and who were reduced to the most abject moral, physical, and mental prostration, removed to hospitals, divested of chains, fetters, and filthy garments; bathed, clothed, nursed, and nourished with careful kindness; whose improvement was, according to constitution and the nature of the disease, more or less rapid, and who in a few months became the most able laborers, under constant direction, upon the hospital farms, in the gardens, shops, and barns; and while these labors engaged the men, the women were no less busily occupied in the washing and ironing rooms, in the seamstress and dress-making apartments, and about various household daily recurring labors. These might never recover the right exercise of reason—might never be able to bear the excitements of society and the vicissitudes of life abroad; but, subject to judicious direction, be as cheerful and comfortable as the malady permits; occasional recurrence of paroxsyms sometimes disqualifying from the exercise of ordinary employments. A few examples may not be without interest. A young man who for ten years had been confined in an out-building of a poorhouse, in Rhode Island, who was chained and neglected, by the interposition of a visitor was released and removed to the McLean Asylum, in Massachusetts. In a few weeks he recovered the use of his limbs, so as to adopt a little voluntary exercise. Gradually he improved so as to follow the gardener; at first merely as an observer, but after a time as an efficient laborer, always cheerful and ready for employment; but he was never restored to mental health. In the same institution a young lady, insane for several years, and classing with the incurables, supports her own expenses by the use of her needle, making the most tasteful and beautiful articles, which find a ready sale. Many besides are employed variously; several draw very beautifully, observing the proportions and rules of art with great exactness.

In 1836, a raving maniac was conveyed to the State Hospital; he refused to be clothed, committed every sort of extravagance, and months passed before he was sufficiently composed to address himself to any useful employment. Gradually, however, he resorted to the carpenter's shop, amused himself with the tools, but finally applied to useful work, and, with few intervals, has since been able to accomplish a large amount of productive labor.

Another patient, who was confined nearly four years in a county prison, had several violent paroxysms: his mind is never entirely free from delusions: he speaks of his excitements--knows he is insane, and unsafe to be at large: is now ordinarily quiet, pleasant, and good tempered. He is an ingenious mechanic; makes correct observations on common things, but exhibits strange fancies and delusions upon all spiritual concerns. He labors diligently and profitably most of the time.

I do not recollect a more satisfactory illustration of the benefits of hospital care upon large numbers of incurable patients, brought under improving influences at one and the same time, than is afforded in the first opening of the hospital for the insane poor at South Boston. Prior to 1839, the insane poor of Suffolk county were confined in a receptacle in rear of the almshouse; or rather all those of this class who were furiously mad, and considered dangerous to be abroad upon the farm grounds. This receptacle revealed scenes of horror and utter abomination such as language is powerless to represent. These wretched creatures, both men and women, exhibited cases of long standing, regarded past recovery, their malady being confirmed by the grossest mismanagement.

The citizens were at length roused to a sense of the enormity and extent of these abuses, matched only, it is believed, (except in individual cases,) by the vile condition of the English private madhouses, as thrown open to the inspection of Parliamentary commissioners, within the last thirty years. The monstrous injustice and cruelty of herding these maniacs in a hall filled with cages, behind the bars of which, all loathsome and offensive, they howled, and gibbered, and shrieked, and moaned, day and night, like infuriated wild beasts, moved the kindling sensibilities of those heretofore ignorant or indifferent. The most sanguine friends of the hospital plan expected no more for these wretched beings than to procure for them greater decency and comfort; recovery of the mental faculties, for such as these, was not anticipated.

The new buildings were completed, opened, and a system of discipline adopted by Dr. Butler, the results of which I witnessed with profound interest and surprise. The insane were removed, disencumbered of their chains, freed from the remnants of foul garments, bathed, clothed, fed decently, and placed by kind nurses in comfortable apartments. Remedial means, medical and moral, were judiciously applied. Behold the result of a few months' care, in their recovered physical health, order, general quiet, and well-directed employments. Now, and since, visit the hospital when you may, at neither set time nor season, you will find this class of *incurable* patients exercising in companies or singly, reading the papers of the day, or books loaned from the library ; some busy in the vegetable, some in the flower gardens, while some are found occupied in the washing and ironing rooms, in the kitchen and in the sewing rooms. Less than one-sixth of those who were removed from the almshouse recovered their reason ; but, with the exception of three or four individuals, they regained the decent habits of respectable life, and a capacity to be useful, to labor, and to enjoy occupation.

No hospital in the United States but affords abundant evidence of the capacity of the insane to work under direction of suitable attendants, and of recovery from utter helplessness to a considerable degree of activity and capacity for various employments.

I have seen the patient attendants, in many institutions, persevere day by day in endeavors to rouse, and interest, and instruct the demented in healthful occupations; and these efforts after a time have found reward in the gradual improvement of the objects of their care, and their acquisition of power to attend to stated healthful labors.

While the interests of humanity, those first great obligations, are consulted by the establishment of well regulated hospitals for the insane, political economy and the public safety are not less insured. The following tables exhibit the advantage of largely extended and seasonable hospital care for the insane. I am indebted chiefly to the reports of Drs. Woodward and Awl for these carefully prepared records.

Table showing the comparative expense of supporting old and recent cases of insanity, from which we learn the economy of placing patients in institutions in the early periods of disease; from the report of the Massachusetts State Hospital, for 1843. By Dr. Woodward.

No. of old cases.	Present age.	Time insane, in years.	Total expense, at $100 a year, before entering the hospital, and $132 a year since; last year $120.	Number of recent cases discharged.	Present age.	Time insane, in weeks.	Cost of support, at $2 30 per week.
2	69	28	$3,212 00	1,622	30	7	$16 10
7	48	17	2,004 00	1,624	34	20	46 00
8	60	21	2,504 00	1,625	51	32	73 60
12	47	25	2,894 00	1,635	23	28	64 40
18	71	34	3,794 00	1,642	42	40	92 00
19	59	18	2,204 00	1,643	55	14	32 20
21	39	16	1,993 00	1,645	63	36	82 80
27	47	16	1,994 00	1,649	22	40	92 00
44	56	26	2,982 00	1,650	36	28	64 40
45	60	25	2,835 00	1,658	36	14	32 20
102	53	25	2,833 00	1,660	21	16	36 80
133	44	13	1,431 00	1,661	19	27	62 10
176	55	20	2,486 00	1,672	40	11	25 70
209	39	16	1,964 00	1,676	23	23	52 90
223	50	20	2,364 00	1,688	23	11	25 70
260	47	16	2,112 00	1,690	23	27	62 10
278	49	10	1,424 00	1,691	37	20	46 00
319	53	10	1,247 00	1,699	30	28	64 40
347	58	14	1,644 00	1,705	24	17	39 10
367	40	12	1,444 00	1,706	55	10	23 00
400	43	14	1,644 00	1,709	17	10	23 00
425	48	13	2,112 00	1,715	19	40	92 00
431	36	13	1,412 00	1,716	35	48	110 40
435	55	15	1,712 00	1,728	52	55	126 50
488	37	17	1,912 00	1,737	30	33	75 90
		454	$54,157 00			635	$1,461 30

From Dr. Awl's reports of the Ohio institution, we extract the following tables:

In the report of 1840, the number of years that the twenty-five old cases had been insane, was 413; the whole expense of their support during that time, $47,590; the average $1,903 60. The time that the twenty-five recent cases had been confined, was 556 weeks; the expense, $1,400; the average $56.

In 1841, whole cost of twenty-five old cases - - -	$49,248 00
Average - - - - - - -	1,969 00
Whole cost of twenty-five recent cases - - -	1,330 50
Average - - - - - - -	52 22
In 1842, whole expense of twenty-five old cases - -	50,611 00
Average - - - - - - -	2,020 00
Whole expense of twenty-five recent cases - - -	1,130 00
Average - - - - - - -	45 20
In this institution, in 1843, twenty old cases had cost -	44,782 00
Average cost of old cases - - - - -	2,239 10
Whole expense of twenty recent cases till recovered - -	1,308 30
Average cost of recent cases - - - - -	65 41
In the Massachuseetts State Lunatic Asylum, in 1843, twenty-five old cases had cost - - - - -	54,157 00
Average expense of old cases - - - - -	2,166 20
Whole expense of twenty-five recent cases till recovered -	1,461 30
Average expense of recent cases - - - -	58 45
In the Ohio Lunatic Asylum, in 1844, twenty-five old cases had cost - - - - - - -	35,464 00
Average expense of old cases - - - - -	1,418 56
Whole expense of twenty-five recent cases - - -	1,608 00
Average expense of recent cases - - - -	64 32
In the Maine Lunatic Hospital, in 1842, twelve old cases had cost - - - - - - -	25,300 00
Average expense of old cases - - - - -	2,108 33
Whole expense of twelve recent cases - - -	426 00
Average expense of recent cases - - - -	35 50
In the Hospital at Staunton, Va., twenty old cases had cost -	41,633 00
Average expense of old cases - - - - -	2,081 65
Whole expense of twenty recent cases - - -	1,265 00
Average expense of recent cases - - - -	63 25

It will be said by a few, perhaps, that each State should establish and sustain its own institutions; that it is not obligatory upon the general government to legislate for the maintenance of State charities, by supplying the means of relief to individual sufferers; but may it not be demonstrated as the soundest policy for the federal government to assist in the accomplishment of great moral obligations, by diminishing and arresting wide-spread miseries which mar the face of society, and weaken the strength of communities?

Should your sense of moral responsibility seek support in precedents for guiding present action, I may be permitted to refer to the fact of liberal grants of common national property made, in the light of a wise discrimination, to various institutions of learning; also to advance in the new

States common school education, and to aid two seminaries of instruction for the deaf and dumb, viz : that in Hartford, Connecticut, and the school at Danville, in Kentucky, &c.

But it is not for one section of the United States that I solicit benefits, while all beside are deprived of direct advantages. I entertain no sectional prejudices, advance no local claims, and propose the advancement of no selfish aims, present or remote.

I advocate the cause of the much suffering insane throughout the entire length and breadth of my country : I ask relief for the east and for the west, for the north and for the south ; and for all I claim equal and proportionate benefits.

I ask of the Senate and House of Representatives of the United States, with respectful but earnest importunity, assistance to the several States of the Union in providing *appropriate care and support for the curable and incurable indigent insane.*

I ask of the representatives of a whole nation, benefits for all their constituents. Annual taxation for the support of the insane in hospitals is felt to be onerous, both in the populous maritime States, and in the States and Territories west of the Alleghanies. Much has been done, but much more remains to be accomplished, as I have endeavored to demonstrate in the preceding pages, for the relief of the sufferings and oppressions of that large class of the distressed for whom I plead, and upon whose condition I am solicitous to fix your attention.

I ask for the people that which is already the property of the people ; but possessions so holden, that it is through your action alone they can be applied as is now urged.

The whole public good must be sought and advanced through those channels which most certainly contribute to the moral elevation and true dignity of a great people.

Americans boast much of superior intelligence and sagacity ; of power and influence ; of their vast resources possessed and yet undeveloped ; of their free institutions and civil liberty ; of their liberally endowed schools of learning, and of their far-reaching commerce : they call themselves a mighty nation ; they name themselves a great and wise people. If these claims to distinction above most nations of the earth are established upon undeniable premises, then will the rulers, the political economists, and the moral philosophers of other and remote countries, look scrutinizingly into our civil and social condition for examples to illustrate the greatness of our name. They will seek not to measure the strength and extent of the fortifications which guard our coast ; they will not number our vessels of war, or of commerce ; they will not note the strength of our armies ; they will not trace the course of the thousands eager for self-aggrandizement, nor of the tens of thousands led on by ambition and vain glory : they will search after illustrations in those God-like attributes which sanctify private life, and in that incorruptible integrity and justice which perpetuates national existence. They will note the moral grandeur and dignity which leads the statesman to lay broad and deep the foundations of national greatness, in working out the greatest good for the whole people ; in effect, making paramount the interests of mind to material wealth, or mere physical prosperity. *Primarily*, then, in the highest order of means for confirming the prosperity of a people and the duration of government must be the education of the ignorant, and restoring the health and maintaining the sick mind in its natural integrity.

I will not presume to dictate to those in whose humane dispositions I have faith, and whose wisdom I cannot question.

I have approached you with self-diffidence, but with confidence in your impartial and just consideration of the subject submitted to your discussion and righteous effective decision.

I confide to you the cause and the claims of the destitute and of the desolate, without fear or distrust. I ask, for the thirty States of the Union, 5,000,000 acres of land, of the many hundreds of millions of public lands, appropriated in such manner as shall assure the greatest benefits to all who are in circumstances of extreme necessity, and who, through the providence of God, *are wards of the nation,* claimants on the sympathy and care of the public, through the miseries and disqualifications brought upon them by the sorest afflictions with which humanity can be visited.

Respectfully submitted.

D. L. DIX.

WASHINGTON, *June* 23, 1848.

Statement of the number of insane and idiots, from the uncorrected census of 1840.

States and Territories.	White persons.		Colored.		Total.	Population.	Proportion of insane and idiots to the whole.
	Public charge.	Private charge.	Private charge.	Public charge.			
Maine -	207	330	56	38	631	501,793	1 to 795
New Hampshire -	180	306	8	11	505	284,574	1 to 563
Massachusetts -	471	600	27	173	1,271	737,699	1 to 580
Rhode Island -	117	86	8	5	216	108,830	1 to 503
Connecticut -	114	384	20	24	542	309,978	1 to 572
Vermont -	144	254	9	4	411	291,948	1 to 710
New York -	683	1,463	138	56	2,340	2,428,921	1 to 1,038
New Jersey -	144	225	46	27	442	373,306	1 to 844
Pennsylvania -	469	1,477	132	55	2,133	1,724,033	1 to 808
Delaware -	22	30	21	7	80	78,085	1 to 976
Maryland -	137	263	108	42	550	470,019	1 to 852
Virginia -	317	735	327	54	1,433	1,239,797	1 to 866
North Carolina -	152	428	192	29	801	753,419	1 to 940
South Carolina -	91	285	121	16	513	594,398	1 to 6,158
Georgia -	51	243	108	26	428	691,392	1 to 1,615
Alabama -	39	193	100	25	357	590,756	1 to 1,655
Mississippi -	14	102	66	16	198	375,651	1 to 1,897
Louisiana -	6	49	38	7	100	352,411	1 to 3,524
Tennessee -	103	596	124	28	851	829,210	1 to 974
Kentucky -	305	490	102	48	975	779,828	1 to 799
Ohio -	363	832	103	62	1,360	1,519,467	1 to 1,117
Indiana -	110	377	47	28	562	685,866	1 to 1,220
Illinois -	36	177	65	14	292	476,183	1 to 1,630
Missouri -	42	160	50	18	270	383,702	1 to 1,420
Arkansas -	9	36	13	8	66	97,574	1 to 1,478
Michigan -	2	37	21	5	65	212,267	1 to 3,265
Florida -	1	9	12	–	22	54,477	1 to 2,476
Wisconsin -	1	7	3	–	11	30,945	1 to 2,813
Iowa -	2	5	4	–	11	43,112	1 to 3,919
Dis't Columbia -	1	13	4	3	21	43,712	1 to 2,081
Total -	4,333	10,192	2,103	829	17,457	17,069,453	1 to 977

MEMORIAL

MISSISSIPPI

1850

MEMORIAL

SOLICITING ADEQUATE APPROPRIATIONS

FOR THE CONSTRUCTION

OF A

STATE HOSPITAL FOR THE INSANE,

IN THE

STATE OF MISSISSIPPI.

FEBRUARY, 1850.

Printed by order of the Legislature.

JACKSON, MISS

FALL & MARSHALL....STATE PRINTERS,

1850.

MEMORIAL

To the Honorable, the General Assembly of Misssissippi.

GENTLEEEN: A sense of moral and social obligation ; a duty created through painful knowledge of the woes of suffering humanity, urges my appeal to you in your Legislative capacity, convened as you are, to deliberate and act upon measures for the advancement of the general prosperity and security of your State, as also for the social, well being and interests of your constituents -and their dependents.

Occasionally in the progress of Legislative councils, questions of grave moral obligation arise, and are urged with more or less earnestness, according to the measure of their importance, or the appreciation of their importance, by those who are required to investigate their merits.

Your memorialist respectfully and earnestly solicits your careful attention to the actual wants of the insane in Mississippi, who, as a numerous and increasing class of sufferers, present peculiar and imperative claims on your care. Suffering under the most distressing malady which can assail our race, they are, by a great and acknowledged law of civil society and social life, made *wards* of the State, and as such claim, liberal and humane restoring cares. The obligation of all governments to extend efficient patronage, or primarily to found and support institutions for the remedial treatment of the insane, has been admitted alike by all civilized nations of modern times, and acted upon with more or less liberality, as ability and circumstances have determined. In the United States especially within the last half century, hospitals for the insane have been multiplied, yet we are startled, almost appalled, by the fact, that the settled portions of our country contain, at the most moderate estimate, 22,000 insane men and women ; and of this most distressed multitude, less than 5,000 are receiving the benefits of appropriate curative or protecting care. The malady is becoming more prevalent ; the cases curable, under prompt and suitable treatment, are yet, through neglect, fast multiplying on the iucurable lists, and more urgent claims indicate that the interests of political economy, no less than the charities due to humanity, call for effectual Legislation in behalf of the insane.

"There are twenty State hospitals, besides several incorporated hospitals, for the treatment of the insane, in nineteen States of the Union, Virginia alone having two government State hospitals. The following is a correct list, omitting several small establishments conducted by private individuals, and several pretty extensive poor-house departments.

The first hospital for the insane in the United States was established in Philadelphia, as a department of the Penn Hospital, in the year 1752. This has been transferred to a fine district near the village of Mantua, in the vicinity of Philadelphia, since 1832 : number of patients 188.

The second institution receiving insane patients, and the first exclusively for their use, was at Williamsburg, Virginia, in 1773 : number of patients 165.

The third was the Friend's Hospital, at Frankfort, near Philadelphia, in 1817 : number of patients 55.

The next was the McLean Hospital, at Charlestown, (now Summerville,) in Massachusetts, in 1818. This valuable institution is second to none in America. Number of patients 180.

Bloomingdale Hospital, near the city of New York, was established in 1821 ; number of patients 126 : South Carolina Hospital, at Columbia, in 1822 ; number of patients 104 : Connecticut Hospital, at Hartford; patients 122, and Kentucky Hospital, at Lexington, patients 247, in 1824.

In 1845–'46, the Legislature of Kentucky passed a bill to establish a second State Institution in the Green River country.

Virginia Western Hospital was opened at Staunton in 1828 ; number of patients 217. Massachusets State Hospital, at Worcester, was opened in 1833, and enlarged in 1843 ; it has 370 patients. Maryland Hospital, at Baltimore, was founded in 1834 ; it has the present year 109 patients. Vermont State Hospital, at Battleborough, was opened for patients in 1837, and enlarged in 1846–'47 ; it has at present 321 patients. New York City Hospital for the poor, on Blackwell's island, was occupied in 1838 ; it is now being considerably enlarged : and has above 400 patients.

Tennessee State Hospital, at Nashville, was opened in 1839. According to an act of the Legislature in 1847–'48, this hospital is to be replaced by one of capacity to receive 250 patients In the old hospital are 64 patients. Boston City Hospital for the indigent, which has 150 patients, and Ohio State Hospital, at Columbus, were severally opened in 1839. The latter has been considerably enlarged, and has now 329 patients. Maine State Hospital, at Augusta, 1840 ; patients 130. New Hampshire State Hospital, at Concord, was opened in 1842, and has above 100 patients. New York State Hospital, at Utica, was established in 1843, and has since been largely extended, and has 600 patients. Mount Hope Hospital, near Baltimore, 1844–'45 : has 72 insane patients.— Georgia has an institution for the insane at Milledgeville, and at present 128 patients. Rhode Island State Hospital was opened, under the direction of Dr. Ray, early in 1848. New Jersey State Hospital, at Trenton, 1848. Indiana State Hospital, at Indianapolis, opened in 1848. State Hospital of Illinois, at Jacksonville, was occupied before 1849. The Lonisiana State Hospital will be occupied perhaps within a year.

It will be seen that Mississippi is one of the few States in which no provision has yet been supplied for the recovery of the demented and the maniac. Such as have received the advantages of hospital treatment have, under very difficult and painful circumstances of fatigue and expense, been conveyed to institutions in other States, more or less remote ; but there are *many* who languish in inappropriate habitations, in wretched poverty-stricken dwellings—in ill-directed poor houses ; in exposed pens, or dreary, unlighted and unventilated cells ; and in those most unfit departments, the solitary strong rooms or the dungeons of your county jails—guiltless of crime, chargeable only with incapacity for self-care, and irresponsible, by reason of sickness—physical infirmity and the breaking down of the fortress of reason !

A wise and enlightened State policy promotes the application of public improvements ; and canals, and plank roads, and railroads, attest the zeal and enterprise which opens the resources of the country, and conducts to every district the channels of inflowing wealth ; yet are the insane suffered to shriek and wail, and wear slowly out an existence of unmitigated misery ; and the blind, and the deaf and dumb sit in mental darkness, and institutions of general and common school instruction struggle on, year after year, with few or no substantial evidences of public fostering care. That this course has no basis in sound, wise policy, is too evident to need demonstration. The chief province of legislators, it is allowed, confines them to the more practical business of the country ; but intelligent humanity has marked other paths, which conduct to noble acts and great and glorious results.

I am not unaware that the legislature of Mississippi, at the close of the session of 1848, recognized the deficiencies and obligations of the State, in connection with the miseries of the insane, by the passage of an act which, no doubt, in all good faith, was designed to accomplish, in part, at least, benefits so imperatively demanded.

Your memorialist must believe that it was want of correct and sufficient information, rather than the want of a just liberality, which determined the amount of the very insufficient appropriation which was made for the construction of hospital buildings. Citizens of Mississippi, surely, cannot be chargeable with narrow parsimony. Fairly understanding the merits of the case, they will not hoard their gold and condemn to a more terrible than physical death, the insane within their own borders—their fellow-citizens, their friends, and their kindred !

In 1840, ten years since, according to the records of the United State census, there were in the State of Mississippi one hundred and ninety-eight cases. These did not embrace the many patients whose kindred, being in affluent circumstances, were able to place them in the hospitals of sister States, as in Tennessee, Kentucky, Ohio, Pennsylvania, and others. According to reliable data, the lowest possible estimate of the insane in this State is four hundred; but there is substantial reason for believing that this esttmate is much below the standard, and that the census of 1850, if correctly made will show from four hundred and fifty to five hundred.

To those who have not investigated facts, these estimates must appear to be greatly exaggerated; but patient inquiry and careful observation will, it is certainly known, afford results no less painful and revolting, than unanticipated and unimagined.

Of the entire number of the insane counted throughout the State, it is not assumed that all, or even one-half, would be essentially benefited by hospital treatment; but, from one hundred to one hundred and seventy-five or two hundred, would be fit subjects for remedial care, or the protecting and *humanizing* influences which appropriate institutions furnish.

An institution for the insane requires peculiar arrangements for the classification, association, or the isolation of the patients, in the various stages of the malady. The violent maniac must be parted from the quiet patient; the convalescent from those whose cases are either hopeless or stationary; those suffering under the access of other maladies, in addition to the general invalidism of insanity; also, the men from the women, and the workers from such as are incapable of pursuing employments and enjoying recreative exercise.

Dr. Zeller observes that, of the first essential considerations, it is needful to prevent the patient from injuring himself or others. He must be placed in a situation which will guard off all violent acts. 2d. His morbid propensities must be controlled, and all his real wants carefully and constantly supplied. In arrangements for hospital buildings, the following rules must be heeded.

" 1st. Those which have reference to general salubrity of climate, supplies of water, light, and air.

" 2d. The most practicable *security* and *preservation* of the patients, especially for the violent and destructive classes; and these considerations involve heavier outlays, in construction of buildings, than in edifices destined for any other purposes."

Institutions for the insane can never be made productive property to States or communities; but, once constructed, furnished, organized and opened to patients, after the first year may be self-supporting—that is, the indigent and pauper patient, paying by counties or townships the *actual cost* only of their support in the hospital, (a sum varying from $1 75 to $2 or $2 50 per week,) and the paying patients, in affluent circumstances, rendering from $3 to $10 and $15 per week, according to the accommodations furnished, and special nursing and watching required, meet the current expenses of the institution.

To illustrate this position, I refer to the annual reports of several State hospitals:

Vermont hospital, at Brattleboro, 312 patients; expenditures, in 1848, $30,975 93; income from the board of patients, $31,-295 34.

Massachusetts State hospital, 1847: number of patients, 396; receipts, $45,662 92; expenditures, $1,235 61 less than the current income. The year 1846 shows upon the books a balance in favor of the hospital of $6,218 47. This was applied to repairs and various improvements.

South Carolina hospital, at Columbia, in 1844: patients, 72; receipts and outlays balanced, being $20,985 95—$8,222 61 being applied to the construction of a new wing.

Connecticut hospital for the insane, with 122 patients, received $23,760 17, which balanced actual expenses.

Pennsylvania hospital, with 208 patients, nett receipts, $40,-180 53; total expenditures, including building a cottage and repairs, $40,150 80.

References might be multiplied, but it is believed that the above will suffice for illustrating the capability of these institutions, when rightly managed, to stand independent of the State treasury.

It may be interesting to note appropriations made in different States from time to time, for extending and improving as well as for establishing in the first instance, hospitals for the insane. It will not be attempted to produce complete records of every institution.

The first appropriation for the Connecticut hospital in 1824, was $26,000. Shortly after, the additional sum of $40,000 was applied; since which, about $60,000 have been expended in additional buildings, and in purchasing a large farm.

The Pennsylvania hospital opened in 1840, cost $325,000: since which a large amount has been applied in extending accommodations. The central buildings and main wings present an eastern front of 436 feet · the dimensions of the two wings I do not certainly recollect; but the detached buildings, and apart from the cottages, are 95 feet in length. The entire institution is completely finished and furnished, and affords excellent accommodations for every class of patients.

The New York State hospital buildings cost the State more than half a million, including furnishing, &c.

The cost of the Bloomingdale hospital, near the city of New York, including all out-buildings, furniture and improvements, was more than $200,000. Number of patients varies; 126 present average-The farm and vegetable gardens are productive, and in a state of high cultivation.

The Rhode Island hospital for the insane, at Providence, cost $81,300. Farm and improvements, $10,648 37. Furniture $6,800. Incidental expenses, $8,334 82.

The McLean hospital, at Somerville, Massachusetts, was established and has been sustained entirely by private benefactions. The largest legacy from Mr. McLean of Boston, whose name it bears, was $100,000 ; the next largest was from **Miss Mary Belknap**, whose name is given to one wing, constructed at a cost of ,$90,000, which sum she gave for that use. The institution can accommodate about 150 patients and has cost in buildings and improvements over $300,000.

The Massachusetts State hospital has cost something less than $280,000 ; it can receive 400 patients. The buildings present a front of 525 feet, with six wings, making a range of 2,000 feet, beside extensive out-buildings, workshops, sundry barns, &c. There is a farm of 150 acres, and gardens in fine cultivation.

New Jersey State hospital, at Trenton, may in all respects be regarded as a model institution ; it cost $153,000, and for the accommodations it affords, and excellence of its construction is one of the best and cheapest institutions in the United States. As is usual in establishing all modern hospitals for the insane, an extensive and productive farm is attached to the establishment.

The buildings, furniture, and improvements of the Ohio State hospital have cost above $230,000. It can now accommodate about 400 patients.

"Friends Asylum," at Frankfort, Pennsylvania, receives irom 40 to 60 patients; has good buildings and nearly 70 acres of land, and the original buildings had cost, in 1816 and 1817, $46,000. Considerable sums have since that time been expended on improvements.

The original cost of the Maryland hospital for the insane, with accommodations for 120 patients, was $200,000. The necessities of the State demand much additional provision for this class of citizens, and Governor Thomas, in the last annual gubernatorial message, refers to the subject as follows .

"Full estimates have been made, pursuant to resolutions, of the cost of additional buildings to the Maryland hospital, suitable for the accommodation of the insane persons in the alms-house, at Baltimore, and for the insane poor, unprovided for in the State. The plan contemplates the erection of two wings, extending two hundred and fifty-two feet each, from either end of the present building, and designed to accommodate one hundred and fifty patients ; the cost of these is accurately estimated at $74,519 ; but if steam is substituted for heating, in place of air furnaces, the cost will be $81,518. It must be recollected that these buildings, if erected for the number of patients above stated, will not accommodate one-half of the insane now requiring hospital care in the State."

Large appropriations, within three years, have been made for adding new wings to the two State institutions at Staunton and at Williamsburg, Virginia ; these are finished and crowded to their utmost capacity, and it is a question if sound State policy does not demand a third hospital capable of receiving 280 patients in that State. Hundreds of insane patients there are still lodged in the dungeons of jails and cells of poor-houses.

North Carolina passed a bill in 1848, appropriating $87,500 46 for hospital buildings, exclusive of all contingent expenses, and with the full understanding, that for 250 patients, the building would cost, when fully completed, $100,000.

South Carolina, in addition to large sums applied to building purposes from time to time, appropriated $8,222 61 to building a small wing in 1844. In 1847, new appropriations were solicited and applied ; in 1848, $15,000 was appropriated for another wing; to this the surplus funds of the hospital were added, and Dr. Trezevant, now at the close of 1849, reports "the hospital inconveniently crowded for some months, the corridors occupied, as well as the lodging rooms, and 140 patients under charge during the year, the average being 104. It must be kept in recollection, that large numbers of paying patients are annually conveyed from the southern States to northern institutions, in which the means of comfort, care, and cure are more amply provided. This should not be necessary, and it would not be, if the outlays by the State legislatures were as ample as the real wants of the people demand. Of 1320 patients in one northern hospital alone, in a few years there have been 131 of the rich paying patients received from the South. In another hospital, of 93 patients under treatment in 1848, only 71 belonged within the State

Of 142 patients in the Maryland hospital in 1843, 39 were from southern borders.

In 1837–'38, Georgia purchased a tract of land near Milledgeville, and adopted a plan embracing two buildings, each 4 stories high, 129 feet long, and 39 wide, parallel to and distant from each other 222 feet, which space was left for the foundation of a third building, touching the corners of each of the two first, and to be 40 feet in width, and connected with the first named wings by a verandah on each. The first appropriation to begin and complete one wing, was $45,000. I have not with me the memoranda to show certainly the appropriations made since 1840, but the second wing was finished and occupied several years since.

Louisiana is building a hospital for the insane at Jackson, upon a well chosen site, and with means to make an excellent institution.

Indiana State hospital is not yet finished, but urgent need demanded the occupation of a part of the institution, and 104 patients were admitted under very disadvantageous circumstances, during the first eleven months from the completion of one wing. This hospital is well managed, and is skilfully directed by an experienced physician. It presents a front of 300 feet, *four* stories high, with attics on the centre, and the extreme ends. Its cubical contents are 820,000 feet ; its cost, not including the farm, the improvements, nor the furniture, $70,000, or 8½ cents per cubic foot. The roof is of slate, and the whole presents a finished and handsome appearnnce highly creditable to the indefatigable and skill-ful architect, Joseph Willis.

The farm, garden, grounds, &c., writes Dr. Patterson, under the judicious management of Mr. Bradshaw, the Steward, have produced abundantly, so far as we have been able to cultivate it during the past season. It has furnished desirable employment for our male patients, and will aid materially in defraying the current expenses of the institution during the year. It has produced during the season:

400 Sheets,

500 cords of Wood,
1000 bushels of Corn,
200 bushels of Potatoes,
200 bushels of Apples
200 bushels of Oats,
5000 lbs. Pork.

Besides a plentiful supply of cabbage, beets, onions, parsnips, tomatoes, beans, peas, and other garden vegetables, and it has also afforded twenty acres of pasture for the use of the hospital. One and a half miles of fence have been constructed, enclosing the front grounds and eighty acres of wood-land, and the farm has been supplied with stock and farming utensils. These have added considerably to the expenses of the year, but as the farm is now supplied with the necessary implements, the expense of managing it during the coming year, will be less than it has been during the past,

The grounds have been marked out, but they are yet to be graded and ornamented with evergreens and other shrubbery; and a hospital cemetery has been selected and neatly enclosed with a board fence

While the male patients have been engaged in agricultural pursuits and other out-door employments, the female patients have been industrious within doors, and, under the direction of the Matron, they have made for the use of the institution,

400 Sheets,
100 Bed-spreads,
160 Comforts,
224 Pillow cases,
120 Under bed-ticks,
50 Window curtains.
40 Dresses,
4 Double mattrasses,
50 Table cloths,
20 Pairs of pantaloons,
130 Pillows,

And besides this, they have done a large amount of mending, some ironing, washing, and other house-work.

Of the 104 patients first received, 79 were natives of other States. Eighty of the one hundred and four patients in this institution, are supported by the State, at the cost of $8,000. A library was purchased for a little less than one hundred dollars, for the use of the patients. Indeed, in the outset, the plan here has been to *cure* the patients, by supplying, at once, all means possible at command, for their comfort and recreation.

While Indiana has been building her hospital for the insane, she has also been making efficient and very liberal appropriations for the blind, and for the deaf mutes. The architect for constructing the State buildings for the residence and education of the latter, reports as follows:

"The buildings consist of a centre 74 by 56, four stories, and a basement, and surrounded by a dome or cupalo, the top being 105 feet from the ground. The whole roofings are of slate. A doric portico is sustained by a platform 30 feet by 11, and like the dome, covered with copper. The wings are 60 feet by 33; attached to these are transverse wings; the entire length is 256 feet. In the rear are the school-house and chapel, two stories high, and 134 feet long, covered with slate and rough-cast with lime and sand, and hydraulic cement. The cubical contents of these buildings are 964,000 feet; the cost of building, without furnishing and improving, $55,000.

"Number of teachers, four; number of pupils, 125; 80 males, 45 females; expenses of the school, $9,369 09. The valuable farm connected with the school is about to be enclosed, and brought under cultivation."

Tennessee is now building a State hospital, which will accommodate 250 patients: as is expedient and invariable in establishing all modern hospitals for the insane, a large farm is attached to the site.

Kentucky has extended her accommodations for patients by constructing new wings at the hospital in Lexington, and is building a new and much needed institution, on a liberal scale, in the Green river country.

All modern experience, both in our own country and in Europe, proves the importance of connecting extensive grounds with hospitals for the insane, as well as establishing these institutions beyond the borders of towns and cities, viz: at a distance varying according to circumstances, of from one to two miles.

Every institution should have sufficient land to furnish the patients with ample employment in its cultivation. Means should be afforded for the cultivation of vegetable and flower gardens, as well as for producing the heavier crops of the farm or plantation. From one to three hundred acres is usually secured. Cases of chronic insanity are especially benefitted by out-door labor, and by daily useful employment of some sort. Whether the attention is directed to the gardens, the plantations, ornamenting the grounds, repairing out-buildings, fences, &c., the advantage to the patient exceeds the value of the mere returns for labor. It often restores the curable, and gives health, cheerfulness, and contentment to the feeble.

"During the past year," writes the physician of the Maryland State hospital, "our efforts to supply the inmates with ample means of *useful employment*, exercise in the open air, and amusements adapted to their tastes and habits, *have been unremitting*. In carrying out the moral treatment, these means *are* indispensible." The reason is obvious; well-timed employments, well selected amusements attract the mind from its delusions and fix it on other objects. The sound faculties are thus called into action and invigorated. Indeed, among all the agents for moral discipline, none supersede manual labor

Of 99 men patients, at the Baltimore hospital, 45 were habitually employed in some useful labor : and of 57 women at the same period, all but 11 were usefully and pleasantly occupied. Regular exercise and amusements, alternating with a suitable amount of labor, promote refreshing sleep, tranquilize the nervous system, and revive cheerfulness, and tend to restore self-control.

Dr. Laborde, of South Carolina, says, in a report of the committee of regents of the State hospital at Columbus, that the beneficial effects of *employments* cannot well be over-rated, and that these must be diversified to suit the health and abilities of the patients; but none takes so high a place as a curative means, as gardening and agriculture. A farm is as necessary as a physician, and more valuable than all the drugs of the apothecary.

Dr. Allen. of Kentucky, and Dr. Stribling of the Western State hospital, at Staunton, Virginia, state in their annual reports, their sense of the value of the farms severally attached to the hospitals, they conduct as assisting, not only largely in meeting supplies for the institution, but much more as aiding the recovery of their patients.

Dr. Chandler, in the 15th annual report of the Worcester hospital, gives as follows, his opinion and experience on the value of farming labor for the patients, as well as the profitable returns, through the same, in favor of the establishment :

"Farming and horticulture, for the past year, have been pursued by us with our customary success. The crops have been abundant, as the subjoined enumeration will show. Our attention has been turned less to the raising of corn and potatoes than to other crops. The tilled soil here is not adapted to produce the potato of the best quality. It is too light and sandy, or it may be that a rotation of crops is needed to resuscitate the soil.

"Such crops as require the most care and labor, which we have in the ready assistance of our patients to bestow, give the largest returns for the number of acres cultivated. We require a large amount of garden vegetables. It would be difficult to purchase our supply of them; but we are, by the situation of our gardens, and by the assistance of patients, conveniently situated for raising them. The following are some of the articles, with their value :—

"122 bushels of corn at 90 cents...............	$ 109 80
300 bushels oats at 50 cents....................	150 00
11 bushels dried beans at $1 25 cents..........	13 75
9 bushels dry peas at $1.....................	9 00
240 bushels beets at 34 cents..................	81 60
186 bushels English turnips at 25 cents.	46 50
30 bushels Swedish turnips at 25 cents.........	7 50
258 bushels potatoes at 50 cents...............	129 00
80 bushels parsnips at 67 cents................	53 60
30 bushels apples at 50 cents.................	15 00
135 bushels onions, at 67 cents................	90 45
1800 cabbages, at 4 cents a piece...............	72 00
12 tons of winter squashes at 1 cent per pound...	240 00
44 bushels of green peas......................	44 00
110 bushels summer squashes..................	55 00
156 bushels cucumbers, at 75 cents............	117 00
oat straw................................	40 00
36500 quarts of milk at 3½ cents..................	1277 50
8461 pounds of beef at 6¼ cents.................	528 81
9313 pounds of pork at 7½ cents.................	698 47
120 pounds of poultry at 10 cents..............	12 00
167 pounds of veal at 6 cents.................	11 82
	$3802 20

"A full supply of summer vegetables, for the use of the establishment, was raised from our two gardens, comprising about six acres of ground.

"There was raised for wintering the stock :—

60 tons of hay at $13.........................	780 80
1176 bushels of carrots at 25 cents..............	294 00
7 loads of pumpkins.........................	10 00
corn fodder...............................	15 00
	$1099 80

"Twenty cows and two oxen were pastured on the farm. There are about one hundred and fifty acres now attached to it, and it is all absolutely needed for, the uses of the hospital.

"The live stock now consists of four horses, four oxen, seventeen cows, twenty-six swine, and seventy fowls.

"In the shoe-shop, from two to five patients have worked daily with Mr. David Hitchcock. They have not at any time been urged to work hard, but they go there as an amusement, and to keep their minds occupied by something besides their own delusions. Some have completed their recovery, and probably hastened it too, by being employed here."

It appears unnecessary to adduce additional evidence of the *necessity* for connecting a considerable tract of arable land with a hospital. Not less absolute is the demand for an *inexhaustible* supply upon the premises of *pure water*. These objects being secured, and a somewhat elevated site chosen, the next essential consideration is a *liberal* appropriation for the *substantial* construction of *well planned, fire-proof buildings*. The recently constructed hospital at Trenton, New Jersey, affords a model from which but few deviations need be made, to adapt it to the wants and accommodation of a like number of patients (about two hundred and fifty) in Mississippi. It is well known that a permanent, solid structure, such as your improving State *now needs*, cannot be built for less than eighty or one hundred thousand dollars. All attempts at abridging expense, in works for these purposes, are eminently mistaken and ill-judged. In support of this unqualified assertion, I refer to the history of *all* institutions for the insane in the United States and in England.

"Liberal outlays," writes Dr. Luther V. Bell, an authority which none will question, at home or abroad, "*liberal outlays* are indispensable to the prosperity and success of the hospitals for the insane." He remarks that, during a recent tour in Europe, for the purpose of visiting the most approved hospitals, he everywhere found "this principle recognized, and declared to be the practical fruits of the experience of institutions brought into existence within thirty years. The principle is this, *that there is no such thing as a just and proper curative or ameliorating treatment of the insane in very cheaply constructed or cheaply arranged institutions. That the measure of expense should never be regarded in providing for the insane.*" If it is worth while to have institutions at all, it is worth while to have such as will accomplish all of care and cure which is practicable.

"*Every State*," writes Dr. Woodward, "should *make ample* provision for the cure of insanity, whether it is found in the rich or the poor classes of society." All so afflicted need this guardian and remedial care, and all should have it. What outlay of dollars can compare with the blessings of restoration to reason? Who can weigh gold against the value of the right use of reason?

The importance of early, prompt hospital treatment, also, cannot be too strongly enforced.

Dr. Trezement, a name of influence in Carolina, commenting on this subject, declared that "nothing could excuse the friends of insane persons, and the commissioners acting for the insane poor, from *early* sending these to receive the benefits of appropriate hospital care;" for, he adds, "it is proved by incontestible facts that it is *cheaper to do so, and far less expensive, in the end,* for those who are charged with the support of these unfortunate persons. *Retrenchment has been the curse of the poor, but especially of the insane poor.*" "When the mind is warped and the reason gone, *no circumstances should be considered valid* in preventing hospital care."

"The great importance of *early* treatment," writes Dr. Fisher, of Maryland, "should be impressed on the public mind with renewed and imperative emphasis. In the treatment of insanity, almost everything depends on the first few months. Of the cases placed in a well regulated hospital, *within the first twelve months* of the invasion of the disease, from eighty to ninety per cent. will be fully restored. After the lapse of this period, the proportion rapidly declines;" and, as writes Esquirlo, "after the third year, no more than one in *thirty* recover."

Dr. Stribling and Dr. Galt, of Virginia, urge, in every annual report from their institutions to the State legislature, the great importance of prompt, efficient care for all classes of the insane, and show by examples too numerous to quote, the obligation of rendering remedial treatment in the *first months* of the attack; but their views are common to all medical men whose cares have been directed to the treatment of insanity.

Dr. Stribling in a recent report, writes as follows:

"Of one hundred and fifty-eight cases now in the asylum, who are in all probability doomed for life to endure the burthen of remediless disease, how many might have been restored to reason, to usefulness, and to happiness, had weeks or only months been permitted to elapse before suitable resources were resorted to for their relief; but years went on, and at last, the anxious and exhausted friends bring to the asylum a long afflicted patient, laboring under a *fixed* malady, and for whom our best cares result in little more than soothing the pathway to the tomb!" In connection with this plain and truthful exposition, I find the following official record: "Received 151 cases of *less* than one year's standing:—of these, 119 recovered; 17 were relieved; 4 wholly unimproved, and 11 have died." What can more forcibly illustrate the value and obligation of early hospital care and treatment for the insane?

The report of the Superintendent of the Pennsylvania Hospital, for 1848, shows—cured, 120; much improved, 23; improved, 24; stationary, 19; died, 17. Total, 203.

The history of a large proportion of cases which may be traced, and which have passed into a chronic state, show that had remedial measures been promptly adopted, many might have been restored to sound health and reason, and thus to ability to share in the duties of life, and those acts which make every rational individual an assistant in sustaining the social and civil organization of society. It is not a theoretical supposition, but a fact capable of absolute demonstration, in every State and country where hospital treatment has been developed, that though the first expense of maintaining a patient in a hospital is greater than in a jail, a poor-house, or a private dwelling; yet, in consequence of the number cured, and the small number of *early* treated cases which remain on charge, the *final* expense is much less than if they are suffered to drag out a wretched existence, laboring under the infliction of a distracted or demented mind.

"A point of great importance," writes Dr. Buttolph, of the New Jersey State Hospital, "and one that should be distinctly understood, and *conscientiously* acted upon by friends of the insane, is that *appropriate curative* treatment be resorted to *early* after the attack. The statistical records of institutions for the insane, in all countries, show that a much greater per centage of recoveries occur of the patients treated within the first few months of the attack, than those in whom it has existed for a longer period."

Dr. Bates, of the State Hospital, at Augusta, Maine, records of cases admitted *within one year after the attack,* 52 recovered ; 25 unimproved, improved, and died. Of those admitted in 1848, after more than one year's duration of disease, only 8 recovered ; 38 remained improved, unimproved and died." In the McLean asylum, the same year, "87 were discharged, restored ; 8 much improved ; 16 improved ; 21 underwent no important change."

Referring to authentic hospital records, too copious to transfer to these pages, I find the following summary : In the Massachusetts State Hospital, in 1843, *twenty-five old* cases had cost $54,157 00; average expense of these $2,166 20. Whole expense of twenty-five *recent cases* till recovered, $1,461 30 ; average expense of twenty-five recent cases $58 48.

In the Western Hospital, Virginia, twenty old cases had cost $41,633 00 ; average cost $2,081 65. Whole expense of twenty *recent* cases, $1,263 00; average expense of twenty recent cases till recovered, $63 23. The cost of supporting 102 cases in five different hospitals, had amounted to $201,336 00, on an average for each to $1,973 88 ; while in the same institntions the cost of *same number of recent cases discharged, cured.* amounted to only $6,068 60, or to an average of $59 49.

In one single institution in New England, three cases of incurable insanity first admitted, have already cost their friends $11,100 00, or $3,700 00 each ; while the three last cases of recovery have cost $170 74, or only $56 96 each. The old cases, so far as is apparent, had they been brought under early treatment, might have been recovered, and not have remained a sorrow of heart and a burthen on the resources of their friends ; the last, which were recent cases, are already sharing in society the duties of life.

In 1844–'45, 104 patients were discharged, recovered, from the Massachusetts Hospital, whose cases were *recent* at the time of admission ; at the same hospital, the per cent. recovery in all recent cases, was 89½ in 1843; 79 in 1846; 72 in 1847; 86 in 1848; and of old cases, 31¼ in 1845; 28 in 1846; 17 in 1847, and 19 in 1848.

In the hospital of Augusta, Maine, the average *time* of recent cases recovered, was 157 days; that of old cases recovered was 229 days.

A Table showing the comparative cost to the State of twenty old and twenty recent cases of insanity, illustrating the importance, in an economical point of view, of placing such persons under treatment at an early period of their disease and of providing every means of treating them successfully in an Asylum, from the Kentucky Hospital records.

	OLD CASES.				RECENT CASES.		
No.	Age.	Time spent in Asylum.	Cost of each case at $65 per annum.	No.	Duration before admission.	Time spent in Asylum.	Cost of each case at $1 50 per week.
1	47	20 years,	$1,300 00	1	1 week,	36 weeks,	$54 00
2	48	20 years,	1,300 00	2	7 weeks,	16 weeks,	24 00
3	52	17 years,	1,105 00	3	3 months,	32 weeks,	48 00
4	54	16 years,	1,140 00	4	2 months,	40 weeks	60 00
5	47	17 yeass,	1,005 00	5	2 months,	20 weeks,	30 00
6	46	15 years,	975 00	6	2 months,	20 weeks,	30 00
7	51	14 years,	910 00	7	3 months,	12 weeks,	18 00
8	31	13 years,	845 00	8	1 month,	20 weeks,	30 00
9	33	11 years,	715 00	9	2 months,	28 weeks,	42 00
10	45	12 years,	780 00	10	3 months,	24 weeks,	36 00
11	37	10 years,	650 00	11	6 months,	24 weeks,	36 00
12	39	10 years,	650 00	12	6 months,	32 weeks,	48 00
13	33	12 years,	780 00	13	4 months,	28 weeks,	42 00
14	45	15 years,	975 00	14	4 months,	12 weeks,	18 00
15	48	16 years,	1,040 00	15	6 months,	8 weeks,	12 00
16	56	12 years,	780 00	16	1 month,	8 weeks,	12 00
17	44	13 years,	715 00	17	2 months,	24 weeks,	36 00
18	47	15 years,	975 00	18	1 month,	20 weeks,	30 00
19	36	13 years,	845 00	19	6 months,	12 weeks,	18 00
20	36	9 years,	580 00	20	1 month,	20 weeks,	30 00
			$18,030 00				$654 00

Aggregate cost of 20 old cases, $18,030 00. | Aggregate cost of 20 recent cases, $654 00·

Average time spent in Asylum by each, 14 years. | Average time spent in Asylum, nearly five months.

Average cost of each case, $901 50. | Average cost of each case, $32 14.

Table (*from Dr. Awl's sixth report for* 1844, *of the State Hospital, at Columbus, Ohio,*) *showing the comparative expense of supporting old and recent cases of insanity.*

No. of old cases.	Present age.	Duration, in years of insanity before admission.	Cost of support before admission, at $2 per week.	Number of recent cases.	Age.	Duration of insanity before admission.	Time, in weeks, spent in the Asylum.	Cost of cure at $3 per week.
1	42	18	$1,872 00	1	29	1 month,	20	$60 00
2	45	11	1,144 00	2	22	6 "	18	54 00
3	35	13	1,352 00	3	35	5 "	15	45 00
4	40	12	1,248 00	4	26	4 "	9	27 00
5	38	15	1,560 00	5	41	8 "	43	129 00
6	38	10	1,040 00	6	37	5 "	16	48 00
7	42	10	1,040 00	7	27	7 "	59	177 00
8	40	15	1,560 00	8	34	4 "	15	45 00
9	40	20	2,080 00	9	31	1 "	18	54 00
10	40	9	936 00	10	22	9 "	13	39 00
11	50	10	1,040 00	11	18	1 week,	11	33 00
12	48	11	1,144 00	12	29	2 months,	52	156 00
13	45	9	936 00	13	23	5 "	25	75 00
14	35	10	1,040 00	14	24	8 "	5	15 00
15	57	27	2,808 00	15	28	2 "	13	39 00
16	57	10	1,040 00	16	45	4 "	14	42 00
17	28	13	1,352 00	17	28	4 "	26	78 00
18	49	21	2,184 00	18	41	1 "	23	69 00
19	43	15	1,560 00	19	24	3 "	15	45 00
20	45	10	1,040 00	20	32	2 "	15	45 00
21	29	14	1,456 00	21	20	5 "	33	99 00
22	33	10	1,040 00	22	20	8 "	29	87 00
23	40	28	2,912 00	23	21	5 "	8	24 00
24	39	10	1,040 00	24	31	5 days,	16	48 00
25	40	10	1,040 00	25	25	10 months.	25	75 00
			$35,464 00					$1,608 00

Average number of years for each case before admission into the asylum. 13¾.

Average number of weeks spent on the asylum, 21½.

Average cost of each case before admission into the asylum, $1,418 56.

Average cost of each recovery in the asylum, $64 32.

Dr. Trezevant, long well known in the Southern States, as the counselling physician of the South Carolina State Hospital, in his report for 1847, presents a painful but exactly correct view of the evils of Alms-house treatment for the insane, and justly deprecates all treatment save that which is provided in rightly managed Hospitals. I quote from his own pages illustrative of this position:

"Much has been done, and much remains to be done, which I flatter myself will be accomplished; but it will be the work of time, and the gradual enlightening of the minds of the community, and satisfying the commissioners of the poor of the actual necessity of sending *early* their insane to the Asylum. I have nothing to do with it politically, but it comes before me so frequently in the acts of some of the commissioners, daily and hourly, that I cannot but feel that it is a wonderful agent of mischief, even in that most humble portion of our State government. The law leaves it in a measure optional with the commissioners, and though imperative in its phraseology, yet it gives a discretionary power, and for fear of increasing the poor rates, many will, with the utmost purity of heart and genuine kindness of feeling, save the parish, but at the fearful sacrifice of the maniac. They will retain him at the poor house, where he can be kept for $50 per annum, and perhaps eventually send him to the Asylum, as it has been done, with the skin literally roasted from his limbs by the fire, for the want of proper attention. Some wretched old crone, half crazed herself, or unable to move about, the partaker of their charity, is installed as the keeper of the insane, and the effect of their injudicious parsimony is very speedily made obvious, by the wanderings of the maniac, the trouble he occasions in the neighborhood, or the injuries inflicted on him by those who, ignorant of his misfortune, deem him an impudent and troublesome vagrant. The law should be positive—for his being placed in the institution erected by the State for his especial benefit—there should be his location, and it should be the pride of every resident of the district, to see that the wretched maniac was sent to the place appropriated for his comfort and happiness."

The last annual report of the Directors of the Baltimore City Alms-house contains an appeal, to which innumerable facts might be added, in support of the plea for hospitals for the relief of the disease.

"Insanity," writes the Secretary, "is an affliction that appeals urgently to the sympathies of a benevolent and enlightened public. To omit providing the means which may contribute to the comfort and recovery of those who are visited by this awful calamity, is like denying the physician to the sick, and medicine to those who must perish without it."

If the Alms-house is an unfit receptacle for the insane, and cure in these institutions hopeless, how much more objectionable are the dungeons of the county jails. To look for suitable care or recovery in these, is to anticipate results which cannot be realized; and who is ready to consign his child, his father, brother, wife or

MEMORIAL

MARYLAND

1852

[Document C.]

BY THE SENATE,
February 25th, 1852.

Read and ordered to be printed.

MEMORIAL

OF

MISS D. L. DIX,

TO THE

HONORABLE THE GENERAL ASSEMBLY

IN BEHALF OF THE

INSANE OF MARYLAND.

MEMORIAL

TO THE

Honorable the General Assembly of Maryland.

Gentlemen of the Senate
and House of Delegates:

THE subject to which your memorialist solicits your candid attention, and on which she urges early and effective legislation, embraces from more than one point of view, the civil and social interests of the State of Maryland; reaching through every community, and penetrating the seclusion of every family.

This proposition, facts, not opinions, must demonstrate.

Your memorialist presents the claims of that portion of a large, and fast increasing class for which appropriate care and protection are not now secured: she asks of Maryland, what has not yet been provided—a State Hospital which shall supply full remedial treatment for the Insane.

This question, with ever strengthening and uncompromising force, acquires, day by day, and year by year, weight and urgency, and now presents a phase so strongly defined, that no eye can be blind to the significance of the sign it exhibits, and no sound mind or humane heart, can be at fault in determining the course which a just legislation must pursue, consulting alike the rights and the necessities of individuals, and guarding the financial interests of the State.

Gentlemen, your memorialist is compelled to deal with severe facts, whose sharp outlines may not be softened by the graces of studied phrases and polished periods. With your permission she respectfully, but plainly and earnestly, brings to your knowledge, records gathered through cautious inquiry, and established by patient investigation. She asks your honest and deliberate examination of the statements and tables, which, without an elaborate preamble, are now presented, and urges impartial and fair discussion of the true merits of the cause she advocates, and which you alone, in your capacity as legislators, have authority to sustain ; and she believes, humanity and justice to conduct to a successful issue.

There are but two institutions in the State of Maryland in which insane patients are brought under curative treatment ; and but one, exclusively devoted to the reception of this class. Neither propose to confine their cares to citizens of Maryland ; the one has at the present time, thirty-five (35) patients from the District of Columbia, sustained by goverment ; thirty-four (34) from the city and county of Baltimore, from the indigent classes ; thirty-seven (37) from other counties in the State, leaving twenty-four (24) remaining paying patients, from this and other States. Total 130, January 1st, 1852. This institution can properly accommodate but 120 patients, but by appropriating two large parlors for lodging-rooms, 15 more can be received ; meanwhile this accession of numbers, diminishes the comfort and trenches on the remedial means of the hospital. This institution, the first movement for establishing which was in 1798—was first opened under charge of "an attending physician and other persons," in 1807, under the title of "The Public Hospital, for the relief of Indigent Sick persons and the cure of Lunatics ;" and, finally, the establishment under various restrictions and conditions at different periods, was leased by the city of Baltimore to private individuals, conditioned on being "exclusively devoted to the treatment of lunatics."

A board of visitors was appointed by the legislature in 1828— Dr. Mackenzie retaining the lease from the city, till the first of January, 1834; at which time, by act of the legislature, the hospital was taken possession of by the president and board of visitors, in the name of the State ; having at the time 26 inmates. At the present date the resident physician pronounces the institution seriously incommoded by receiving a larger number than 120 ; and positively suffering disadvantages with 135 patients which is the maximum.

The message of the Executive for 1849, contains the following paragraph in relation to the wants of the Insane :

"Although the Hospital is now filled to its utmost capacity, there are hundreds of insane persons in the State, one hundred and twenty three of whom are in the Baltimore Alms-House, and eight in the Penitentiary, without the means of proper treatment for the mitigation or cure of the awful malady with which they are afflicted. However urgent may be the demands of humanity in behalf of this unfortunate class of persons, and however clear the obligations of society to provide for their wants, in view, never theless, of the proximity of the Hospital to the city of Baltimore, and the limited extent of its grounds, it is questionable whether instead of enlarging the present building, it would not be wiser and better to dispose of the establishment and employ the proceeds, with such appropriation as the Legislature may choose to make, in the purchase of a sufficient quantity of land and the erection of an Asylum upon the most modern and approved plan, adapted in all its arrangements for the comfortable accommodation, treatment and cure of insane patients, and of a style and character worthy the munificence of the State."

1852, Jan. 13. The President and Board, in a report to the. General Assembly, declare their opinion, that it is not expedient to enlarge the present Hospital; which, however, they recommend to be preserved as an auxiliary institution.

Dr. Fonerden renders testimony in behalf of a new hospital in the report for 1852, from which the following paragraph is an extract.

"It has been mentioned in previous reports, that our accommodations are not sufficient to receive all the patients ordered to be sent by the courts and commissioners. Applications from Baltimore city and from the counties are constantly on file for the admission of public patients. When persons are admitted at the public expense by order of a court, they are retained and provided for during life, if not restored, with scarcely an exception. The rooms set apart for this permanent class are therefore generally occupied. Vacancies take place slowly, and sometimes months elapse without one. Hence new cases cannot be promptly admitted, and some of them while waiting their turn are placed in jails and alms-houses."

I ask your attention, in closing the presentation of the above facts, illustrating the inability of the Board of Visitors of the Maryland Hospital, to afford admission for the fast increasing numbers of applicants, to the Institution at Mount Hope, established and conducted by a band of the Sisters of Charity. The ninth Annual Report reaches the public, embodying an earnest claim on Legislative interposition, to protect it from encroachments which threaten its very existence. A petition, sustained by such arguments, as are feelingly and emphatically therein set forth, merits impartial consideration.

Mt. Hope Hospital is not exclusively, nor mainly occupied for the treatment of insanity;—but according to its report, a majority of the patients are of that class; we make exception to 56 cases during the past twelve months, of *mania a potu*, a malady not coming rightly under the statistics of insanity, of the 102 cases admitted during the past year under varying forms of mental disease, 54 were recorded under the division of *mania a potu.* Two already were in the Hospital at the commencement of 1852. So that we have before us the record 52 discharged recovered, 2 remaining at the present date, and 2 deceased. In 1850 and '51, 70 cases were treated at Mount Hope, for this malady. The whole number of patients of all classes now remaining, is stated to be 115. Thus is shown the insufficient and sole provision had in Maryland for cure of the insane.

On the first of January, 1850, according to the most correct tables I possess, we find within the limits of Baltimore city alone, 348 insane individuals: this does not include the insane in private families, either in the city or county at large, nor does it include idiots, simpletons, and epileptics,—a large class to omit.

January 1st, 1850, there were—

In the Maryland Hospital, - - -	133
In Mount Hope Hospital, - -	74

Total, under curative treatment,- -	217
In the Alms House, were - - -	123
In the Penitentiary, - .. - -	8

Total, recorded cases in Baltimore city alone,	348

Cases in private families not noted here.

I have shown in part, the insufficiency of the Hospital Institutions at Baltimore, for meeting the wants of the citizens of Maryland, in relieving and affording curative treatment for the insane, and that these Hospitals are the sole resource of the citizens within their own borders. Briefly, that which is needed, is a new Institution capable of receiving *two hundred and fifty* patients, which is the maximum for any first class curative Hospital, and *in it* should constantly reside the medical Superintendent, whose whole time and care should be devoted to the pursuit of means for securing the comfort and recovery of his patients. Well-timed employment, alternating with repose, useful labor, and suitable diversions, should be successively provided. What contrasts from these appropriate cares are presented in the condition of very many, though not the largest portion of this class throughout this State! The largest part, indeed, wear out life in adverse situations, but not in extremest abandonment to misery ; that any abuses and unnecessary sufferings exist, is a sufficient argument for assuring now at once, such remedies as shall spare the repetition and perpetuation of these sore distresses.

Your memorialist knows, and all may know, that confined apartments, narrow cells, dungeons, and not seldom chains and manicles—both in private dwellings, in poor-houses, in county jails, and in the penitentiary, are the miserable alternatives, (in default of adequate Hospital provision for these unfortunates,) upon which every sentiment of justice and humanity stamps a negative. It is asked, how I know that any extreme examples of misery exist? I reply, that I have traversed the State with this express object to incite my search. I do not propose to detain you upon the detailed history of the prisons and poor-houses of Maryland, nor to break down the screen which shuts out from general inspection and curious gaze, the troubles and sufferings of many respectable but indigent families, who hide their insane in their own dwellings—for—what remedy have they? Nothing, save extremest necessity, and that only as a temporary expedient, can justify the incarceration of the insane in jails. In poor-houses, the objections though differing are equally urgent. The trustees and medical attendants, uniting with successive superintendents, in the Baltimore Alms-House, have, for years, earnestly and faithfully presented in their Annual Reports, the inhumanity and mischief re-

sulting to all parties from this association of the demented, and
the raving maniac, with the aged and the infirm; the feeble and the
sick; the young and the helpless; your memoralist can but add
another voice of remonstrance against the perpetuation of this
great abuse. I have said that the sufferings of the insane, exposed in unfit situations are great;—language, however strong, is
feeble to describe them,—but I would not be understood to cast
blame on superintendents of poor-houses, and keepers of jails:
either they have not the means, or they have not the knowledge to
conduct rightly, one may almost say decently, the cares required
by the unfortunate maniac; they abide a necessity of which they
do not know how to rid themselves; and become hardened to
sufferings which since they cannot remedy, they strive to forget.
These men who govern poor-houses and prisons, are not cruel and
brutal,—but they are wrongly *forced* to a work which every hour
sears the better feelings, and which almost converts them to the
rude, hard guardians, which they sometimes, by the hasty observer, are charged with being.

The establishment of a State Hospital would put an end to the
continual repetition of scenes and conditions of existence which
should not be suffered for a day to blemish the history of any
community, nor any civilized and christian people. That this
condition of things is not confined to one, three, six, or any dozen
of the States, nay, that it is found now at this day, in every one
of these United States, is no excuse for its toleration in any of
them. Much has been done for the relief of the insane, and for
lessening, by contrast, what is of minor consideration, the cost of
their support to the public;—but much more remains to be accomplished. It is a fact known to all experience, that the longer
a necessary work is delayed, the greater the trouble and expense
in effecting it. In this case, it is beyond estimate; for who can
show how many of the unhappy Insane are now but *commencing*
an *existence*, in which the reason is merged in delusions and
vehement ravings, and for how many dreary years life may be
protracted; and, for what purposes, it becomes those who enjoy
health and reason to inquire :—"Perhaps," as long since wrote a
deep thinker and close observer of the course of human affairs,
" these poor maniacs are a particular rent—charge on the great
family of mankind;—left by the Maker of us all, like younger
children, who though the estate be given from them, yet the *Father*
expected that the heir should take care of them."

The insane cannot be left in charge of their families, nor to the
ordinary charities which flourish more or less freely in all communities; they require arrangements specially adapted to their special
necessities. No domestic cares, no common modes of treating the
sick; no accustomed practice of accomplished medical advisers
reaches their necessities. In what these necessities consist, none
can understand, except they have paused to search out the states
of suffering, the entire disqualification for self-care which this

malady often creates and perpetuates in the management of the unskilful and uninformed. No helpless infant can be more helpless, no wild animal of the desert more uncontrollable, than are many of these unfortunates, in different states and stages of the disease. Yet this malady, the result, in almost all instances of physical ailments, and so distressing in its effects upon the sufferer, and all with whom he is connected, is less hopeless than two-thirds of the same diseases which attack mankind. The tabular returns of all well conducted Hospitals of these times; and the whole experience of society establishes my position.

Referring to the United States Census for 1840, we find the insane and idiot population of Maryland, recorded as 550, the entire number of citizens being 470,019. An interval of ten years has closed, and in 1850 we derive from the United States Census the following record:—Insane, 946, (it is not shown what proportion of these are a private charge,) total population 583,-035 ; showing an increase, supposing the returns approximate to accuracy, of 406, a ratio far exceeding the increase of the whole population, and offering the most persuasive argument for early and effectual care of recent cases; but even this large increase we know, falls within the actual amount. The supposition, that this increase, so disproportionate, may be explained by the influx of emigrants, is unsubstantial. Of the 946 which are contained in the tables of the seventh census, 63 only are foreigners by birth. And, again, 104 only are free negroes, and 96 slaves, so that we have still in Maryland 683 Anglo Americans disqualified for all the offices of civil and social obligation, by reason of mental disease;—or a total of 746 whites. The statistics of all the States exhibit rapid and fearful increase of this terrible malady. The entire number in the United States, according to the census of 1840, was 17,457, to a population of 17,069,453.

The census of 1850 gives, in a total population of 23,267,498 an insane population of above 27,000. Not only is this great increase of insanity an alarming fact, but tracing the tabular statements, sent abroad annually, from all hospitals for the reception and treatment of insanity in the United States, we note year by year, the increase, if not predominance of insanity in the *youthful* classes of society. Medical men of sound minds and rare skill urge vainly on the dull ear of society, that *prevention* is in its power to a vast extent, and of infinite worth before *cure*, or, alas, the hazard of no cure—but the timely warnings are unheeded, and individuals, as communities, rashly multiply exciting causes, and too late deplore the inevitable results consequent on transgression of the physical laws of health and life.

I offer two tables, the first borrowed from Dr. Stokes' last Report; that which follows is taken from the last Annual Report of the Western Hospital, at Staunton, Virginia, and prepared by Dr. Stribling. I only add, that the records of other institutions exhibit large numbers of patients comparatively youthful, or in the very prime of life.

TABLE

*Showing the Ages of Insane Patients, from January 1st 1851,
to January 1st, 1852:*

	Males.	Females.	Total.
Between 10 and 15, - -	2	1	3
" 15 20, - - -	0	13	13
" 20 30, - - -	30	32	62
" 30 40, - - -	26	31	57
" 40 50, - - -	7	16	23
" 50 60, - - -	4	8	12
" 60 70, - - -	1	4	5
" 70 80, - - -	2	3	5
" 80 90, - - -	1	1	2
	73	109	182

This table furnishes a view of the ages of all the insane patients treated in the course of the year. No one can pass through this institution without being forcibly struck with the large number of young females, and young men, evidently belonging to the middle and higher walks of life, who are here the subjects of insanity. The question at once presents itself to every reflecting mind, whence comes it, that so many at the tender ages of *fifteen to twenty five* are stricken with this heavy calamity?

*Shews the Age at which Insanity is supposed to have commenced
with Patients who have been in the Asylum during the year:*

	Males.	Females.	Total.
Of those under 15 years, - -	10	7	17
between 15 and 20 years, -	23	24	47
20 and 25 " -	35	28	63
25 and 30 " -	38	28	66
30 and 35 " -	26	20	46
35 and 40 " -	14	12	26
40 and 45 " -	23	16	39
45 and 50 " -	4	9	13
50 and 60 " -	7	9	16
60 and 70 " -	2	2	4
over 80 years, - -	1	0	1
Unascertained, - - -	45	23	68
	228	178	406

Dr. Ray states in the Report of the Butler Hospital, for 1851, "that the increasing prevalence of insanity cannot be denied;"—

2

"of the causes which appear, in answer to our earnest inquiries, we cannot speak in detail, but there is much in our political, religious, and social usages,—calculated to disturb the balance of the mental powers, and prepare the way for unequivocal
insanity ;—also the eagerness, the hurry, the vehemence which
constitute such prominent traits in our national character, produce
a morbid irritability of the brain, but a single remove from overt
disease." " The gross neglect of correct family education and
discipline, and the neglect of the moral powers—those which guide
the passions and determine the motives, is the crowning defect of
the education of our times, ruinous in its consequences to the
health both of the body and of the mind." I am compelled to
omit the pages which follow these remarks ; rich and strong in
wisdom and truth; they are, so to say, a code of sound instructions which all need to study with care and reflection.

In adverting to one very fruitful cause of cerebral disease, I find
no little difficulty, but shall adduce one example, which I might
follow with a thousand, to show the *wickedness and ill-conse-
quences of the intermarriage of blood-relations*. In a community composed of 300 families, 34 heads of families were known
to be nearly allied by the ties of consanguinity. There were born
to these parents *ninety-five* children, of whom 44 were *idiotic*,
12 *scrofulous*, 1 was *deaf*, and 1 was a *dwarf*. In one family of
8 children, 5 were idiots. Not one of the 95 could be called perfectly sound in body and mind.

Increase of Insanity amongst the younger classes of society,
furnishes another argument for *early* treatment of the malady, before disease has fastened for life, on its victim. The public safety,
equity, economy and lastly humanity, require adequate, appropriate provision for the insane before the malady assumes a chronic
character, and the hapless being becomes a life-care to his friends,
or a heavy burthen upon the public. Every man and woman
possessed of sound health is wealth to the State; every individual
diseased and disabled is a draft, both directly and indirectly, on its
riches and prosperity. It is *cheaper to cure than it is to support*,
even at the very lowest rates. I ask to show you, by positive estimate, results reached by examining, collating, and contrasting
accounts gathered with careful labor.

In the Hospital at Staunton, Va., in 1842, twenty old cases had
cost, $41,633 00
Average expense of old cases, 2,081 65
Whole expense of curing twenty recent cases, 1,265 00
Average expense of curing these cases, 63 25
In the Ohio State Hospital, in 1842, the whole expense of twen-
ty-five old cases had been $50,611 00
Average do., 2,020 00
Whole expense of twenty-five recent cases cured, 1,130 00
Average of twenty-five cured, 45 20
In the Massachusetts State Hospital, in 1843, there remained
twenty-five old cases, the periods of whose insanity had varied,

and all in sufficiently rigorous physical health to authorise the expectation of their living many years longer, and the cost of whose support to the public had already reached the sum of $54,157 00

Average expense of do., 2,166 20

The whole expense of twenty-five cases of indigent patients recovered, was 1,461 30

Average, 58 45

Thus it is seen that while the interests of humanity, those first great obligations, are consulted by the establishment of well regu- lated hospitals for the insane, political economy and the public safety are not less insured.

Dr. Trezevant, (Report of the South Carolina Lunatic Asylum for 1842 and '45,) observes, "Many sunk from chronic diseases of the lungs and bowels, *engendered by exposure during their wan- derings, or the want of attention, when confined in the jails or work houses.*" He complains of their being kept five or six months under care of the family physician, and asks, "Is it right that the patient should be placed under the care of those, *who are unac- customed to the care of Lunatics?* How often is the case aggravat- ed either by the foolish indulgence of friends, the restraints of gross ignorance, or the injudicious treatment of the medical advisers?"

Dr. Ray (Medical Jurisprudence of Insanity) argues thus, "In case of homicide and other acts of violence, if the subject be insane, it is an act of humanity to afford him the refuge. *If he be crimi- nal* and pleads insanity as a means to elude the law, then the *re- straint* of the Asylum, guards the community from the further commission of crime."

Dr. Allen, of the Kentucky State Hospital, makes in a late re- port the following practical remarks :

"Cases of recent occurrence, which have been treated this year, have, as usual, very generally recovered.

"After several years constant and close observation of insanity, in its various forms and indications, I am more and more confirm- ed in the opinion, that the only grounds upon which a cure can be, with any degree of confidence expected, is a prompt applica- tion of proper treatment in the early stages of the disorder. True some recover from the chronic forms of the malady ; but I must own, that were it has occurred, I claim little credit for the science of medicine. Nature, by some evolution in the system, effecting it, aided, no doubt, to some extent, by the wholesome discipline of the Institution.

"There is no affection so little understood by the community, and I may say, perhaps by medical men generally, as insanity cases of years duration are often brought here by friends, under medical advice, who ask and expect us to 'feel the pulse and tell them when a cure may be effected.'"

The following tables exhibit the advantage of largely extended and seasonable hospital care for the insane. I am indebted chiefly to the reports of Drs. Woodward and Awl for these carefully pre- pared records:

TABLE

Showing the comparative expense of supporting old and recent cases of insanity, from which we learn the economy of placing patients in Institutions in the early periods of disease:

No. of old cases.	Present age.	Time insane, in years.	Total expense, at $100 a year, before entering the hospital, and $132 a year since; last year $120.	Number of recent cases discharged.	Present age.	Time insane, in weeks.	Cost of support, at $2 30 per week.
2	69	28	$ 3,212 00	1,622	30	7	$ 16 10
7	48	17	2,004 00	1,624	34	20	46 00
8	60	21	2,504 00	1,625	51	32	73 60
12	47	25	2,894 00	1,635	23	28	64 40
18	71	34	3,794 00	1,642	42	40	92 00
19	59	18	2,204 00	1,643	55	14	32 20
21	39	16	1,993 00	1,645	63	36	82 80
27	47	16	1,994 00	1,649	22	40	92 00
44	56	26	2,982 00	1,650	36	28	64 40
45	60	25	2,835 00	1,658	36	14	32 20
102	53	25	2,833 00	1,660	21	16	36 80
133	44	13	1,431 00	1,661	19	27	62 10
176	55	20	2,486 00	1,672	40	11	25 70
209	39	16	1,964 00	1,676	23	23	52 90
223	50	20	2,364 00	1,688	23	11	25 70
260	47	16	2,112 00	1,690	23	27	62 10
278	49	10	1,424 00	1,691	37	20	46 00
319	53	10	1,247 00	1,699	30	28	64 40
347	58	14	1,644 00	1,705	24	17	39 10
367	40	12	1,444 00	1,706	55	10	23 00
400	43	14	1,644 00	1,709	17	10	23 00
425	48	13	2,112 00	1,715	19	40	92 00
431	36	13	1,412 00	1,716	35	48	110 40
435	55	15	1,712 00	1,728	52	55	126 50
488	37	17	1,912 00	1,737	30	33	75 90
		454	$54,157 00			635	$ 1,461 30

When it is remembered, in addition to these facts, that there are very few acute diseases from which so large a proportion of persons attacked, fully recover, as from insanity, brought under *early and appropriate hospital treatment,* the positive obligation to meet fully this great want throughout the United States, as well as in Maryland, is too plain to admit a question. *Entire and early cure of cases which are functional, not organic; early cared for, and not protracted,* is the *rule;* duration of the disease, the *exception.* Recovery, implies *a complete* restoration of the mental powers.

TABLE

Showing the comparative curability of a given number of cases healed at different periods of insanity, as introduced to hospital care :

	Total cases.	Total of each sex.	Cured or curable.	Not cured, or incurable.
Less than one year's duration,	232			
Men, - - -		123	110	13
Women, - -		109	100	9
From one to two years' duration,	94			
Men, - - -		49	31	18
Women, - -		45	32	13
From two to five years, -	109			
Men, - - -		65	18	47
Women, - -		44	18	26
From five to ten years, -	76			
Men, - - -		40	5	35
Women, - -		36	4	32
From ten to fifteen years, -	56			
Men, - - -		35	2	33
Women, - -		21	1	20

An author of profound research and high intellectual endowments, in a work which was first published some years since in several foreign languages, and has since been reproduced in this country, states that " *the general certainty of curing insanity in its early stage* is a fact which ought to be universally known, and then it would be properly appreciated and acted upon by the public."

Dr. Ellis, director of the West Riding Lunatic Hospital, England, stated in 1827, that of 312 patients admitted within three months after their first attack, 216 recovered ; while, in contrast with this, he adds that of 318 patients admitted, who had been insane for upwards of one year to thirty, only 26 recovered. In La Salpetriere, near Paris, the proportion of cures of recent cases was, in 1806-'7, according to Dr. Veitch's official statement, as nearly *two* or *three* cured, while only five out of 152 old cases recovered. Dr. Burrows stated, in 1820, that of recent cases under his care, 91 in 100 recovered ; and in 1828, that the annual reports of other hospitals, added to his own larger experience, confirmed the observations. Dr. Willis made to Parliament corresponding statements. At the Senavra hospital, near Milan, the same results appeared upon the annual records

But *cure* alone, manifestly, is not the sole object of hospital care: secondary indeed, but of vast importance, is the secure and comfortable provision for that now large class throughout the country, the incurable insane. Their condition, we know, is susceptible of amelioration, and of elevation to a state of comparative comfort and usefulness.

Perhaps no more substantial proof can be adduced of the value of well organized hospital cares, than is shown in the following extracts from Dr. Stribling's report for 1851, of the institution he directs in Western Virginia ; an institution liberally sustained by the State, (as is also her other and senior hospital at Williamsburg,) and of which she may well be proud.

Among the many moral means there are none which, whilst it conduces more than any other to the contentment, health and recovery of the insane, promotes in so high a degree the pecuniary interests of the asylum, as occupation in the way of manual labor. The garden, the farm, and the work shops are to the males, and the needle and ordinary housework are to the females, sources of decided benefit, both intellectually and physically; and the burthen to the State of supporting so large an establishment is materially lessened by the products of labor thus employed.

Believing that abstracts from the books of the asylum, furnishing items in reference to these matters, might not be uninteresting or unprofitable, we have taken some care to have them properly made out, and herewith present them. The prices affixed are the estimates of the steward, and we consider them, to say the least, not too high.

"The products of the garden from the 1st day of October, 1850, to the 30th September, 1851, were as follows:

2,700 heads of early cabbage, at 4 cents per head,	108 00
3,775 heads of late cabbage, at 4 cents per head,	151 00
1,200 heads of celery, at 3 cents per head,	36 00
241 bushels tomatoes, at $1 per bushel,	241 00
45 bushels green peas, at $1 per bushel,	45 00
95 bushels turnip salad, at 50 cents per bushel,	47 50
49 bushels beets, at 50 cents per bushel,	24 50
57 bushels snap beans, at $1 per bushel,	57 00
20 bushels Lima beans, at $2 per bushel,	40 00
10 bushels carrots, at 50 cents per bushel,	5 00
51 bushels lettuce, at 25 cents per bushel,	12 75
34 bushels turnips, at 50 cents per bushel,	17 00
20 bushels salsify, at $1 per bushel,	20 00
12 bushels parsnips, at 50 cents per bushel,	6 00
4 bushels late onions, for sets, at $3 50 per bushel,	14 00
404 dozen early onions, at 6¼ cents per dozen,	25 25
422 dozen summer squash, at 12½ cents per dozen,	52 75
395 roasting ears, at 12½ cents per dozen,	49 37½
40 gallons raspberries, at 50 cents per gallon,	20 00

$ 972 12½

In addition to the above, the hands employed on the garden have taken care of a green house containing a large number of plants, have attended to the transplanting of trees and shrubbery, and bestowed much labor in other ways of which no note has been taken.

The products of the farm, including carpenters' work done by the farmer and those patients entrusted to his care, were as follows :

500 bushels corn, at 50 cents per bushel,	- -	250 00
240 bushels potatoes, at 50 cents per bushel,	-	120 00
103 bushels buckwheat, at 50 cents per bushel,	-	51 50
9 loads fodder,	- - - - - -	20 00
126 loads wood, at $1 75 per load,	- - -	220 50
300 dozen sheaf oats, at 25 cents per dozen,	-	75 00
8,000 lbs. pork, at $4 50 per hundred	- - -	360 00
266 lbs. veal, at 6 cents per lb.,	- - - -	10 64
3 calf skins, at $1 each,	-	3 00
6,570 gallons milk, at 20 cents per gallon,	- -	1,314 00
37 head of stock hogs, at $2 each,	- - -	74 00
5 head young cattle, at $10 each,	- -, -	50 00
Making 115 panels plank fence, at 30 cents each,	-	34 50
Making and hanging 3 large gates, at $7 each,	-	21 00
Remodeling horse stable,	- . - - -	50 00
Erecting a building 80 feet long by 26 feet wide, for barn, corn crib, flour house, cow stable, &c. &c.,		276 50
		$2,930 64

The farmer and his assistants have done much that was useful and necessary, such as clearing woodland, hauling stone, &c. &c., not included in this statement.

The female patients have in their appropriate sphere been no less industrious, and their labor attended with proportionate profit, as the following statement will shew :

277	men's	coats, made at $1 each,	- -	277 00
310	"	pantaloons, made at 50 cents each,	155 00
257	"	vests, made at 50 cents each,	-	128 50
25	"	drawers, made at 25 cents each,	-	6 25
216	"	shirts, made at 37½ cents each,	-	81 00
77	"	roundabouts, made at 75 cents each,	38 50
192	female's	dresses, made at 37½ cents each, ..	72 00
212	"	under dresses, made at 25 cents each,	53 00
154	"	aprons, made at 12½ cents each, -	19 25
71	"	caps, made at 17 cents each, -	6 83
88	"	collars, made at 12½ cents each, -	11 00
32	"	night gowns, made at 25 cents each,	8 00
60 pair stockings, knit at 37½ cents each,			22 50

Carried forward, $878 83

		Brought forward,	$878 83
360	pair socks, knit at 25 cents each, - -		90 00
98	pair socks, footed at 18¾ cents each, -		18 37½
408	hankerchiefs and towels, hemmed at 6¼ cents each,		25 50
11	mattress ticks, made at 75 cents each, -		8 25
68	mattress slips, made at 25 cents each, -		17 00
142	pillow ticks and cases, made at 12½ cents each,		17 75
4	bed ticks, made at 37½ cents each, - -		1 50
84	bolster ticks and cases, made at 12½ cents each,		10 50
213	sheets and bed spreads, made at 25 cents each,		53 25
25	comforts, made at $1 each, - - -		25 00
8	bed quilts, pieced and quilted, at $3 each,		24 00
94	curtains for windows, made at 25 cents each,		23 50
7	carpets, made up at $1 50 cents each, -		10 50
2,974	pieces of clothing, mended at 3 cents each,		89 22
	Amount of fancy work, made and sold, proceeds to be applied to completing chapel, - - -		77 00

	Total, - - - -	$1.370 07½

SHOE SHOP.

The new work and mending done amounts to $1,021 73

Contra.

The cost of material used, - - -	$ 414 21	
The wages of foreman 12 months, - -	252 00	
The dieting of do. do. at $8 per mo.,	96 00	
		762 21

	Profit, - - -	$259 52

This statement cannot exhibit the *saving* to the institution, as from the convenience of having such a shop, shoes are often mended so soon as they need it; whereas, if they had to be sent elsewhere it would be deferred, notwithstanding the admonition of Dr. Franklin, that "a stitch in time saves nine," until the expense of repairing would be greatly increased or the shoe be rendered useless. Our patients, both male and female, have uniformly been well supplied with shoes. The servants, numbering about thirty, get, under a rule of the institution, two pair each per annum; and the whole cost for the year of having supplied the wants in this respect of more than four hundred patients and thirty servants, has only been seven hundred and sixty-two dollars and fifty-two cents.

HAT SHOP.

The hats for patients who are supplied by the State, and for the servants, are made by one of the attendants, with such aid as his patients can afford him. Not less than two hundred and fifty patients and thirty servants have been provided for during the year, at a cost to the institution of not more than one hundred and thirty-five dollars. The hats are made of coney and cotton—are neat, durable, and comfortable—superior greatly in all respects to the wool hat, which, if purchased at wholesale, would cost considerably more than is expended under our present arrangement.

It is not *occupation* alone, but *useful employment*, that so eminently assists other remedial moral means for the restoration of the patient. Hence the value of a productive farm or plantation, on which those who are able, and whose early habits permit, may find in labor, not the curse, but the inestimable blessing of well-directed toil; due exercise of the physical powers, and occupied attention, recalling the disturbed and distracted mind to the integrity of sound health.

I have endeavored to prove the advantages to be possessed by hospital treatment for the insane. I have tried to illustrate the disadvantages of domestic care and prescription for this suffering class of our fellow-beings. I have glanced at the inefficiency and cruelty of a poor-house and prison residence for the epileptic and the maniac. In imagination for a short time, place yourselves in their stead. Enter the horrid noisome cell; invest yourselves with the foul tattered garments which scantily serve the purposes of decent covering; cast yourself upon the loathsome pile of filthy straw, find companionship in your own cries and groans, or in the wailings and gibberings of wretches miserable like yourselves; call for help and release, for blessed words of soothing, and kind offices of care till the dull walls weary in sending back the echo of your moans; then, if your self-possession is not overwhelmed under the *imagined* miseries of what are the *actual* distresses of the insane, return to the consciousness of your sound intellectual health, and answer if you will longer refuse or delay to make adequate appropriation for the establishment of a hospital for the care and cure of those who are deprived of the use of their reasoning faculties, and who are incapable of exercising a rational judgment.

Of all men, they are to be accounted most miserable, who are reduced to mere animal existence.

In asking for the establishment of a State Hospital for the Insane in Maryland, located to assure, through *salubrity of air, abundance of pure water, a productive farm*, and *open access*, by *far reaching lines of travel*, the largest good to the largest numbers, your memorialist is sustained by the opinions of all the citizens of the State *who have had time and opportunity of studying the subject fully*, and of examining its claims. By none is this more earnestly desired than by the Physician of the Maryland Hospital, and by the President of that Institution, that good man and good citizen, who for 24 years, without reward or recompense, "hoping all things, and seeking not his own," has spared neither time, nor labor, nor that which most men give least readily and latest, large

3

pecuniary aid to keep in existence and useful operation the oldest charitable and humane institution in the State of Maryland. *Non immemor tanti beneficii!*

It is not improbable, that some members of your Honorable Body, men, too, of good hearts and liberal minds, will hesitate, if not seriously demur to a measure they will admit to be important, and opening strong claims on their efficient support and official action, but who will urge the large indebtedness of the State as an argument against new plans for the application of the public funds. I respect their cautiousness and hesitation. The monetary obligations of the State are heavy; taxation is already onerous; but will these be lessened by the omission to provide by creating a State Hospital for the Insane of the State, for those *who must be supported* in some way during the period of their natural lives. In hundreds of cases, if not thousands, it rests on *your* decision, Legislators of Maryland, whether this shall be accomplished at *heavy* or *light* cost to the State. The time-worn adage, —"Honesty is the best policy," Maryland has engraven on her shield, and the citizens stand firm, as honest men, on the strong rock of Integrity, honored and honorable, each lends his strength to redeem the State from the heavy burthens of her debt. And is the rich man less affluent, or the poor man the poorer, for coming up boldly to this work? No, no, they have struck the vein of the pure gold of virtue, and are enriched by treasures that "moth and rust do not corrupt." And does the legislator argue that being true to the principles of honesty, he may stand acquitted of other obligations? No, there is another law to which he will pay tribute;—in "doing justice," he will "*remember mercy.*" And, again, he will not consent that Sister States, younger and feebler, by reason of earlier years, should take precedence of his maternal Maryland. See Alabama—honest and resolved, she provides for full payment of her monetary obligations, and at the same time assumes cheerfully the debt she owes humanity. Owning the wardship of her insane children,—she appropriates $100,000.00 for a State Hospital, and is earnest only to advance to completion the work so well and wisely commenced. Look at Indiana—noble, clear-sighted Indiana,—honest and true; liberal and wise!—But few years since, Indiana made provision for the gradual payment of nearly twelve millions of dollars of her public debt, and being instructed in the necessity of timely provision for the insane, the deaf mutes, and the blind within her borders,—she adopted a wise and noble policy, equally prudent and humane; and levied a special tax for the erection of edifices for the insane, for the deaf mute, and the blind, at a cost of more than $200,000, and provided for the ample support of all these;—and a section in the new Constitution lays down a principle, and establishes a law for the perpetual support of these three charities by the State.

There, in the young State of Indiana, almost within the shadow of her Capitol at Indianapolis, stand these monuments of a christian and enlightened age, recording a forethought and munificence, which, under the circumstances has no parallel, though Illinois, ranging side by side geographically, almost completes a corresponding page in *her* history. Shall Maryland falter, solicited by more urgent incentives to determine her decisions and to quicken her energies?—Surely she will not!

No truth in ethics is more surely established than this;—not one human being, whether of high or low degree, strong or weak, learned or unlearned, conspicuous or humble, old or young, in the full fresh vigor of health, or feeble through weakness, but is vulnerable to the attacks of maniacal insanity. The man of most mighty intellect, the woman endowed with rarest virtues, may in an hour become the beneficiary of humanity ;—the hapless ward of heart stricken kindred, helpless alike to restore and cherish. The precious home no longer offers health giving influences; the cares and caresses of dearest friends but enhance the miseries of this terrible malady. "Lover and friend it puts far away, and acquaintances into darkness." The well-organized, well-sustained Hospital alone opens its portals for shelter and relief. The skill which directs appropriate care, here dissipates the delusions which distract; and heals the sicknesses which other direction could not arrest.

Legislators of Maryland, importunity urged by the sacred voice of unerring Duty, presses this cause upon your notice ;—you who fill places of authority,—forget not, amidst the heat of debate, the clash of opinions, and the sometime strife for political distinctions, forget not the majesty of your station, the dignity and sacredness of that trust confided to you by your constituents; forget not that you have the right and the means of exercising the ennobling offices of justice, humanity, and civil obligation. Becoming through your station as legislators, benefactors of the needy, whose mental darkness, through your action, may be dispersed, how many prayers and blessings from grateful hearts will enrich you! As your work on earth shall be measured, and your last hours shall be slowly numbered; when the review of life's deeds becomes more and more searching, amidst the flashes of uncompromising memories, how consoling will be the remembrance that of many transactions—often controlling, transient and outward affairs,—frequently conducting to disquieting results,—possibly sometimes to those of doubtful good, you have accomplished a work whose results of widely diffused benefits, create a light brightening your path through " the dark valley," and leading to those "gates of eternal life" which open upon "the blessed mansions" in which the finite faculties are beyond the reach of blight, and advance continually in knowledge, to perfection!

Respectfully submitted,

D. L. DIX.

ANNAPOLIS, February 24th, 1852.

APPENDIX.

—

1841—Admitted 4,366 : Restored to family perfectly cured 1,493. Discharged improved, 913. 1843—Admitted, 258 : Cured, 68. In three years, admitted, males, 288; females, 181—439 : Cured, males, 97 ; females, 61—158. 1844—Admitted, 285 : Cured, 75. 1850—Admitted, 228 : Cured, 106.—[*Sundry Reports by Dr. Kirkbride.*

TABLE (from Dr. Awl's sixth report for 1844, of the State Hospital, at Columbus, Ohio,) showing the comparative expense of supporting old and recent cases of insanity:

No. of old cases.	Present age.	Duration, in years, of insanity before admission.	Cost of support before admission, at $2 per week.	Number of recent cases.	Age.	Duration of insanity before admission.	Time, in weeks, spent in the asylum.	Cost of cure at $3 per week.
1	42	18	$1,872 00	1	29	1 month	20	$ 60 00
2	45	11	1,144 00	2	22	6 "	18	54 00
3	35	13	1,352 00	3	35	5 "	15	45 00
4	40	12	1,248 00	4	26	4 "	9	27 00
5	38	15	1,560 00	5	41	8 "	43	129 00
6	38	10	1,040 00	6	37	5 "	16	48 00
7	42	10	1,040 00	7	27	7 "	59	177 00
8	40	15	1,560 00	8	34	4 "	15	45 00
9	40	20	2,080 00	9	31	1 "	18	54 00
10	40	9	936 00	10	22	9 "	13	39 00
11	50	10	1,040 00	11	18	1 week	11	33 00
12	48	11	1,144 00	12	29	2 months	52	156 00
13	45	9	936 00	13	23	5 "	25	75 00
14	35	10	1,040 00	14	24	8 "	5	15 00
15	57	27	2,808 00	15	28	2 "	13	39 00
16	57	10	1,040 00	16	45	4 "	14	42 00
17	28	13	1,352 00	17	28	4 "	26	78 00
18	49	21	2,184 00	18	41	1 "	23	69 00
19	43	15	1,560 00	19	24	3 "	15	45 00
20	45	10	1,040 00	20	32	2 "	15	45 00
21	29	14	1,456 00	21	20	5 "	33	99 00
22	33	10	1,040 00	22	20	8 "	29	87 00
23	40	28	2,912 00	23	21	5 "	8	24 00
24	39	10	1,040 00	24	31	5 days	16	48 00
25	40	10	1,040 00	25	25	10 months	25	75 00
			$35,464 00					$ 1,608 00

Average number of years for each case before admission into the asylum, 13⅔.
Average number of weeks spent in the asylum, 21½.
Average cost of each case before admission into the asylum, $1,418 56.
Average cost of each recovery in the asylum, $64 32.

POVERTY, U. S. A.

THE HISTORICAL RECORD

An Arno Press/New York Times Collection

Adams, Grace. **Workers on Relief.** 1939.

The Almshouse Experience: Collected Reports. 1821-1827.

Armstrong, Louise V. **We Too Are The People.** 1938.

Bloodworth, Jessie A. and Elizabeth J. Greenwood.
The Personal Side. 1939.

Brunner, Edmund de S. and Irving Lorge.
**Rural Trends in Depression Years: A Survey of
Village-Centered Agricultural Communities, 1930-1936.**
1937.

Calkins, Raymond.
**Substitutes for the Saloon: An Investigation Originally
made for The Committee of Fifty.** 1919.

Cavan, Ruth Shonle and Katherine Howland Ranck.
**The Family and the Depression: A Study of
One Hundred Chicago Families.** 1938.

Chapin, Robert Coit.
**The Standard of Living Among Workingmen's Families
in New York City.** 1909.

**The Charitable Impulse in Eighteenth Century America:
Collected Papers.** 1711-1797.

Children's Aid Society.
Children's Aid Society Annual Reports, 1-10.
February 1854-February 1863.

Conference on the Care of Dependent Children.
**Proceedings of the Conference on the Care
of Dependent Children.** 1909.

Conyngton, Mary.
How to Help: A Manual of Practical Charity. 1909.

Devine, Edward T. **Misery and its Causes.** 1909.

Devine, Edward T. **Principles of Relief.** 1904.

Dix, Dorothea L.
On Behalf of the Insane Poor: Selected Reports. 1843-1852.

Douglas, Paul H.
**Social Security in the United States: An Analysis and
Appraisal of the Federal Social Security Act.** 1936.

Farm Tenancy: Black and White. Two Reports. 1935, 1937.

Feder, Leah Hannah.
**Unemployment Relief in Periods of Depression:
A Study of Measures Adopted in Certain American
Cities, 1857 through 1922.** 1936.

Folks, Homer.
**The Care of Destitute, Neglected, and
Delinquent Children.** 1900.

Guardians of the Poor.
**A Compilation of the Poor Laws of the State of
Pennsylvania from the Year 1700 to 1788, Inclusive.** 1788.

Hart, Hastings, H.
Preventive Treatment of Neglected Children.
(Correction and Prevention, Vol. 4) 1910.

Herring, Harriet L.
**Welfare Work in Mill Villages: The Story of Extra-Mill
Activities in North Carolina.** 1929.

The Jacksonians on the Poor: Collected Pamphlets.
1822-1844.

Karpf, Maurice J.
Jewish Community Organization in the United States.
1938.

Kellor, Frances A.
Out of Work: A Study of Unemployment. 1915.

Kirkpatrick, Ellis Lore.
The Farmer's Standard of Living. 1929.

Komarovsky, Mirra.
The Unemployed Man and His Family: The Effect of Unemployment Upon the Status of the Man in Fifty-Nine Families. 1940.

Leupp, Francis E. **The Indian and His Problem.** 1910.

Lowell, Josephine Shaw.
Public Relief and Private Charity. 1884.

More, Louise Bolard.
Wage Earners' Budgets: A Study of Standards and Cost of Living in New York City. 1907.

New York Association for Improving the Condition of the Poor.
AICP First Annual Reports Investigating Poverty. 1845-1853.

O'Grady, John.
Catholic Charities in the United States: History and Problems. 1930.

Raper, Arthur F.
Preface to Peasantry: A Tale of Two Black Belt Counties. 1936.

Raper, Arthur F. **Tenants of The Almighty.** 1943.

Richmond, Mary E.
What is Social Case Work? An Introductory Description. 1922.

Riis, Jacob A. **The Children of the Poor.** 1892.

Rural Poor in the Great Depression: Three Studies. 1938.

Sedgwick, Theodore.
Public and Private Economy: Part I. 1836.

Smith, Reginald Heber. **Justice and the Poor.** 1919.

Sutherland, Edwin H. and Harvey J. Locke.
Twenty Thousand Homeless Men: A Study of Unemployed Men in the Chicago Shelters. 1936.

Tuckerman, Joseph.
On the Elevation of the Poor: A Selection From His Reports as Minister at Large in Boston. 1874.

Warner, Amos G. **American Charities.** 1894.

Watson, Frank Dekker.
The Charity Organization Movement in the United States: A Study in American Philanthropy. 1922.

Woods, Robert A., et al. **The Poor in Great Cities.** 1895.